THE THERAPIST'S GUIDE
TO PSYCHOPHARMACOLOGY

The Therapist's Guide to Psychopharmacology

WORKING WITH PATIENTS, FAMILIES, AND PHYSICIANS TO OPTIMIZE CARE

REVISED EDITION

JoEllen Patterson
A. Ari Albala
Margaret E. McCahill
Todd M. Edwards

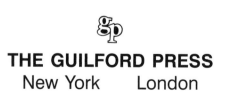

THE GUILFORD PRESS
New York   London

© 2006; revisions © 2010 The Guilford Press
A Division of Guilford Publications, Inc.
72 Spring Street, New York, NY 10012
www.guilford.com

Printed in the United States of America

This book is printed on acid-free paper.

As with every work dealing with science, the contents of this book are subject to evolving standards and advancements. Being apprised of such changes and advancements is an important part of the informed consent to which patients are entitled. In addition, any summary treatment of a subject so complicated can omit details such as rare or newly discovered but unconfirmed contraindications. Because medications should only be administered according to the most current guidelines available, practitioners are strongly reminded to consult and review carefully the product information sheets that accompany each drug administered, in light of the patient's history.

The authors have checked with sources believed to be reliable in their efforts to provide information that is complete and generally in accord with the standards of practice that are accepted at the time of publication. However, in view of the possibility of human error or changes in medical sciences, neither the authors, nor the editor and publisher, nor any other party who has been involved in the preparation or publication of this work warrants that the information contained herein is in every respect accurate or complete, and they are not responsible for any errors or omissions or the results obtained from the use of such information. Readers are encouraged to confirm the information contained in this book with other sources.

Last digit is print number: 9 8 7 6 5 4 3 2

Library of Congress Cataloging-in-Publication Data is available from the Publisher.

ISBN 978-1-60623-700-7 (paperback)
ISBN 978-1-60623-713-7 (hardcover)

For David.
For all that has been,
Thanks.
For all that shall be,
Yes.
(Dag Hammarskjold)

— J. E. P.

I dedicate this book to the memory of my parents,
Américo and Juanita, who showed me the love of learning;
to my wife, Barbara, who showed me the love of caring;
and to my children, Johanna, Keren, and David,
who every day show me what's meaningful.

— A. A. A.

I dedicate this work to my wonderful children and their spouses;
my grandchildren, sister, brother, mother, and most especially
my dear husband. We are fortunate to have been blessed
with a deeply devoted and loving family, and I thank you all
for your work and commitment to keeping it that way.

—M. E. M.

I lovingly dedicate this book to my family, close and extended,
and especially to my wife, Kyle, and our children,
Grayson, Cole, and Quinn Edwards.

—T. M. E.

About the Authors

JoEllen Patterson, PhD, is a Professor in the Marital and Family Therapy Program at the University of San Diego. She is also an Associate Clinical Professor of Family Medicine and Psychiatry at the University of California, San Diego School of Medicine. Besides receiving a Rotary International Scholarship to work at Cambridge University, Dr. Patterson has had two Fulbright Scholarships to work in Norway and New Zealand. She serves on the editorial board for *Family Systems and Health* and the *Journal of Marital and Family Therapy*. This is her third book.

A. Ari Albala, MD, received his medical education at the University of Chile and the University of Tel-Aviv, Israel, and completed a psychiatry residency and a research fellowship at the University of Michigan. He is currently Clinical Professor of Psychiatry at the University of California, San Diego School of Medicine; Clinical Director, Quality Improvement, Aurora Behavioral Health; and Medical Director at Psychiatric Centers at San Diego. Dr. Albala has received numerous distinctions in his career as both an educator and practitioner, including a Teaching Excellence Award from the University of California, San Diego; an Education Award from the San Diego Psychiatric Society; and the status of Distinguished Life Fellow of the American Psychiatric Association.

Margaret E. McCahill, MD, is a Health Sciences Clinical Professor of Family Medicine and Psychiatry at the University of California, San Diego (UCSD) School of Medicine. Dr. McCahill has practiced both family medicine and psychiatry in the U.S. Public Health Service/Indian Health Service, at a U.S. Naval Hospital, as a university faculty member, and in a free clinic that serves the homeless. She is the Founding Director of the UCSD Combined Family Medicine–Psychiatry Residency Training Program and the Medical Director of St. Vincent de Paul Village in San Diego, California. Dr. McCahill has received many teaching awards as a teacher of resident physicians for more than 20 years, and she also provides classroom instruction and practicum supervision for mental health care trainees in clinical social work, marital and family therapy, and clinical psychology.

Todd M. Edwards, PhD, is an Associate Professor and Director of the Marital and Family Therapy Program at the University of San Diego. He is also a Voluntary Assistant Clinical Professor in the Department of Family and Preventive Medicine at the University of California, San Diego School of Medicine. Dr. Edwards received his doctorate in marriage and family therapy from Virginia Tech and completed a medical family therapy internship in the Department of Family Medicine at the University of Rochester.

Contents

Introduction

Several years ago, we were supervising student therapists working in community clinics. During the students' case presentations, they would frequently mention, almost as an afterthought, that their patients were taking medication X. Being therapists, we knew little about **psychotropic medication**.[1] It was not our domain, after all. Instead, we refocused the discussion onto the "important" material—the topics we understood.

At that time, "important" material could include the patient's diagnosis, family problems, stressors, previous mental health history, or therapeutic relationships. As clinicians, however, we prided ourselves on not being wedded to one particular model, theory, or treatment protocol. We were open to almost all material, as long as it pertained to the patient's psychological or social experiences.

At the same time that we were ignoring information about psychotropic medication usage or biological history, there were increasing references to medications in daily life. Reading book reviews (notably *Listening to Prozac* [Kramer, 1993]), having friends and family members who began taking antidepressants, and having our own patients asking about medication as a treatment option, we soon realized that psychotropic medication was a burgeoning approach to treatment. And to stay

---

[1]Terms in **boldface** type are included in the glossary at the end of the book.

1

current, we had to gain a rudimentary knowledge about these medications and how they were used, as did our students (Patterson & Magulac, 1994).

EMBRACING THE "BIO" IN BIOPSYCHOSOCIAL

While espousing the biopsychosocial model in our work as therapists in medical settings, we did not have enough knowledge of human biology, genetics, and neuroscience to consider our patients' biological influences and needs. Regardless of our knowledge or interest, neurobiological research was creating a revolution by offering treatments for psychological disorders that sometimes involved simply taking a pill every morning. These new treatments were less intrusive than traditional, weekly psychotherapy, and they were frequently being delivered by primary care physicians, not psychiatrists. In addition, new research suggested that psychotherapy could affect biological systems such as the brain (Kandel, 1995, 1998, 2006). These combined research initiatives demonstrated that cause and effect within the biopsychosocial model is a multidirectional process.

The biopsychosocial model was originally created for physicians, to help them have a more balanced view of patients' needs. Engel (1980) suggested that the biomedical model was flawed because it ignored the patient's context and even the patient him- or herself. Instead, Engel suggested that the organized whole (the patient), as well as the component parts (the patient's brain, immune system, family, etc.), should be considered. According to systems theory, every unit is at the same time both a whole and a part. Nothing exists in isolation. Thus, physicians must take into account not only the patient's physical body and the disease but also the patient's reported inner experiences (feelings, sensations, memories) as well as his or her reported and observable behavior.

Similar to the physician's myopic view, we as therapists were equally short-sighted. We focused on our patients' experiences and feelings to the extent that we ignored their biological systems. Not acknowledging or understanding the importance of these systems meant that we ignored possible treatment options that targeted them—that is, we failed to consider psychotropic medications. And by failing to consider psychotropic medications in treatment, we were possibly failing our own patients.

Realizing that our therapeutic knowledge had to expand if we were going to truly follow a biopsychosocial model, we learned everything we could about medications and started encouraging our students to do the same. Textbooks for nonphysicians about psychotropic medications were published (Beitman, Safer, Thase, Blinder, & Riba, 2003; Gitlin, 1996; Riba & Balon, 1999; Sammons & Schmidt, 2001). Courses about neurobiology, medications, and genetics were added to mental health training programs. A paradigm shift was occurring: the dissolving of mind–body dualism.

However, this revolution in the academic mental health community did not necessarily lead to better patient care. Although we could explain the basic neurobiological mechanisms of medications, we could not get our patients to keep taking them if their spouses did not like the way the patients' sex drive was affected, if the medications made the patients gain weight, or if the medications were taken off an insurance company's reimbursed medications list. The books we collectively read on combining psychotherapy and medications or simply educating nonphysicians and patients about medications led us to believe that providing knowledge to mental health professionals would be enough to create change. This assumption was not true. In addition, there was virtually no communication between the prescribing physician—regardless of his or her medical discipline—and the therapist. And family members, who may be most affected by patients' responses to medication, were completely ignored. The impact of payors, employers, health care system providers, and others was never mentioned along with the discussion of the neuromechanisms of the medications. But these impediments were the everyday challenges that we faced with our patients. Even if our patients were open to the idea of medication, structural impediments, especially the lack of communication between the prescribing physician and the therapist, limited the medications' effectiveness.

Engel (1980) had originally focused on the biological, psychological, and social systems of his patients. But we were discovering that other systems were also affecting the care we could offer. The organizational and financial structures of the health care systems, as well as the divisions among the different mental health disciplines, meant that patient care was often fragmented and uncoordinated.

THE COLLABORATIVE CARE MOVEMENT

At the same time that we were struggling with these issues, there was a growing movement in health care that had as its goal the collaboration of physicians and therapists in assessing, planning, and providing patient care. A growing group of health professionals had been attempting to repair both the fragmentation in health care services and the conceptual split between mind and body. In fact, there were already several organizations and groups devoted to this model of care, especially in the United States, Canada, the United Kingdom, and Australia.

Defining Collaborative Care

Collaborative care has many definitions. It does not refer to split care, which usually implies that the physician treats the biological part of the patient by prescribing medication, and the therapist does the rest. Although split care may be attractive in terms of cost and ease for the provider, it is inadequate care. Patients need their therapist and physician to communicate, particularly in the creation and maintenance of a treatment plan.

Collaboration also differs from consultation. Consultation implies an event rather than a process. It is possible that a psychiatrist, for example, could conduct an evaluation and offer suggestions without prescribing medication, which may negate the need for ongoing contact. However, in most cases, the physician ideally becomes a treatment team member, not simply a consultant who offers expert advice and disappears.

One definition of collaboration is "the concurrent use of medical and mental health services" (Roesler, Gavin, & Brenner, 1995). Although this definition is absolutely correct, it obscures the diversity in how collaborative treatment is delivered. Collaboration can include phone calls, hallway discussions, exchanges of letters, participation by a physician—primary care or otherwise—in part or all of a therapy session, and meetings that involve all professionals, the patient, and his or her family. Nor does this definition suggest the difficulty in practicing collaboratively. Even with good intentions to "work together" and "share care," good collaboration is hard work.

Several excellent works on collaboration have been published (Blount, 1998; Doherty & Baird, 1983; Seaburn, Lorenz, Gunn, Gawinski, & Mauksch, 1996). Doherty (1995) developed a model that defines five levels of collaboration. The levels range from minimal collaboration, in which professionals work in different sites and rarely communicate about a case, to close collaboration in a fully integrated system, in which professionals from different disciplines practice in the same site and hold team meetings regularly to discuss collaboration issues. For most physicians and therapists, level 5 is more of a dream than a reality. Because of the structure of health care today, most professionals probably practice at levels 1 or 2.

If levels 3 or 4 are not possible for therapists because of the location of their practice, we advocate a model that is a modified version of level 2, which we call "close collaboration at a distance." Such a model provides health care services that focus on coordinated assessment and treatment by providers from different disciplines, so that all aspects of the patient's health—whether biological, psychological, spiritual, or social—can be addressed. Successful collaborative care presumes shared treatment planning and decision making by interdisciplinary teams. Shared care over time and across disciplines results in comprehensive care. Although the primary focus is on the integration of biomedical problems and mental health problems, all variables related to the patient's quality of life are considered, most notably the patient's family. The importance of family in both treatment and the collaborative effort is highlighted later in the text. Under the collaborative model, there are regular interactions to discuss patients and an appreciation for each other's professional culture (Doherty, 1995).

Although lofty in its expectations, in practice this model provides the best possible care for patients and their families. Sharing care also decreases the isolation that therapists and physicians commonly experience, which can further complicate the work with complex patients. Sharing responsibility for managing mental health crises, generating fresh ideas, expressing frustration, and carrying the emotional burden of serving these patients are only a few of the benefits that such care provides to the professional.

Collaborative Care: An Integrated Conceptualization

As clinicians, we were beginning to understand that a collaborative care model addresses gaps and fragmentation in the health care delivery system. It means that we do not have to know every fact about every system that might affect the patient's care. Instead of viewing ourselves as the sole deliverers of treatment, we have become the purveyors of possibilities in a system that extends beyond our own personal limitations, in addition to offering the patient our clinical expertise.

All treatment options are equally plausible, regardless of whether we can deliver the treatment ourselves. We might provide the treatment, or we might serve as a conduit of information and resources so that our patient can receive the best possible care. When psychotropic medications are used, we consider their impact beyond the patient's biological system. In a collaborative care model, it has become our job to understand the impact that psychotropic medications could have on the patients and their families, at home or in their work environment, even though as therapists we do not deliver the medication ourselves.

TRENDS IN MENTAL HEALTH CARE

We have also been reading about important trends in patient care such as the following:

- The U.S. Surgeon General declared that ensuring that treatments were available (minus problems of access) for patients with depression was a more significant problem than developing more efficacious treatment.
- There was a marked increase in the proportion of the population who received outpatient treatment for mental health problems, but this care was often provided by primary care physicians.
- There was greater involvement of physicians in patient mental health care and greater use of psychotropic medications.
- Over one-half of all patients who were prescribed psychotropic medications failed to complete the treatment course.
- With the exponential growth of the Internet, there was a dramatic increase in the use of self-help groups.
- Also, many patients used multiple venues to treat their mental health problems—self-help groups, human services (school counselors and ministers), primary care, and specialty mental health services.
- In general, this care was uncoordinated (Kessler, Zhao, & Katz, 1999; Olfson et al., 2002).

It has become clear that training in collaborative care and the development of supportive systems are essential initiatives if future patients are going to receive optimal care. We have realized that we have to train our students not only in traditional practice and technique but also in the principles of collaborative care. We also have to play a part in building support for collaborative care models within health care systems.

PREPARING THE NEXT GENERATION OF THERAPISTS

Despite our immersion in the collaborative care movement, we were doing training as usual in our family therapy master's program. That is, we were training future therapists to work independently, using the tools that we gave them, including theory and popular treatment techniques. At best, working with other colleagues meant providing a referral for some special treatment, such as psychological testing.

Eventually my colleagues and I realized that our training models would no longer work. Using the ideals of the collaborative care movement, we began creating new treatment goals. Believing that psychotropic medication could be an essential treatment and that many of our patients would be obtaining medication from their physicians, we considered what new knowledge future therapists (our students) would need.

We began experimenting with collaborative care models of patient care and thinking about how to train students in their use. The four of us—two psychiatrists and two family therapists—began to share patient care. That is, we began to provide joint clinical supervision to family medicine residents and family therapy interns, and we began to teach each other's students.[2]

This book is the result of our collective search for better ways to care for patients with mental health problems. Its purpose is to provide the information a non-MD therapist needs to know about psychotropic medication and collaborative care. It is intended for nonprescribing clinicians who work in mental health. We wrote it with two objectives in mind: to give readers a basic sense of pharmacotherapy for various mental health disorders, and, more important, to provide a conceptual framework, a mind-set, and specific approaches for working in a collaborative care environment with medical professionals who *do* prescribe psychotropics.

Many books about psychotropic medications have been written for psychotherapists, and some recent books discuss split treatment models. As clinicians we found that these books, although helpful, did not meet our needs. We recognized that there are many effective treatments, including combined therapy and medications. However, many of these treatments never reach the people who need them most. We became increasingly interested in the efficacy of the delivery of mental health ser-

---

[2]For example, in a specific week, Dr. Albala and Dr. Patterson might exchange e-mails about a shared patient, jointly conduct live supervision for family medicine residents who are interviewing challenging patients; Dr. Albala might lecture to Dr. Patterson's students about basic antidepressant medication.

Dr. Edwards and Dr. McCahill might meet to talk about further developing treatment protocols at the collaborative clinic they are developing and might engage in a problem-solving session to figure out ways to help their homeless, indigent patients get access to appropriate care, including medication.

vices. What obstacles exist for the typical clinician and patient who seek optimal treatment?

Our goal in this book is to provide basic scientific information about psychotropic medications and, even more important, to offer pragmatic advice on helping patients benefit from these medications. Although there are many potential concerns, such as a family's response and insurance issues, we believe collaboration is the cornerstone of efficacy.

There are many models of care in addition to the psychotherapist–physician collaboration. For example, there is a movement to provide psychologists with prescription-writing privileges. As reported by the American Psychological Association (2002), New Mexico was the first state to give psychologists prescription-writing privileges, followed by Louisiana. Some psychiatrists suggest that it is cost-effective for the psychiatrist to provide both medication and psychotherapy, thus eliminating the need for a nonphysician provider. In addition, some patients do not want therapy and simply seek medication from their primary care providers. Other patients would never consider medication and seek therapy only. Finally, some people seek informal help only through Internet searches or talking to a friend, member of the clergy, or human resources employee.

This book does not focus on these other treatment modalities. It simply focuses on a non-MD therapist and a physician working together to care for their common patient. However, the non-MD therapist could be a psychologist, a social worker, a marriage and family therapist, a psychiatric nurse, or a counselor. When we refer to physicians, we could mean a family physician, a psychiatrist, an internist, a pediatrician, or an obstetrician–gynecologist. To simplify matters, we refer to "the therapist" and "the physician" throughout this book. This book is primarily intended for therapists who want to build collaborative relationships and learn the biological information they need to communicate with physicians.

In writing this book, we made a few assumptions:

1. We want this book to be theory-neutral. Each model and every therapist makes unique contributions to the therapeutic process. You might be an expert in cognitive-behavioral therapy, family systems theory, interpersonal therapy, or another model; your expertise is a critical component of healing. However, because we assume that you already have expertise in some type of psychotherapy, that is not the focus of this book.

2. Rather, we assume that you want to improve your collaborative relationships with physicians. We suggest you can do this by knowing more about psychotropic medications and how they work in the brain.

3. In addition to promoting more collaboration with physicians, we also advocate for more family involvement in health care. We urge you to think about not only your individual patient but also his or her family. This need became strikingly clear to us when a seriously depressed mother went to her primary care doctor because she "didn't know what else to do." She had seen several mental health professionals during the last year, yet none of their treatments had helped her. The physician enlisted the aid of an on-site therapist, and they interviewed the patient together. Fifteen minutes into the interview, it became clear that the patient was a single mother of a 6-year-old and an 8-year-old. She tearfully reported that the 8-year-old had taken on all household responsibilities: walking her younger brother to and from school, preparing all meals, and doing all the shopping and other "parenting" responsibilities that the mother could not do—given that she could not get out of bed most days. The patient reported that she had never given this information to any other health care professionals simply because none had asked. Often, health care professionals are focused only on the individual patient who is present during the interview. As a result, they can miss important information about other family members and the repercussions of the problem throughout the entire family.

4. Some readers, particularly those already trained in neuroscience and biological treatments, may find specific parts of this book too simplistic. We have tried to write the book so that you can skip the parts that are not helpful and turn instead to the sections that offer new information. You may find the chapters on collaboration or the appendices especially useful.

5. We assume that you are pressed for time, that the physicians you work with are pressed for time, and that the payors (including employers and insurance companies) want the patient to get better as quickly as possible. The physicians you work with might have little knowledge or interest in your contribution to the shared treatment—namely, the therapy. They may even have little time or interest in working or communicating with you. Although it is helpful if both professionals share a commitment to collaborative care, it is not essential.

6. Biological treatments are changing at a rapid pace, and this book can quickly become dated. Thus, we have tried to write in terms of general ideas or principles. In general, we talk about classes of medications, not specific drugs. In addition, we talk about the process of how drugs

are created and tested. We know that you need to find your own methods of staying abreast of trends in psychopharmacology and collaborative care. We hope this book serves as one foundation for the ongoing process of learning about biology, neuroscience, psychotropic medications, and collaborative care.

We now narrow our focus to the information you need to effectively collaborate with your medical colleagues. That information includes the following:

- Basic neuroscience information on how the brain works and how drugs affect the brain.
- The biomedical information that you need to understand about psychotropic medications, one of the key treatments the physician might utilize. This is organized by specific disorders.
- An action plan for building collaboration: For example, we discuss what a therapist might consider when deciding to refer a patient to a generalist physician or a psychiatrist. The basics tenets of collaborative care are discussed (beyond collaborating about the patient's psychotropic medication). Whether you are currently in a private practice or in a hospital-based interdisciplinary team, this section provides tools to enhance collaboration.

We recognize that your professional experiences may be significantly different from ours. But we surmise that you share some of our frustrations as we try to provide excellent care in a rapidly changing health care world. Your training may not have provided all of the tools you need for optimal care, and you may be frustrated with the limits of your work setting. We hope this book supplies some knowledge and ways to help you overcome the limits you have faced in caring for your patients.

PART I

The Mind–Body Connection

In this section, we discuss some basic concepts about how the brain works and how psychotropic medications affect it. We believe you should have some understanding of these issues for four reasons:

1. To further develop your understanding of the biological component in the biopsychosocial model. You will more readily include biological issues in your thinking about your patients if you know some specifics about the brain's biology. And with that knowledge, you will probably better understand the later chapters on specific disorders and medications.

2. To help you communicate with physicians. The physicians you collaborate with, by training, have a detailed and sophisticated understanding of these issues. You will be better able to understand and talk with them if you are familiar with terms like "neurotransmitter," "serotonin," and "anticholinergic."

3. To help you explain medications to patients and family members. Some patients may feel more comfortable taking their medications if they understand a little bit about what the drugs do. Although the prescribing physician is the ideal person to provide

this information, not all physicians have the time or inclination to discuss basic biology with their patients. It will often strengthen your relationship with your patients and their confidence in your collaboration with their physicians if you can answer some of their questions and help them understand the information their physicians give them (within the limits of your professional scope of practice and personal knowledge). You may also find that educating your patients about their brain biology can provide them with more productive ways to think about their medications—for example, by replacing "I must be crazy if I need to take drugs" with "My brain doesn't make or use enough serotonin for it to function at its best, but my medication can correct that problem."

4. To improve your assessments. In contrast to the physician's view, you may have a differing opinion about the importance of using the *Diagnostic and Statistical Manual of Mental Disorders* (**DSM**) criteria as the primary means to assess and treat the patient. Most physicians rely on the DSM criteria to make a diagnosis. Their specific diagnoses often lead, naturally, to specific psychotropic medication recommendations. In this way, assessment by a physician may be more specific and, at times, more reductionistic than an assessment by a therapist, who, for example, might prefer a narrative of the patient's complaints.

These viewpoints are not mutually exclusive, and in fact they can be complementary. Physicians often need the therapist to provide a set of symptoms and also offer a holistic perspective on the patient's situation. Problems can occur when either professional is wedded to a singular perspective, especially if the patient is confused by two differing providers. We hope that basic information on a biological perspective will help you understand the physician's unique contributions to your patient's care.

Depending on your training and clinical background, the information in this section may be familiar, or it may seem like a foreign language. We have written it for the latter, the person whose last foray into biology may have been a dimly remembered high school class. On the other hand, if you already know this information and have developed effective ways of communicating it to patients, feel free to skip this section. We leave it up to you to decide how this book can be most helpful.

CHAPTER 1

How the Brain Works

THE HUMAN BODY

... for I am fearfully and wonderfully made.
—PSALMS (139:14)

As we see ourselves and each other, alive and vivacious, we witness an incredible principle in action: that of *the preservation of* **homeostasis**, the tendency of a living organism to maintain balanced, constant conditions in its internal environment. For example, if we drink too much water, our kidneys will help preserve the balance in our internal environment by having us pass that extra water out as urine. Millions of checks and balances are going on at every moment in a human body, and all of the body's components must be healthy for it to go exactly right. When a body is ill, some of the compensatory mechanisms are not working well, and, for example, there may be a fever, diarrhea, diabetes, high blood pressure, or mental illness. If the attack on the body (or its deterioration) is severe enough to overwhelm its compensatory mechanisms, homeostasis cannot be preserved and the body dies. The preservation of homeostasis is essential to the continuation of life. Medications used to treat various maladies often affect the homeostatic compensating mechanisms in the body, and we always hope that the medications' influence is for the better. When we treat mental illness, whether through therapy and/or medication, we are attempting to assist in the brain's and the body's tendency to restore homeostasis and healthy functioning.

CELLS, ORGANELLES, NEUROTRANSMITTERS, AND RECEPTORS

The basic building block of the human body is the **cell**, and a typical adult has approximately 100 trillion cells. Each cell has an outer envelope, or **cell membrane**, and a **nucleus** (see Figure 1.1).

That cell membrane is very complicated, governing what gets into and leaves the cell, among many other tasks. The nucleus contains all of the genetic information (DNA or *genes*) to tell the cell what to do and how to make its contribution to the homeostasis of the total body. Cells (e.g., **neurons**) are organized into **organs** (e.g., the brain), which are organized into **systems** (e.g., the central nervous system, or CNS). At every level of organization in the body, each cell, organ, and system has one priority: maintain homeostasis; keep the balance that is essential to survival.

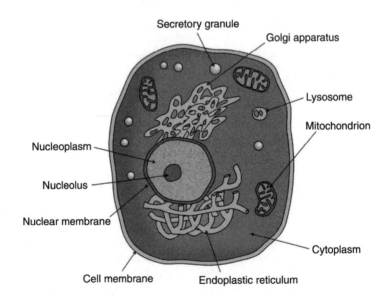

FIGURE 1.1. The anatomy of a cell. Illustration copyright 2004 by James P. McCahill. Used with permission.

Many tiny structures reside in the **cytoplasm** (the liquid interior) of the cell; these **organelles** are responsible for making proteins and other substances that enable the cell to do its job. Other organelles (**mitochondria**) provide energy to other cell parts. Without healthy mitochondria, cells cannot function. For example, in a nerve cell (a neuron; see Figure 1.2) there are components that make chemicals called **neurotransmitters**, which allow one neuron to transmit an impulse to another.

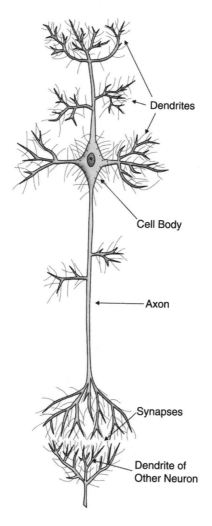

FIGURE 1.2. The neuron, or nerve cell. Illustration copyright 2004 by James P. McCahill. Used with permission.

The **presynaptic neuron** makes the neurotransmitters, puts them into little sacs called **vesicles**, and moves the filled vesicles to the cell membrane in order to **secrete** or dump the neurotransmitters out of the neuron into the right place at the right time. The right place is a tiny space between one neuron and another, called a **synapse** (Figure 1.3), and the right time is when the neuron wishes to activate or inhibit its neighbor neuron.

The **postsynaptic neuron** receives the neurotransmitter when the neurotransmitter engages a **receptor site** on the neuron's cell membrane. Each type of neurotransmitter will react with one specific type of receptor site and no other, similar to a lock and key. But it would not do to just let neurotransmitters sit there in the synapse causing unending activity, so there are other components in presynaptic neurons that take the extra neurotransmitters in a particular area back into the cell (this is called **reuptake**). Sometimes the neurotransmitters that have been taken back are broken down in the presynaptic neuron (by **enzymes,** such as monoamine oxidase, or MAO), and then are recycled in the vesicles for later use. There are at least 40 different chemicals that have been shown to act as neurotransmitters; some of the most common are listed in Table 1.1.

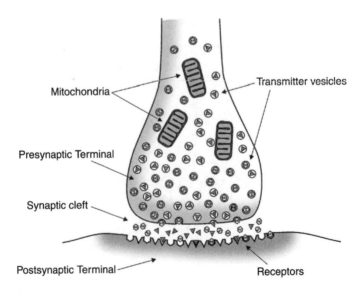

FIGURE 1.3. The nerve synapse. Illustration copyright 2004 by James P. McCahill. Used with permission.

TABLE 1.1. Some of the Most Common Neurotransmitters

Neurotransmitter	Function/biology	Disorder if malfunction	Medications used to influence this neurotransmitter
Acetylcholine	Usually excitatory, except for some parasympathetic nerve endings where it is inhibitory (such as the effect on the heart by the vagus nerve). Secreted by many neurons, including those in the motor area of the brain, basal ganglia, skeletal muscle motor neurons, all preganglionic autonomic nervous system neurons, all postganglionic parasympathetic neurons, and some postganglionic sympathetic neurons.	A complex, diffuse symptoms affecting all bodily systems. This is a complex, widespread neurotransmitter, the receptor sites of which are affected (usually adversely) by some psychotropic medications (anticholinergic side effects).	Very diffusely affected by many medications. In particular, antihistamines, anti-Parkinsonian drugs, and medications for dementia affect this system, as do numerous medications for general medical conditions. Many psychiatric medications have side effects that occur because of their influence on the acetylcholine receptors.
Dopamine	Usually inhibitory. Secreted by neurons in substantia nigra onto neurons of the basal ganglia, both subcortical areas of the brain.	Disorder in the dopamine system has been hypothesized to be important in psychotic disorders, and many antipsychotic medications work on dopamine receptors, of which there are several subtypes. affects cardiovascular system and has other widespread effects.	Diffusely affected by many medications. Antipsychotic medications and some antidepressants have some dopaminergic effects; certain medications, used for general medical conditions also affect dopamine receptors.

(continued)

TABLE 1.1. *(continued)*

Neurotransmitter	Function/biology	Disorder if malfunction	Medications used to influence this neurotransmitter
GABA (gamma-aminobutyric acid)	Inhibitory. Secreted by neurons in the cerebral cortex, subcortical area, and spinal cord.	Anxiety states, also involved in chemical dependency.	Diffusely affected by many medications. Many antianxiety medications work on GABA receptor sites, especially in the frontal lobe of the brain. Alcohol, benzodiazepines, and barbiturates all affect GABA receptors, as do other drugs.
Norepinephrine	Mostly excitatory, but inhibitory in some areas. Secreted by neurons in the locus ceruleus (subcortical area) to widespread areas of the brain, controlling wakefulness, overall activity, and mood. Also diffusely secreted in the sympathetic nervous system.	Diffuse and widespread symptoms, including depression, changes in blood pressure, heart rate, and diffuse physiological responses, among many others. An important transmitter in the sympathetic branch of the autonomic nervous system.	Diffusely affected by many medications. Several antidepressants work specifically on this neurotransmitter and its receptor sites. Many medications for general medical conditions affect this neurotransmitter as well.
Serotonin	Usually inhibitory; helps control mood, influences sleep, and inhibits pain pathways in the spinal cord. Secreted by subcortical structures into hypothalamus, brain, and spinal cord. There are many subtypes of serotonin receptors.	Diffuse and widespread symptoms: depression, headache, diarrhea, constipation, sexual dysfunction, and other medical symptoms.	The selective serotonin reuptake inhibitors (SSRIs), the most commonly used antidepressants, work specifically on this neurotransmitter system.

18

Also important in understanding the function of the nervous system are the **one-way flow** of information across synapses and stimulatory versus inhibitory impulses Most synapses in the CNS will conduct an impulse (usually via a neurotransmitter) in one direction only; that is, from the **axon** of the presynaptic neuron to the **dendrite** or cell body (**soma**) of the postsynaptic neuron (see Figures 1.2 and 1.3). This unidirectionality is critical in preserving the integrity of the information flow in the CNS. A particular postsynaptic neuron will have anywhere from 10,000 to 200,000 terminals, or receptor sites, that interact with presynaptic neurons. These terminals are activated by neurotransmitters. Activating some terminals will cause the postsynaptic neuron to fire an impulse to its neighbor neurons. When other terminals are activated, the same postsynaptic neuron will be especially quiet and will not fire off any impulses. This concept of stimulation versus inhibition and inhibitory impulses from one neuron to another is key in our discussion of mental illness and its treatment.

In sum, most of the words in boldface type above represent areas of active research and knowledge about how medications are used to treat mental illness. How synapses function, the types of receptor sites, the secretion of neurotransmitters from vesicles, the reuptake process, the MAO inhibitors, and the process of neuron inhibition are all referred to often in the chapters on mental illness and psychopharmacology.

ORGANIZATION OF THE HUMAN NERVOUS SYSTEM

There are approximately 100 billion nerve cells, or neurons, in the human body. They are organized into **peripheral nerves**; the ANS; and the CNS, which includes the spinal cord, subcortical brain, and **cerebral cortex**.

The peripheral nerves in the various regions of the body, such as hands, arms, legs, the torso, and so forth, come in two types: those that send information to the *spinal cord* about what is going on (**sensory neurons**) and those that carry orders from the spinal cord and brain telling the body part to move or do something else (**motor neurons**). Depending on how important the sensory information is, it may or may not be sent up from the spinal cord to the brain. The sense of pressure of your shirt on your skin is not considered important, and the brain is typically not bothered with that information. If you are in a conversation, your brain is generally focused on that and does not pay attention to the ventilation fan that may be running in the background. In fact, more than 99% of incoming sensory information is screened out by the CNS (spinal cord and brain) as not being significant enough for the higher parts of the brain (the cerebral cortex) to focus on. This important skill is called **sensory gating,** and it is severely impaired in some patients who suffer from a psychosis. Touching a hot flame is *very* important, much too important to waste time sending it to the brain to think about before acting. So the spinal cord sends a **reflex message** via the motor nerves to get the hand out of the flame, then tells the brain later. The brain then tells the mouth to say "ouch!" and maybe other things.

The ANS governs life-sustaining functions that are critical and too complicated for the CNS to spend time on. If we had to think about how fast our heart should beat minute to minute, how high our blood pressure should be, or when the sandwich we ate for lunch is ready to move from the stomach to the small intestine, we would be too busy to do anything else. So the ANS controls all of these activities. It is divided into two parts: the **sympathetic nervous system** and the **parasympathetic nervous system.** Some effects of the sympathetic versus parasympathetic stimulation on various organs are listed in Table 1.2.

In general, sympathetic system activity usually has a multiorgan impact, such as the fight-or-flight response. On the other hand, the parasympathetic system usually causes a focused response of a particular organ—for example, emptying the bladder (a very complex affair)—without causing other organs or systems to be affected. Each of these systems uses different neurotransmitters. The sympathetic nervous system secretes **norepinephrine** primarily, and the parasympathetic nervous system secretes **acetylcholine.** When we talk about medications used to treat mental illness, we will refer to **anticholinergic side effects** of some

TABLE 1.2. Some Effects of Sympathetic and Parasympathetic Stimulation on Various Bodily Organs

Organ	Sympathetic stimulation	Parasympathetic stimulation
Eyes—pupil	Dilated	Constricted
Eyes—focus	Relaxed (distance vision)	Constricted (near vision)
Heart	Increased heart rate	Decreased heart rate
	Increased contraction force	Decreased contraction force
Gut	Decreased food movement	Increased food movement
	Increased tone of muscles	Mostly relaxed muscle tone
Bladder	Hold urine	Void urine
Penis	Ejaculation	Erection

drugs, which are those side effects that interfere somehow with the normal function of the parasympathetic nervous system. A medication that causes anticholinergic side effects would be expected to cause blurry vision, dry mouth, heart rate disturbance, constipation, and difficulty in voiding urine, among other symptoms.

The CNS includes the spinal cord (which deals with basic reflexes, walking movements, and control of information to and from the brain), the subcortical brain (which deals with such matters as coordination; balance and equilibrium; wakefulness; respiration and heart rate; and basic emotions such as anger, excitement, sexual response, and response to pain and pleasure), and the cerebral cortex (which receives sensory input; controls motor functions; and deals with higher functions of thinking, memory, integration of information, learning, and executive function (see Figure 1.4).

The cerebral cortex is a large memory storehouse, and it is essential for thought processing. However, it relies on the subcortical brain centers to keep it awake, focused, and free of distracting stimuli and tasks. The medications that we use to treat mental illness work in the synapses

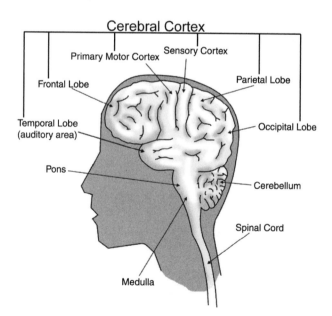

FIGURE 1.4. The brain, brainstem, and upper spinal cord. Illustration copyright 2004 by James P. McCahill. Used with permission.

of both the cerebral cortex and subcortical levels. They also go everywhere else in the body, however, and they have effects, usually referred to as side effects, in many other organ systems.

Modern psychopharmacology works by delivering chemical compounds to the neurons of the brain and the synapses that will alter the activity in those synapses. Research suggests that some drugs work by one or more of the following mechanisms:

- Increasing the amount of neurotransmitter produced by presynaptic neurons and released into a synapse.
- Blocking the reuptake of a neurotransmitter from the synapse.
- Binding to the receptor site on the postsynaptic neuron, disabling the activity of the neurotransmitter present in the synapse.
- Inhibiting the enzymes that break down neurotransmitters.
- Changing the sensitivity of postsynaptic neurons to neurotransmitters.

CHAPTER 2

How Psychotropic Drugs Work

Why can suddenly stopping some antidepressants result in withdrawal symptoms, yet stopping others does not? Why should some medications be taken on an empty stomach? Why is the status of the liver important for some medications, whereas kidney function is relevant for others? Why do some psychotropic medications have noticeable effects minutes to hours after ingestion (e.g., the antianxiety benzodiazepines), whereas others (e.g., antidepressants) take days or weeks for their effects to become apparent? The answers to these questions lie in several pharmacology factors, especially (but not restricted to) **pharmacokinetics** and **pharmacodynamics**. Medications differ in the way they are processed once inside our bodies. They also differ in the way they affect our bodies. These differences confer unique pharmacological "profiles" that make medications produce a unique set of clinical characteristics. When physicians—who more often than not have several medications to choose from for a particular disorder—select a drug, they consider all these characteristics and attempt to match them to the specific needs, sensitivities, and preferences of each individual patient. The purpose of this deliberate decision-making process is to offer the patient an optimal **risk–benefit ratio**. That is, the goal is to select a medication that will produce the strongest possible therapeutic effect with the fewest possible negative side effects.

HOW THE BODY HANDLES DRUGS: PHARMACOKINETICS

The ultimate target for psychotropic drugs is the brain—in fact, specific areas in the brain. Ideally, clinicians would be able to deliver a drug to the desired target and only to that target. This, of course, is not possible, at least not at the current level of clinical biotechnological development. Drugs must use a rather nonspecific method of "public transportation" to reach the brain: the bloodstream. Drugs transported by our bloodstream do make it to the intended targets. Unfortunately, they also reach many unintended areas in the brain, as well as elsewhere. This process, known as **distribution**, will be affected by various factors, including characteristics of the drug. Side effects usually result from this lack of specificity in the delivery system. But first, drugs must reach the bloodstream, and they do so through a process called **absorption**. Different routes can be used: swallowing a pill is the most common. The pill is dissolved in the stomach or in the intestines, a phenomenon mediated by specific "juices" that prepare the drug to cross the microscopic pores that allow entry into the bloodstream. Certain properties of a particular drug will result in faster or slower absorption and, as a result, increase or decrease the time required to reach an appropriate **concentration** of the medication in the bloodstream. The presence of food in the stomach may, in some cases, interfere with the speed of absorption. Conversely, certain drugs have an irritating effect on the lining of the stomach that may lead to adverse consequences, namely, inflammation and pain. Thus, some drugs have instructions to "take with food" and others have instructions to "take on an empty stomach."

In certain clinical situations, we want the beneficial effect of the drug to occur as quickly as possible. For example, an acutely agitated or anxious patient must be given relief very quickly, so getting the drug into the bloodstream as quickly as possible would be of great benefit. For these situations, certain drugs may be given **parenterally**—that is, via routes other than the digestive system—such as **intramuscular** injections of antianxiety or antipsychotic drugs. Intravenous injection of a drug delivers it directly into the bloodstream, causing an immediate effect.

Another way to get a drug into the bloodstream quickly is inhalation. In fact, the short time between the inhalation and the desired effect can sometimes be exploited, with hazardous consequences, as with recreational drugs. For example, nicotine and cocaine, which are very quickly absorbed through the nasal mucosa and the lung tissue, reach the brain in a matter of seconds. Other routes and techniques may be used to deliver drugs to the brain in a controlled fashion. Injections directly into the spinal fluid may be used for certain neurological conditions. Other drugs, after being administered, are released very slowly over a period of days or weeks. Certain antipsychotic preparations (i.e. haloperidol [trade name Haldol], fluphenazine [trade name Prolixin], and risperidone [trade name Risperdal Consta]) can be injected intramuscularly, and they are formulated to release the drugs over a period of several weeks. This "depot" method of administration can provide an essential, consistent baseline concentration of medication for patients who otherwise would not take their medications reliably on a daily basis. Slow-release patches applied to the skin also enable the gradual absorption of certain medications. Nicotine patches, for example, have become useful aids for smoking cessation programs. Selegiline (trade name Emsam), a patch-based antidepressant, has recently been released for clinical use.

Once a drug is in the bloodstream, it is subjected to various factors that can influence how much of it will get into the brain. Some drugs have great affinity for fatty tissue and will be retained in areas of the body where such tissue is in abundance. Such medications need to be taken in higher doses in order to achieve therapeutic concentrations in the blood. Some drugs become tightly bound to proteins found in the bloodstream. For these drugs, part of the administered dose is just ballast (we also call it a "loading dose" in medical terms) since the protein-bound fraction of the ingested medication will not reach the brain.

If a second medication is added—whether for psychiatric purposes or for a concurrent medical problem—there is always the possibility of drug interactions. If the new medication is highly protein-bound, it can compete for the proteins occupied by the first medication and in fact displace some of it, which then becomes free in the bloodstream. Effectively, the concentration of the first medication is now larger, so more of it reaches the brain, with potentially toxic results.

If, following absorption, medications were undisturbed by the body, we would need to take only one dose for an eternal effect. Of course, this is not the case. As soon as drugs enter the bloodstream, the process of **metabolism** ensues. The body recognizes the drug as a foreign substance and eliminates it outright (say, via the kidneys, as in the case of lithium) or transforms it chemically, using a complex enzyme mechanism located in the liver. This chemical transformation enables the medication to be eliminated from the body. In some cases, the chemical transformation produces a new compound that may also have therapeutic effects (or, in some rare instances, a toxic effect). For example, fluoxetine (trade name Prozac) is transformed into norfluoxetine, which is also an antidepressant. A similar situation occurs with the old tricyclic antidepressants (amitriptyline—trade name Elavil—to nortriptyline; the latter, in fact, is "transformed" in the laboratory and marketed as a separate antidepressant, with the trade name Pamelor).

All these different factors—absorption, distribution, metabolism, and excretion—interact with each other and together determine various pharmacological parameters that have clinical significance:

- **Peak concentration:** the time required for the drug, once it is administered, to reach maximum concentration in the blood stream. For those medications that have an "immediate" effect and in which the magnitude of the effect is proportional to the dose (curiously, this is not the case with all medications), knowing the peak concentration will enable us to predict, approximately, the time required for maximum intensity of the desired effect (i.e., how long it will take to feel better).
- **Trough levels:** the point at which the concentration of the medication in the bloodstream is at its lowest. Trough levels that are very low, say, because of lengthy intervals between doses, may actually result in a loss of benefit or may even result in withdrawal symptoms.
- **Half-life:** the time required for the concentration of a medication to decrease by 50% in relation to its peak level. This is the result of metabolism and excretion.
- **Steady state:** the amount of time required for a drug to reach a stable concentration level in the bloodstream. This means that the amount entering the body (repeated doses) matches the amount being eliminated (metabolism and excretion). Typically, for most drugs this time is estimated to be about five half-lives for the medication in question (assuming, of course, no interactions with other medications and other phenomena). So a medication with a half-life of 24 hours will take 5 days to reach steady state. The range of half-lives for psychotropic medications is quite wide, measured from hours (e.g., some benzodiazepines) to many days (norfluoxetine, the active metabolite of fluoxetine). The concepts of steady state and half-life are critical when evaluating clinical results (including the assessment of need for dose adjustments), adverse events, and medication discontinuation phenomena.
- **Plasma levels:** for some psychotropic medications, certain correlations have been established between plasma levels (the concentration of a drug in the liquid portion of the blood) and therapeutic benefit. Using this method, the prescribing physician can make adjustments to the doses with the goal of reaching drug concentrations in the blood that are associated with optimal response. In a few instances—for example the antiobsessional clomipramine (trade name Anafranil) and the antide-

pressant nortriptyline (trade name Pamelor)—clinical research and experience have established a **therapeutic window**, that is, the boundaries of a minimum concentration that must be reached and a maximum concentration that must not be exceeded for the drug to work well. If a patient's blood level is outside the window, in either direction, the benefit is diminished.

HOW DRUGS AFFECT THE BODY: PHARMACODYNAMICS

What are the effects of the medication on our systems, in particular, on the intended targets? Given our current understanding, the intended targets are usually the receptors found in the surfaces of the neurons in the brain. For example, some antidepressants interact with norepinephrine and/or **serotonin** receptors; some antipsychotics exert their effect on **dopamine** receptors. These effects may enhance the function normally carried out by the receptor or inhibit it. Other, more complex interactions can also occur in the neuron. Pharmacodynamics describe the therapeutic and adverse effects of medication. An effect on the desired target will result in symptom relief, but it may produce side effects on unintended targets. Ideally, one would want a medication with high selectivity, that is, affecting the desired target with no or minimal effects on other systems. Second best, a desirable drug will produce a therapeutic benefit at a dose substantially less than that required to produce serious side effects. This is often referred to as the drug's **therapeutic index**. Lithium is an example of a psychotropic drug with a low therapeutic index; small amounts in excess of the doses needed to control manic symptoms may produce serious or even life-threatening side effects. Throughout these medication processes of pharmacokinetics and pharmacodynamics, the body's organ systems are reacting by working to maintain homeostasis. For example, the kidneys detect the lithium as an excess salt in the blood, and they strive to eliminate it. There is a tremendous orchestration of activity going on everywhere in the body (not just the brain) in response to any psychotropic medication, as this is added to the daily physiology of health or disease in that person. Every time a medication is taken, those mechanisms of homeostasis come immediately into play: Every time one neurotransmitter is altered, it sets off a string of counterreactions throughout the body. All of the neurotransmitters affect functions throughout the body and, at the current level of biotechnological development, it is simply impossible to give a medication that does only one thing in one area of the body.

DIVERSE POPULATIONS

To make things a little more complex, different population subgroups with unique pharmacokinetic and pharmacodynamic profiles may require adjustments in dosing and scheduling in order to achieve optimal risk–benefit ratios with certain medications. Children and the elderly are common examples. During their training, many physicians have been admonished to "start low and go slow" when prescribing for geriatric patients. The elderly have absorption, distribution, metabolic, and excretion rates that in many cases differ significantly from those of younger adults. In addition, the elderly often suffer from a number of other medical problems, which in some cases may affect the way they respond to and tolerate medications. Moreover, treatments that they may be receiving for these other medical conditions may interact with the psychotropic medications being prescribed.

An emerging area in clinical pharmacology that promises to produce some clinically meaningful guidelines is **ethnopharmacology**. It has been suspected for a long time that different ethnic groups metabolize and respond to medications differently. These differences appear to be, by and large, genetically determined. However, other factors, such as dietary predilections, may be at play as well. This means that "standard" doses for specific medication might require adjustments when prescribed for members of specific ethnic groups. For example, some data suggest that tricyclic antidepressants are metabolized differently among African Americans (higher blood levels, more side effects, and faster response), Asians (longer elimination times), and native Puerto Ricans (similar response with lower doses and increased side effects) (Preskorn, Feighner, Stanga, & Ross, 2004). Differential responses among some ethnic groups have been reported also for SSRIs, lithium, clozapine (trade name Clozaril), risperidone (trade name Risperdal), and olanzapine (trade name Zyprexa), to name a few. The next few years of research should result in recommendations for specific dose adjustments or, better yet, specific tests that will serve as guidelines for dosing and monitoring the use of psychotropic medications in different populations. The management of all of these factors in psychotropic medication management often constitutes some of the most complex challenges in the practice of medicine.

PART II

Psychiatric Disorders and Their Treatment

In this section, we discuss the various psychiatric disorders and the medications that have been proven effective in treating them. Each chapter focuses on a specific category of disorder and includes the following:

- A definition of the disorder and a summary of the symptoms it gives rise to.
- The biology of the disorder.
- The medications that are commonly used to treat the disorder.
- Issues related to the disorder that may be important in therapy with the patient and/or collaboration with the physician.

To establish a relationship and join with a physician–collaborator, it is necessary to understand his or her way of thinking and talking about patients. Depending on your theoretical orientation, making a diagnosis according to DSM criteria may play a greater or lesser role in how you ordinarily conceptualize your patients' difficulties. For the physician, accurate diagnosis based on criteria in the DSM is the linchpin of treatment, and for good reason. In general, psychotropic medications are developed and approved by the U.S. Food and Drug Administration (FDA) to target the symptoms or symptom clusters of a specific DSM diagnosis. What works for one diagnosis may not work for another; for example, medications that are helpful for social phobia in general are not very effective for specific phobias. So the physician needs to make a diagnosis before he or she can begin to think about what medications are appropriate for the patient. The physician will usually be appreciative if you can assist him or her by communicating your working diagnosis and the symptoms that led you to it in terms of DSM criteria.

Often the **target symptoms** are just as important as the diagnosis in deciding which medication would be most helpful. The target symptoms are those **symptoms** that are interfering with the patient's life and function. They are often (but not always) part of the diagnostic criteria, such as insomnia, poor concentration, and fatigue. Although the diagnosis is very important, the target symptoms will assist the physician in deciding which medication within a class would be the best choice.

These chapters will also help you understand any therapeutic effects and unwanted side effects your patients have when they are taking psychotropic medications. Because you will usually see the patient more often than the physician does, you may be the first professional to whom the patient brings these issues. Although these concerns should be communicated to the physician—and any medication changes must be made by the physician—your knowledge can often reassure the patient, for example, that it is normal for many antidepressant medications to take a few weeks to begin alleviating symptoms. We have designed these chapters to provide you with the basic information you will need to discuss your patients in terms physicians will be familiar with and to alert you to therapeutic issues that may arise in the process of diagnosis and medication.

CHAPTER 3

Mood Disorders

Of all psychiatric disorders, mood disorders (depression, in particular) are probably the most familiar to the general population. The universality of sadness, loneliness, and dejection, all found in different forms and intensities as clinical manifestations of depressive **syndromes**, enables us to understand and empathize with what a depressed person must feel. Also, the pervasive nature of the syndrome, coupled with educational and marketing efforts made in the past decade by mental health organizations and by the pharmaceutical industry, have resulted in some destigmatization. Stigmas of mental illness and of the mentally ill have long been recognized as serious obstacles to access to proper psychiatric care. Progress in CNS research has provided some explanation of the mechanisms underlying psychiatric **symptomatology** and has strongly emphasized the biopsychosocial interplay in mood disorders. The relative widespread availability of effective treatments, essentially nonexistent about 50 years ago, certainly contributes to this improved understanding. A similar shift has occurred in how bipolar disorder and certain anxiety disorders are perceived and understood.

Happily, this evolution in the public's perception of mood disorders has contributed to some improved recognition and treatment, especially of depressive disorders. A large number of patients obtain relief from the unbearable misery of depression in the offices of therapists, primary care physicians, and psychiatrists. And yet we still reach only the minority of those with mood disorders. As epidemiological studies have shown (Kessler et al., 1994), more than half of those suffering from depression in the United States suffer in silence, their condition undiagnosed and untreated. We still have much to learn about how we provide treatment to those with mood disorders. Even diagnosed patients often receive inadequate and/or insufficient treatment. The most common causes of unsuccessful antidepressant medication treatment are suboptimal dosing and insufficient duration of treatment. Guidelines on how to prevent the underdiagnosis and undertreatment of depression are well established but not widely disseminated. And much additional research is needed in order to establish the optimal use of agents that are currently available.

DEPRESSIVE DISORDERS

Epidemiology and Costs

How common is depression? What is its impact on our daily lives and on society? The World Health Organization (WHO) forecasted not long ago that depression would be the main cause of disability in the world within the next several decades. It is estimated that in the United States the lifetime prevalence for major depressive disorder (MDD) is about 17% (Kessler et al., 1994, 2003). The 12-month prevalence is about 6.5%. For dysthymia, the lifetime prevalence is about 6.4%. This means that about one in every five Americans will suffer, at some point in their lives, from a depressive condition that will temporarily render them fully or partially disabled and that will have a serious impact on the lives of their loved ones. About 20 million Americans suffer from clinical depression—not just feeling "down"—on any given day.

By virtue of its severity and clinical impact, major depression is the primary focus of this chapter. However, given its prevalence in outpatient settings, dysthymic disorder—a mild but long-lasting depression—merits additional comments as well. Dysthymic disorder receives less attention from clinicians and less intellectual investment by researchers than major depression, although recently this trend has been somewhat reversed. Dysthymia is not as severe and disabling as MDD, yet it inflicts considerable psychological pain and personal and social burdens.

The principal features of dysthymia are chronicity (duration of at least 2 consecutive years) coupled with some of the symptoms of MDD, although usually of lesser intensity. It often has an early (childhood and adolescence) onset and an ill-defined beginning, slowly evolving into its mature clinical form. Boys and girls are equally affected, but as they enter adult life, dysthymia appears to occur twice as often among women. Frequently, a dysthymic disorder will progress to MDD (for specific diagnostic criteria for each diagnosis, see the DSM). Diagnostic differentiation between the two disorders is not easy. In some cases the same patient will meet criteria for dysthymia at one time and for major depression at another time, a condition sometimes called "double depression." From a pathophysiological perspective, it is unclear whether these are two different mood disorders or some variant therein.

Treatment for dysthymic disorder is similar to that for major depression. When a specific precipitating or sustaining stressor is present (medical, marital, interpersonal, occupational, etc.), as is often the case with these patients, this stressor must be addressed. Treatment includes specific forms of therapy—cognitive-behavioral and interpersonal, in particular—and medication. The clinicopharmacological concepts and techniques discussed in the treatment of major depression later in this chapter are generally valid as well for dysthymia.

Depression is an illness that "maims" and kills. It kills by suicide and it kills by making medical conditions worse or less responsive to treatment. It maims in the sense that it disables individuals socially and occupationally, causes somatic symptoms itself, and contributes to the development of medical conditions that are disabling. Suicide is a major complication of depression and by no means rare. Approximately one out of seven individuals with recurrent major depression will commit suicide. The large majority—about 70%—are suffering from major depression at the time of the act (Ezzell, 2003).

We are gaining considerable understanding about the close relationship between mind and body and their impact on each other. Given that the brain is the organ in which the mind lives—as Hippocrates taught us more than two millennia ago—it is surprising that we ever considered the notion that these two essential realms were separate from and oblivious to each other. Although there is plenty of evidence to support a unitarian construct, we mention here only some examples relevant to depression and its medical significance. Consider, for example, cardiovascular disease. Mental stress is associated with an almost threefold increase in **mortality rates** in certain patients with coronary artery disease. Studies have shown that, following heart attacks, patients who also suffer from depression fare much worse than nondepressed patients. In particular, they die at higher rates (three times higher, during a 6-month follow-up period; Frasure-Smith, Lesperance, & Talajic, 1993). Depression turns out to be the number-one risk factor for people who have suffered a heart attack (even more influential than the ejection fraction, a measure of the heart's pumping function, or **hypertension**) for having a future heart attack. Patients who undergo coronary bypass graft surgery, if depressed at the time of discharge, experience in the subsequent 12 months three times more chest pains, heart failure requiring hospitalization, repeat heart attacks, and need for repeat heart surgery, than individuals who are not depressed after bypass surgery.

This influence is also seen in many other medical conditions, and it is very likely that research will show that the phenomenon probably affects most diseases. We know that depression adversely affects the functional status of patients with chronic obstructive pulmonary disease (COPD); it negatively affects treatment and diet adherence, functional status, and medical-related costs in patients with diabetes; it negatively affects **treatment adherence** in a host of medical and psychiatric disorder patients; it has even been shown that psychological factors are independent predictors of responses in patients receiving chemotherapy for advanced local breast cancer. Finally, from an administrative and cost-containment perspective, undiagnosed and/or untreated depression is associated with longer stays for patients hospitalized for *medical* problems and a higher rate of complications, including a higher rate of mortality.

The cost in suffering is clearly significant. There is, of course, a financial impact as well. For depression alone, this is a staggering figure. It costs our society approximately $12 billion to treat this disease (this includes, among others, costs for hospitalization, psychiatric care, and medications). When indirect costs (i.e., absenteeism, decreased productivity, and increased utilization of medical resources for nonpsychiatric medical problems) are factored in, the total reaches $40 billion or more. It is clear, therefore, that recognition and proper treatment of depression can have a massive impact on individuals and public health efforts. Although the following case is a singular example, considering it against the backdrop of potentially millions throughout society demonstrates the massive impact depression can have on the health care system.

CASE: MAJOR DEPRESSIVE DISORDER, ANXIETY, AND GRIEF

Case Description

Mr. A called Dr. P on the recommendation of another man in his men's Bible study group who had seen Dr. P himself. Mr. A made an initial appointment for himself and gave little explanation of why he wanted it except to say he was "stressed."

During the initial session, Mr. A recounted a painful story, describing the death of his 3-year-old daughter. Mr. A had reluctantly gone on a business trip, leaving his wife with his child, who had flu-like symptoms. His daughter quickly became worse, and Mr. A realized there was an emergency and returned home. Within 24 hours after returning home, Mr. A's beloved daughter died.

Her death had occurred approximately a year earlier. Mr. A recounted the grief and loss he and his wife felt. But he also shared the strength his Christian faith had provided and the tremendous support they had obtained from their friends at church. Mr. A said that he and his wife didn't know how they would have coped without the caring of their friends and their strong faith.

Nevertheless, Mr. A felt it was becoming increasingly difficult to get up every morning and go through the day. He was having trouble concentrating, and it was affecting his business. He was very reluctant to travel, and yet his job required frequent travel. Mr. A became increasingly somber, sad, and discouraged as he described his current situation. When Mr. A had shared these same thoughts with his men's Bible study group, a dear friend had recommended that he come see Dr. P.

It was easy for Dr. P to ascertain that Mr. A's grief had become a major depressive disorder. Both the amount of time and the loss of daily functioning suggested that Mr. A could benefit from treatment. Nevertheless, Dr. P could tell that Mr. A was uncomfortable with the idea of "therapy" and much preferred the support of his church friends. In fact, Dr. P doubted that Mr. A would have ever even considered therapy if his trusted, Christian friend hadn't personally recommended it. Although Dr. P knew that medication might help, she initially decided not to recommend a medication referral because she hoped Mr. A could first become comfortable with therapy. Instead, she spent time listening to Mr. A, building rapport and encouraging the positive coping skills that he already had in place. She also invited him to bring his wife with him to therapy.

Mrs. A accompanied Mr. A to the next few therapy sessions, and she appeared equally depressed. In fact, Dr. P noticed that she felt sad and exhausted herself after each session with the A's. Dr. P felt that her own responses to the A's indicated that the depression was not improving. After careful assessment and attentive empathy to the A's pain, Dr. P felt that they needed additional resources. She brought up the idea of a medication evaluation. Initially, the A's were reluctant. But after discussing the idea of medication for an entire therapy session, they consented to be seen by Dr. P's colleague, Dr. R.

Beginning Collaboration

Dr. R set aside two consecutive hours to evaluate both Mr. and Mrs. A. She let them decide how the sessions would be run—individually or conjointly. Similar to Dr. P, she allowed the A's the opportunity to tell the story of the loss of their daughter before she focused the session on clinical symptoms. Both Mr. and Mrs. A agreed to begin taking medication.

Mr. and Mrs. A continued working with Dr. P, and within a few weeks, Dr. P noted improvement. The A's were able to participate more fully in the therapy, and they were able to complete the homework assignments between the sessions. Within a few weeks, the A's were feeling better and able to complete the tasks of daily living with renewed energy. Dr. P found it easier to conduct the therapy sessions. She called Dr. R to thank her for her critical help with a very difficult family situation.

Questions for Consideration

• *What symptoms did Mr. A present that led to recommendations for both therapy and medication?* It is important to note that environmental events—such as the death of a loved one—while stressful and painful, may not require therapy and/or medication. Dr. P noted the length of time that the A's had been dealing with their grief and the fact that they seemed to be getting worse, not better. In addition, their productivity and ability to complete the tasks of daily life had deteriorated. These were all signs to her that the A's needed therapeutic interventions. In addition, Dr. P noted her own responses to the A's—a sense of sadness and loss that she felt as the end of each of their sessions. Her own sadness helped her understand and empathize with the overwhelming grief.

• *How did the therapist utilize the patient's natural coping skills and the supportive resources he already had in place when he came to therapy?* Dr. P noted how helpful the social support that the A's had received from their church had been to them. She wanted to reinforce the coping strategies and resources that the A's already had. She tried to demonstrate respect for all that the A's had already addressed and tried to keep the therapy in synchrony with the work the A's were doing through their church.

• *What circumstances prompted Dr. P to refer to a physician? Why did she wait a while before she made the referral?* The timing of the medication referral was critical. Since the A's were reluctant to come to therapy in the first place, Dr. P was hesitant to send them to one more doctor. She wanted to establish rapport. In addition, she wanted to explore the possibility of addressing the grief and depression through therapy alone. However, it became clear that the A's were not improving during therapy. Furthermore, the therapy was hard to conduct because the A's had so little energy, motivation, and concentration during the sessions. A medication referral was necessary.

• *How did Mr. A's therapy facilitate the therapeutic experience of his wife and vice versa?* As a therapist, Dr. P was trained to consider other family members even when they did not appear at the initial session. Dr. P knew that Mrs. A must be equally affected by the loss of their daughter and wondered aloud how Mrs. A was doing. Mr. A was enthusiastic about including his wife in the therapy. Dr. R created one long conjoint medication evaluation—in essence a "family medication evaluation." Dr. R and Dr. P were convinced that the A's would improve faster if they improved together instead of in isolation. Thus, the entire treatment was couple-based.

Risk Factors

Although the ultimate causes of depression are unknown, research has contributed substantially to our knowledge about the interaction among biological, psychological, and social spheres of influence. A number of factors, when present, are thought to increase the risk that a specific individual would experience depression (see Table 3.1).

It is well known that individuals with prior episodes of depression are at a much higher risk for **relapse** (see Table 3.2). In fact, the more prior episodes, the higher the risk. If the 45-year-old patient sitting in your office is presenting with her first episode of depression, in general, the risk of a future episode sometime during her lifetime will be about 50%. As you take further history, it becomes apparent that when she went to college this patient had an unequivocal (albeit untreated) episode of major depression.

TABLE 3.1. Some Risk Factors for Depression

- Prior episodes of depression
- Family history of depressive disorder
- Prior suicide attempts
- Female gender
- Early age of onset (< 40)
- Postpartum period
- Menopause
- Current/past marital status
- Medical comorbidity
- Lack of social support
- Stressful life events
- Current alcohol or substance abuse

TABLE 3.2. Risk Factors for Recurrence of Depressive Episodes

- Insufficient treatment duration
- Insufficient maintenance dose
- Poor treatment compliance
- Postpartum period
- Menopause
- Early (< 20 years) or late (> 60 years) age of onset
- History of multiple previous episodes
- History of dysthymia
- Psychosocial stressors (job loss, bereavement, financial distress, etc.)
- Long duration of recent episode
- High severity of recent episode
- History of seasonality of depressive episodes
- Alcohol and/or substance abuse
- Medical comorbidity

Now you are in the presence of a patient on her *second* episode of depression. The estimated risk for a subsequent episode in her case has now increased to about 80%. Now your clinical curiosity is really stimulated. You probe further (in reality, it takes several sessions and questioning to assemble a solid history, as patients simply do not readily remember all details), and it becomes apparent that this patient had an episode of postpartum depression after the birth of her second child 9 years ago. And now, statistically, the risk for a fourth episode sometime in the future is increased to almost a certainty—90% or more.

Other factors include gender (women are nearly twice as likely [1.7:1.0 ratio] to suffer from major depression), marital status (higher risk for separated or divorced individuals living alone), the presence of medical conditions (especially seriously disabling conditions), and a history or current diagnosis of alcohol and/or substance abuse (Kessler et al., 1994). Stressful life events (bereavement, financial loss, and employment changes affecting self-esteem) are notoriously noxious in individuals predisposed to depressive illness (Caspi et al., 2003). This finding, replicated by Kendler, Kuhn, Vittum, Prescott, and Riley (2005), but not confirmed in a recent study (Risch et al., 2009), will continue to fuel the debate on whether genes and the environment interact in such a way that the effect of the environmental stress will be dependent, to some extent, on the individual's genetic predisposition. If confirmed, conversely, one could speculate that environmental manipulation—early or even "preventive" psychotherapy, for example—may attenuate the effect of a genetic makeup that would make an individual particularly vulnerable to depression. Clinicians should always take a detailed clinical history in order to identify the possible presence of these risk factors. Some risk factors are not controllable at the present time (e.g., genetic predisposition), whereas others are subject to intervention (e.g., stress, social support, and substance abuse).

Although the risk factors that are subject to intervention are characteristically universal and cross-demographic, symptomatic depression among the elderly is particularly notable, given that it is the one population in which collaborative care models of treatment have demonstrated the most initial success (Bruce, Ten Have, & Reynolds, 2004; Unützer, Katon, & Callahan, 2002). Several studies, including the PRISMe study, the PROSPECT study, and the IMPACT study (Caton et al., 2005), have demonstrated that collaborative care has better results than the usual care. In particular, collaborative care improves access to mental health services and improves detection rates of commonly missed mental health problems. Usual care, in this case, refers to traditional health care provided by a primary care physician or traditional mental health care. The results of these studies are motivating policymakers to push for more collaborative care on a national level (Boschert, 2004). The goal of policymakers is to promote interdisciplinary team care and ensure continuity of care. An equally important goal is to find ways to include the fundamentals of collaborative care in the training of health care professionals and to ensure ongoing research that examines the best models and applications of collaborative care.

Suicide

Suicide is the ultimate price of severe undetected or untreated depression. The fact that suicide *appears* to be a fully willful act (which it is not, when committed by an individual whose judgment is affected by a severe depression) contributes to the mistaken perception that the mortality factor in depression is low. What makes the act of suicide particularly painful is that in the great majority of cases, it is fully preventable with appropriate treatment and monitoring. Many patients, reflecting on their now resolved depressive episode, regard with horror their struggle with suicidal thoughts and the notion that, without treatment, they would have carried out the act. Important suicide facts are summarized in Table 3.3.

Assessment of suicidal risk is an inherent component of every psychiatric evaluation and should be conducted during the initial visit or

TABLE 3.3. Some Facts about Suicide

- Suicide is the 11th leading cause of death in the United States, accounting for 1.2% of all fatalities.
- A person dies by suicide roughly every 18 minutes in the United States.
- Someone attempts suicide every minute.
- Four males die by suicide for every female, but at least twice as many women as men attempt suicide.
- Approximately 85 Americans take their own lives every day.
- The suicide rate for white males ages 15–24 has tripled since 1950.
- Between 1980 and 1996, the suicide rate for African American males ages 15–19 increased 105%.
- Suicide is the third-ranking cause of death for teens ages 10–19.
- White men 85 and older die by suicide six times the overall national rate.
- Suicide rates for women peak between the ages of 45 and 54 and surge again after age 85.
- Alcoholism is a factor in roughly 30% of all completed suicides.
- Approximately 7% of people with alcohol dependence will die by suicide.
- Eighty-three percent of gun-related deaths in the home are the results of suicide.
- Death by firearms is the fastest-growing method of suicide.
- Suicides outnumber homicides two to one every year in the United States.
- Suicide accounts for nearly 57% of all firearm deaths in the United States; 60% of all suicides involve firearms.

Note. Data from Ezzell (2003), Anderson and Smith (2003), and the CDC National Center for Health Statistics (2006).

contact. Perhaps the most common misconception about suicide is the fear that inquiring about it will "plant" the idea in the patient's mind. In fact, suicidal thoughts are so common among persons suffering from depressive symptoms that individuals consulting a professional most likely have been assailed by them at least in passing. Once a proper assessment has been conducted (see Table 3.4), the clinician can then take the appropriate measures, depending on the results of the assess-

TABLE 3.4. Components of an Evaluation for Suicidal Risk.

- Presence of suicidal or homicidal ideation, intent, or plans.
- Access to the means for suicide and the lethality of those means.
- Presence of psychotic symptoms, command hallucinations, or severe anxiety.
- Presence of alcohol or substance abuse.
- History and seriousness of previous attempts.
- Family history of or recent exposure to suicide.

ment. This may range from simple monitoring to the most protective measure of admitting the patient to a hospital (against the patient's will if the situation so requires, adhering, of course, to all necessary legal requirements).

The Biochemistry of Depression

The discovery in the 1950s of medications capable of modifying the course of some mental illnesses injected enormous energy into the research of their biological causes and mechanisms. These discoveries, coupled with data strongly suggesting the influence of genetic factors in the genesis of mental disorders, led to the inescapable conclusion that biology, in addition to environmental factors, had to play a critical role. In the case of depression, certain medications used for other medical purposes, notably arterial hypertension (high blood pressure), were found to induce psychiatric symptoms. Researchers hypothesized that if chemical compounds were capable of producing such symptoms (or, in some cases, of relieving them), they must result from an underlying biological mechanism.

In the 1960s researchers formulated, and later refined, the so-called monoamine hypothesis of depression. This hypothesis states that symptoms of depression are due to alterations in the functioning of certain neurotransmitters known as monoamines, notably norepinephrine, serotonin, and to a lesser degree, dopamine. Roles for other neurotransmitters have been identified in recent years. The foundation of this hypothesis rests on the finding that all antidepressant medications known at the time had, to some extent, the ability to increase the availability of these neurotransmitters at the synaptic level. Patients and the general public often refer to this hypothesis as "chemical imbalance."

Some antidepressants—specifically, tricyclics like imipramine (trade name Tofranil) and amitryptiline (trade name Elavil)—are thought to exert their antidepressant effect through inhibition of a reuptake mechanism that "sucks" back the neurotransmitters from the synapse into the neuron for storage and future use, a process mentioned in Chapter 1. The resulting net effect is an increase of these molecules at the synapse and thus a more robust neurotransmission. A different category of antidepressants—monoamine oxidase inhibitors (MAOIs)—display a different mechanism of action but with the same net effect of increasing norepinephrine and serotonin neurotransmission: they inhibit the metabolism (breakdown) of the molecules stored in the neurons, thus creating more abundant supplies for neurotransmission.

Once armed with this understanding, pharmaceutical researchers went back to their labs and developed molecules capable of replicating these effects. Adjusting the structure of the molecules and submitting these new compounds to various tests, they produced the "second generation" antidepressants, the SSRIs (selective serotonin reuptake inhibitors; as their name indicates, they selectively inhibit the reuptake of serotonin from the synapse back into the neuron from which it was originally released) and several others.

As research has progressed, it has become apparent that the biochemical mechanisms underlying depression are infinitely more complex than the simple deficiency of monoamines at the synaptic level. It has been hypothesized, for example, that the deficiency may actually be not in a shortage of a specific neurotransmitter (e.g., serotonin) but actually in the mechanism of communication (transduction) between the pre- and postsynaptic neurons. Furthermore, recent research has suggested that the problem may be "downstream" in the cascade of molecular events that convey neural signals. Specifically, a substance called brain-derived neurotrophic factor (BDNF), which is involved in sustaining the viability of neurons, may be deficient in depressed individuals (Karege et al., 2001), thus causing atrophy (or even death) of cells in certain areas of the brain, like the hippocampus. Hippocampal atrophy has been observed in depressed patients (Sapolsky, 2001). Also, stress and its associated elevation of cortisol—a "stress" hormone—are known to reflect limbic hypothalamic–pituitary–adrenal (HPA) axis dysregulation and also cause hippocampal atrophy and deep changes in mood and behavior. All these issues are poorly understood, and their relationship to the antidepressant effects of medications is still unknown. Thus, the proposed mechanism of action for antidepressants that we use on a daily basis does not provide a full explanation of the biochemical mechanisms underlying depression. Does this invalidate the legitimacy of using these medications? Not at all. Many quite effective treatments used in medicine have obscure or unknown mechanisms of action. Aspirin, for example, has been used for a century for a number of purposes, yet its mode of action was only discerned relatively recently. Table 3.5 lists selected antidepressants classified by their proposed mechanisms of action.

In addition to the presumed antidepressant mechanism of these drugs, they exert a multiplicity of effects on other neurotransmitters and neuron receptors, both in the areas that control mood symptoms and elsewhere in the central and peripheral nervous systems. Because medications have effects not only in the areas thought to be related to the disorder being treated but also in other areas in the brain and peripheral nervous system,

TABLE 3.5. Classification of Antidepressants According to Their Presumed Mechanism of Action

Presumed mechanism of action	Examples[a]
Norepinephrine–serotonin reuptake inhibitors	Amitriptyline (Elavil) Clomipramine (Anafranil) Duloxetine (Cymbalta) Imipramine (Tofranil) Venlafaxine (Effexor)
Selective serotonin reuptake inhibitors (SSRIs)	Escitalopram (Lexapro) Fluoxetine (Prozac) Paroxetine (Paxil) Sertraline (Zoloft)
Selective norepinephrine reuptake inhibitors	Desipramine (Norpramin) Nortriptyline (Pamelor, Aventyl) Reboxetine[b]
Serotonin antagonist reuptake inhibitor	Nefazodone (Serzone)
Alpha$_2$ antagonist + noradrenergic/ specific serotonergic	Mirtazapine (Remeron)
Dopamine–norepinephrine reuptake inhibitors	Bupropion (Wellbutrin)
Monamine oxidase inhibitors (MAOIs)	Phenelzine (Nardil) Selegiline transdermal (Emsam) Tranylcypromine (Parnate)

[a]Trade names are in parentheses.
[b]Available in Europe.

it is not surprising that they usually (in fact, almost always) cause side effects. This also explains why some medications may be effective in more than one clinical condition. If a **neurotransmitter** function is linked to depressive symptoms, obsessive–compulsive disorder (OCD), and, say, motor control, one would expect that a medication affecting that particular neurotransmitter might have antidepressant effects and anti-OCD effects but would also cause tremors as a side effect.

The following is useful as an illustration of this common clinical situation. Let us consider a depressed patient with the typical clinical picture, including the target symptoms of mood disturbance, anxiety, recurrent and brooding thoughts, and decreased concentration. Assume, applying the monoamine hypothesis, that this patient has a dysfunction of both norepinephrine and serotonin (incidentally, no clinical test exists yet to determine which neurotransmitters are affected in a particular individual). Our treatment goal is to restore both these neurotransmitters to normal range. Let us say that we use a norepinephrine–serotonin reuptake inhibitor. Since mood is primarily modulated in the frontal cortex (norepinephrine and serotonin) and anxiety in the limbic system (norepinephrine and serotonin), with a single medication we would see clinical improvement in both these areas. Attention and concentration would improve by virtue of similar mechanisms. Side effects would occur as well in other areas of the body where specific functions are regulated either centrally (i.e., in the brain) or peripherally by norepinephrine and/or serotonin. Tables 3.6 and 3.7 summarize the potential effects on the hypothetical patient.

TABLE 3.6. Side Effects Commonly Associated with Antidepressant Therapy

System	Effect
CNS	Activation • Insomnia • Anxiety • Nervousness • Agitation • Tremor • Seizures • Sedation • Somnolence • Fatigue
Gastrointestinal system	Nausea Constipation Diarrhea Dyspepsia Weight gain (rarely, weight loss) Anorexia
Sexual function	Decreased libido Impotence Ejaculation disorder Anorgasmia
Cardiovascular system	Hypertension Orthostatic hypotension Arrhythmias
Other	Dry mouth Increased sweating Asthenia

Note. Data from Depression Guideline Panel (1993a).

TABLE 3.7. Benefits and Side Effects on Hypothetical Patient Treated with a Norepinephrine–Serotonin Reuptake Inhibitor

Location	Neurotransmitter	Function affected	Symptom/side effect examples
Frontal Cortex	NE–SE	Mood	Depressed mood
Frontal Cortex	NE	Attention	Concentration deficits
Limbic system	NE–SE	Emotions, agitation, anxiety, energy	Anxiety, tearfulness
Hypothalamus	SE	Appetite	Anorexia, hyperorexia
Sleep centers	SE	Sleep	Insomnia, hypersomnia
Cerebellum	NE	Motor function	Tremors
Brainstem	NE	Blood pressure	Hyper- or hypotension
Brainstem	SE	Digestion	Nausea, vomiting
Heart	NE	Heart rate	Tachycardia
Bladder	NE	Urinary (bladder) control	Urinary retention
Basal ganglia	SE	Motor function	Compulsions, agitation, restlessness
Spinal chord	SE	Sexual function	Anorgasmia, impotence, ejaculatory delay
Intestine	SE	Digestion	Gastrointestinal cramps, diarrhea

Note. NE, norepinephrine; SE, serotonin.

Clinicians will readily recognize in Table 3.7 the experiences reported by many of their patients when receiving treatment for depression or other related psychiatric disorders. By looking at the "Function affected" column, it is possible to understand why some medications (say, SSRIs) are effective in variable degrees in several conditions associated with serotonin dysfunction (depression, OCD, social anxiety disorder, posttraumatic stress disorder, generalized anxiety disorder, panic disorder, and bulimia nervosa).

As mentioned before, antidepressants affect a variety of neurotransmitters, some having no apparent relation to the depressive syndrome at all. These medications are less specific or less "clean." The effects on these other neurotransmitters will make no contribution to the desired antidepressant goal. Moreover, they may complicate the treatment by causing side effects that may be so uncomfortable or troubling that patients stop taking the medication. Some examples of side effects resulting from activation or inhibition of certain neurotransmitters include the following:

- Blocking acetylcholine receptors (dry mouth, blurred vision, constipation, tachycardia, memory problems).
- Blocking alpha$_1$ norepinephrine receptors (low blood pressure, sedation).
- Blocking histamine receptors (sedation, inattention, low energy, weight gain).

Antidepressant Medications and Clinical Practice

In spite of the dramatic advances in research on depression and the medications used for its treatment, it is important to remember that our understanding of the underlying mechanisms is still relatively elementary. So a clinician must utilize all available scientific information, yet bear in mind that it is incomplete. The application of scientific knowledge to the management of clinical situations has traditionally been referred to as a successful combination of science and art. What Leonardo da Vinci stated centuries ago—"First study the science, then practice the art"—is as valid today as it was then. The "rules" that may emanate from current medical knowledge are peppered with multiple exceptions and unexpected clinical developments. Every capable clinician knows that no two patients are fully alike. Moreover, as research advances, revisions of accepted practices will inevitably occur. With this caveat in mind, let us explore some elements that are often incorporated into the treatment selection and medication monitoring of a depressed patient.

Differences among Antidepressants

Are all antidepressants the same? No. Does it make any difference which one is selected? Yes. In general, when the efficacy of antidepressants is compared, all seem to perform equally, with response and **remission** rates ranging from 40 to 60%. It has been suggested that certain antidepressants—those with robust norepinephrine and serotonin effects—may have an edge in this regard, but a definitive answer to this issue awaits specifically designed replication studies. In fact, a review study examined, among other questions, whether different antidepressant medication mechanisms of action resulted in different levels of antidepressant efficacy, and it found no differences based on pharmacological activity. That is, all antidepressants were equally efficacious regardless of the mechanism of action

(Freemantle, Anderson, & Young, 2000). A recent meta-analysis (Cipriani et al., 2009) found that when both efficacy and patient acceptability are considered, two antidepressants are favored (sertraline and escitalopram). These findings are intriguing—confirmation will be necessary—and may potentially impact clinicians' choices of antidepressant medications. At the present time, it is not the efficacy of a medication but rather other factors (chiefly, side-effect profiles) that the physician looks at when selecting a drug for a specific patient.

Richelson (1994) proposed a set of characteristics for the ideal antidepressant. This medication does not exist, of course. However, the list gives the reader a flavor for the critical elements that physicians look for when making a selection (Table 3.8).

Side Effects

The appearance of side effects in the course of medication treatment is inevitable. The old, paternalistic attitude displayed by many physicians toward their patients—"Take the medicine, and you'll be just fine"—provided little patient education and dispensed with patient autonomy. Fortunately, this attitude is gradually being abandoned, and for good reason. We have learned that for treatment to have the best chance of success, an alliance must develop between the physician and the patient, with each contributing to the effort to treat the disorder. A well-informed patient will fulfill his or her role in this alliance more efficiently. A discussion between the prescribing physician and the patient about potential side effects is a must in this context. Since side effects will almost always occur, patients should be aware of them and told what to expect. Such disclosure will generally promote treatment adherence (also commonly referred to as "treatment compliance").

TABLE 3.8. Pharmacological Characteristics of the Ideal Antidepressant

- Rapid onset of action
- Intermediate half-life
- Defined therapeutic blood level
- No side effects
- Minimal drug interactions
- Low toxicity associated with overdose
- Broad spectrum of efficacy
- No withdrawal syndrome

Note. Data from Richelson (1994).

Inconsistent or nonexistent adherence to treatment is among the most important causes of treatment failure in depression (Lin et al., 1995). Studies have shown that within the first month of treatment, roughly one third of patients will abandon medication treatment! At the conclusion of four months, approximately half of patients will do the same (Lin et al., 1995). This is an unfortunate result for a treatment that in most patients should last at least a year. There are many reasons patients choose to discontinue medication treatment in spite of their physicians' advice to continue. The issue is complex and multifactorial (Table 3.9).

As this study illustrates, side effects are the most common reason for discontinuing medication, both early and late in treatment. In cases where side effects are intolerable (say, severe and sustained diarrhea or frequent and disabling headaches), there is no alternative but to search for a different medication that the patient might tolerate better. However, in many cases, side effects are transient and tend to disappear gradually after a few days to weeks of treatment (a phenomenon sometimes referred to as **habituation**). A common example is nausea, which can be quite bothersome initially but will wear off within 2–3 weeks of treatment with many antidepressants. Most experienced clinicians will agree that telling patients about the potential side effects early in the course of treatment will greatly increase the chances that the patient will be willing to adhere to it. When side effects occur and their intensity goes beyond

TABLE 3.9. Patient Report of Most Common Reasons for Discontinuation of Antidepressant Medication

Reasons for discontinuation	% early quitters ($n = 41$)	% late quitters ($n = 25$)
Disliked side effects	62	67
Didn't need medication	56	46
Felt better	50	44
Felt medication wasn't working	32	52
Ran out of pills	10	0
Doctor's orders to stop	12	24
Friend recommended stopping	7	0
Weight gain	5	16
Forgot to take medication	5	4

Note. Early = first month; late = within 3 months. Data from Lin et al. (1995).

mild nuisance levels, intervention becomes necessary to ensure that the patient does not drop out of treatment.

A very common and (to patients) significantly bothersome side effect of antidepressant medications is sexual dysfunction. Not all sexual dysfunction reported or detected in a depressed patient is necessarily due to medications. Table 3.10 lists some of the frequent causes. Remember that certain forms of sexual dysfunction—notably, loss of libido—are often core symptoms in depression. Coexisting medical conditions (e.g., arteriosclerosis and hardening of the arteries) and medical treatments (e.g., antihypertensives, drugs used to treat high blood pressure) sometimes cause impotence. It could be that the patient suffers from a primary sexual disorder that preceded the onset of the depressive episode by many years and has been hitherto unreported or undiagnosed. It is not uncommon in clinical practice to see patients who, as they begin to experience relief from depression and regain sexual interest, reveal the presence of sexual problems. It is incumbent on the clinician to take the appropriate history so that sexual dysfunction is not automatically attributed to the medication.

Antidepressants do constitute the main cause for new sexual dysfunction seen in the average outpatient (Balon & Harvey, 1995). Although various kinds of sexual dysfunction may be seen in the context of antidepressant therapy (Table 3.11), the most common manifestations seen in clinical practice are erectile dysfunction, partial or complete anorgasmia, and delayed ejaculation. Resolution of these side effects is critical to ensure treatment adherence and remission and to reduce the stress of the depressive episode on the patient's relationship with a spouse or significant other. When an antidepressant treatment achieves symptom remission but is complicated by sexual dysfunction as a side effect, several strategies have been used to deal with the problem, although the success of each varies from patient to patient (Table 3.12).

TABLE 3.10. Causes of Sexual Dysfunction in Depressed Patients

- The depressive syndrome itself
- Comorbid medical illness
- Comorbid psychiatric illness
- Primary sexual dysfunction
- Side effect of antidepressant medication
- Side effects of other concomitant medications
- Combination of some or all of these factors

TABLE 3.11. Types of Sexual Dysfunction Induced by Antidepressant Medications

- Changes in libido (decreased or increased)
- Impaired erectile capacity
- Delayed ejaculation
- Painful ejaculation
- Priapism
- Impotence
- Partial or complete anorgasmia
- Clitoral enlargement

Note. Data from Harvey and Balon (1995).

OPTIMIZATION

Optimization, perhaps the least drastic strategy, consists of adjusting the dose and administration schedule of the medication. A conservative approach would wait for the passage of time, perhaps several weeks, to see if the sexual side effects disappeared with habituation to the medication. Although other side effects such as nausea do tend to go away in most patients during the first weeks of treatment, spontaneous resolution of sexual side effects is not as common, but when it happens there is no need to change the medication or dose.

Reducing the dose of the antidepressant is also an alternative. Since most side effects are dose-related, a decrease in the dose would be expected to result in amelioration of side effects, and indeed, this is often the case. The problem with this approach is that there is an inherent risk

TABLE 3.12. Managing Antidepressant-Induced Sexual Dysfunction

Intervention	Example
Optimization	Anticipate habituation Reduce dose Consider drug holidays
Substitution	Bupropion, mirtazapine
Antidote	Buspirone, bupropion, gingko biloba, sildenafil, cyproheptadine, yohimbine, methylphenidate, etc.

of relapse with dose reductions, meaning clinicians who choose this approach will have to monitor patients closely.

A third conservative approach is the **drug holiday.** Anticipating planned sexual activity, the patient temporarily discontinues the drug, say, for a day or so. The sharp reduction in antidepressant blood levels sometimes results in temporary disappearance or at least reduction of the sexual dysfunction. This method has several limitations as well: it precludes spontaneous sexual activity; it may lead to relapse of depressive symptoms; it may produce antidepressant withdrawal symptoms (see Table 3.13), which can be severe enough to squelch the desire of even the most passionate of lovers; and it is restricted to patients on antidepressants with a short half-life (blood levels of long half-life compounds such as fluoxetine [Prozac] would not drop quickly enough to create the planned holiday).

SUBSTITUTION

Even in the presence of a robust antidepressant effect, the burden of sexual dysfunction sometimes makes it impractical to continue with the same treatment. In these situations, the offending antidepressant is substituted for another one expected to have a much lower potential for causing sexual dysfunction (e.g., bupropion, mirtazapine, and nefazodone). This approach is also fraught with certain risks, as the response to one antidepressant does not guarantee a response to the new one, and thus relapse may occur. It is important to remember that not all antidepressants work with equal efficacy in all patients, and many times responses are idiosyncratic. Also, the introduction of a different antidepressant may result in the appearance of a new set of side effects— intolerable agitation, excessive sedation, or fatigue, to cite some com-

TABLE 3.13. Symptoms That May Occur during Acute SSRI Withdrawal

Physical symptoms	Psychological symptoms
• Lightheadedness	• Anxiety/agitation
• Headaches	• Depression
• Nausea, vomiting	• Spontaneous, uncontrollable crying
• Tremors	• Irritability
• Muscle pain	• Restlessness
• Sensations of electric shock	• Decreased concentration
• Insomnia, vivid dreams	• Derealization, depersonalization
	• Confusion
	• Memory difficulties

mon ones—that may turn out to be even more bothersome than the sexual dysfunction that prompted the substitution.

ANTIDOTE STRATEGIES

Essentially, with antidote strategies, the patient continues with the effective, albeit side-effect-prone, antidepressant but adds another medication that is expected to reverse the sexual dysfunction. No single compound is guaranteed to achieve this goal in all patients. Many different medications have been tried, with mixed results. In essence, antidote strategies require trial and error. One of the most common approaches uses the addition of bupropion (trade name Wellbutrin), an antidepressant in its own right with a known low-risk profile for sexual dysfunction. In some cases it can counteract the sexual dysfunction induced by SSRIs. Many other compounds are thought to be effective in some cases, mostly based on data presented in a few case reports. A handful of controlled studies have produced some promising data, but replication is needed. Among the antidote strategies, gingko biloba is a nonprescription substance sold as a nutritional supplement. There are reports of its effectiveness in reversing sexual side effects in some patients. Your patient may learn of it from the Internet or other sources and ask you about it. Gingko biloba itself has physiological effects, including side effects and undesirable, sometimes dangerous, interactions with some prescription drugs, so it will be essential to include your physician collaborator in any decision about using gingko biloba as an antidote strategy. The main drawback of most antidote methods is the need to take the medication daily rather than restricting its use to the time of sexual activity. The antihistamine cyproheptadine (trade name Periactin) has also been anecdotally reported to help alleviate delayed orgasm due to SSRIs. It is important to stress that all of these medication approaches to SSRI-related sexual dysfunction represent "off-label" use of those medications, and they are not approved by the FDA. However, sildenafil (which is FDA-approved for the treatment of erectile dysfunction in men only) has been reported effective in some cases of SSRI-induced sexual dysfunction in both men and women when used prior to sexual intercourse.

Although it may be necessary to try more than one of these strategies before finding the one that will work for a particular patient, sexual dysfunction as a side effect must not be passively accepted during the treatment of individuals with depression. In fact, ignoring the importance of this side effect—or any others, for that matter—will greatly risk treatment nonadherence and the very real probability of relapse. Also, a clinician's indifference to the presence of sexual dysfunction is likely to affect the patient's self-esteem and the relationship with his or her spouse or partner.

The Phases of Treatment

It is useful to conceptualize drug treatment of depressive illness as occurring in phases. This approach is based on observations made in the natural course of the disorder and on the knowledge gained during the first decades after the introduction of antidepressant medications. Depression is a chronic, episodic, remitting, and relapsing disease.

Left untreated, episodes will come and go over the years, with a general tendency to become more frequent and more severe with each subsequent relapse. The average length of a depressive episode—although there is great variability—is between 8 months and 2 years.

In general, it can take several weeks for the response to the medication to become apparent ("response" is arbitrarily defined as a 50% reduction in the severity of symptoms, as measured by certain rating scales). Several more weeks may still elapse before full symptom remission occurs. This phase of treatment has been termed "acute treatment" (Figure 3.1).

Once remission has taken place, many patients are naturally inclined to discontinue treatment. In fact, in the early days of antidepressant treatment, most physicians would discontinue medications as soon as remission occurred. It quickly became apparent that the risk of relapse was quite pronounced when medications were discontinued

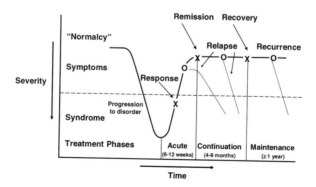

FIGURE 3.1. Phases of treatment for depression: The five R's. Data from Kupfer (1991) and Depression Guideline Panel (1993b).

shortly after remission. The hypothesis proposed to explain this phenomenon is that medications are "masking" the symptoms while the underlying pathophysiological alteration caused by the disease continued its natural course. When medications were removed, the illness manifested itself again. To prevent this relapse, it is now standard to continue treatment for a period of time equivalent to the assumed natural duration of a typical depressive episode. Several time frames have been proposed for the duration of this second phase of treatment, termed the "continuation phase" (Table 3.14).

Accordingly, treatment should last, at the very least, for about 9 months (up to 3 months to reach full symptom remission and 6 months to drastically reduce the risk of relapse). Equally important, dose reductions should be avoided during this period of treatment. In the past, it was assumed that full doses were unnecessary to sustain remission, but observations of high relapse rates led the field to abandon this approach. In practical terms, most patients today receive antidepressant treatment at the same dose required to achieve remission for a total of 1 year before consideration is given to discontinuation.

The third phase of treatment is called the "maintenance phase." As mentioned earlier, recurrence (the reappearance of symptoms reflecting a *new* episode) is the hallmark of many depressions (see Table 3.15). This pattern dictates the clinical strategy. If the patient has completed treatment for a first episode ever, most physicians—cognizant of the fact that the lifetime recurrence risk is approximately 50%—will discontinue medication once a year has been completed. This appears the sensible

TABLE 3.14. Guidelines for Duration of Antidepressant Treatment *after* Acute Treatment Response

Organization	Continuation treatment (months at same dose)	Number of episodes for long-term maintenance treatment
U.K. "Defeat Depression" consensus statement	4–6 months	Two?
U.S. Agency for Health Care Policy and Research	4–9 months	Three?
British Association for Psychopharmacology	6 months	Three? in past 5 years (or six? in total)
American Psychiatric Association	4–5 months	Not specified

Note. Data from Geddes et al. (2003).

TABLE 3.15. Guidelines for the Maintenance Phase in the Treatment of Depression

Three major depressive episodes or two episodes and a risk factor:
- Family history of bipolar disorder or recurrent MDD
- Psychotic or severe prior episode
- Closely spaced episodes (two in < 3 years)
- Incomplete interepisode recovery
- Onset of first episode < 21 or > 60 years old
- Antecedent dysthymia ("double depression")
- Major depressive episode of > 2 years' duration

Note. Data from Depression Guideline Panel (1993b) and Rush (personal communication, 1999).

thing to do, considering that half of the patients would otherwise receive unneeded treatment. And of those in the other half, the second episode may not occur for a decade or more.

When patients have a history of three or more episodes—including the present one—the recurrence risk would predict that a future episode, more likely sooner than later, is a virtual certainty. For this group of patients, it is appropriate to implement the maintenance phase of the medication treatment. The duration of this phase is currently a matter of debate. Some clinicians advocate continuing treatment for several years; others regard lifetime treatment as a must for those with three or more previous episodes. Definitive conclusions will have to await the publication of incontrovertible data to guide the clinician's decision making on this issue. Many patients will be distressed to hear their doctors tell them that they ought to expect to take their medications for the rest of their lives. Given some uncertainty in the field and the likelihood of patient ambivalence about staying on a medication indefinitely, the issue demands careful attention both by the prescribing physician and the psychotherapist so that the selected treatment will enjoy the full support and commitment of the patient.

Individuals completing treatment for a second depressive episode present the psychopharmacologist with somewhat of a conundrum. Although a large proportion will be at risk for relapse, many will not, and it would be desirable to avoid unnecessary treatment. The physician must evaluate each patient's unique situation, with particular emphasis on factors that may pose a risk of recurrence. When one or more of these factors are present, maintenance treatment is preferred. Table 3.15 shows a useful set of guidelines to assist in the selection of patients for whom maintenance phase treatment after a second episode is highly desirable.

In this patient population, the risk of relapse, with its resulting consequences of suffering, disability, loss of income, potential need for hospitalization, and suicidal risk, to mention some, greatly outweighs the possible side-effect burden and cost of maintenance treatment.

Within these clinical guidelines, the unique characteristics of each patient will dictate the course to follow. Side effects, variations of clinical course, the presence of life stressors, economic considerations, relocation, concurrent illnesses, and other factors will affect the formulation of a specific plan that is suitable for a particular patient.

What If There Is No Response to the First Antidepressant Used?

Although antidepressant medications have made a dramatic difference in the outcome of depressive illness, they are by no means the panacea that some would like to believe. The overall *response* rate to antidepressants is thought to be in the vicinity of 60–70% after the first attempt. Response, it will be remembered, is defined as a 50% reduction in the severity of symptoms, usually as measured in research studies with the HAM-D (Hamilton Rating Scale for Depression; Hamilton, 1960) or the MADRS (Montgomery–Asberg Depression Rating Scale; Montgomery & Asberg, 1979).

Although this represents a considerable reduction in suffering and disability, it is not, by any means, the ultimate goal of treatment. If we apply the more stringent—and more logical—standard of remission (i.e., HAM-D scores of less than 8, at worst, more or less the equivalent to the feelings experienced by the average individual on a given Monday morning), then the efficacy of antidepressants drops to 35–50%. This limited performance leaves a considerable number of patients in need of supplemental or alternative treatment. Several factors are thought to be at play in those patients obtaining less than desirable clinical benefit (see Table 3.16). We discuss them briefly.

WRONG DIAGNOSIS

Several subtypes of depression require specific treatment strategies that go beyond a simple course of conventional antidepressant therapy (these subtypes include bipolar depression, major depression with psychotic features, seasonal depression, atypical depression, comorbid anxiety disorder, comorbid substance abuse, double depression [major depression

TABLE 3.16. Considerations for Nonresponse to Treatment

* Reassessment of clinical status
* Reconsideration of the diagnosis
* Core residual symptoms or side effects
* Dose and duration
* Drug interactions
* Augmentation
* Substitution
* Treatment nonadherence

plus dysthymia], and persistent psychosocial stressors). In the presence of **nonresponse**, the clinician will be well advised to reevaluate the patient for the presence of depressive subtypes and unique circumstances that require a specific approach.

INADEQUATE TREATMENT

Even when the diagnosis is correct, certain minimal parameters of dose and time are necessary for satisfactory clinical outcomes. When tricyclic antidepressants were the mainstay of antidepressant treatment, their side effects required starting doses much lower than therapeutic doses. The physician had to increase doses slowly in order to minimize and manage the emerging side effects. It typically took 1 to 3 weeks to reach therapeutic doses. Because this requirement was not always understood, many patients ended up receiving subtherapeutic doses, and an insufficient clinical response was not uncommon. Since the introduction of the generally better tolerated SSRIs, physicians sometimes titrate up the dose rapidly, and sometimes they even start patients immediately at the typical therapeutic dose. Still, a sizeable minority of patients requires higher than average doses. As a result, the potential benefit of these medications may not be fully realized at the typical doses and the patient's depression is erroneously labeled "**refractory**" to treatment, when in fact all that is needed is a higher dose to achieve an appropriate response. Table 3.17 shows dose ranges for selected antidepressants. These ranges are for general reference only. Often, physicians will exceed FDA-approved doses when unique clinical situations so require.

A second important factor in nonresponse is insufficient duration of treatment. All antidepressant medications have a lag period between the time treatment starts and the time when a clinical response is readily

TABLE 3.17. Dose Ranges for Selected Antidepressants

Drug name	Dose range (mg/day)
• Amitriptyline	50–300
• Bupropion	200–450
• Bupropion SR	150–400
• Citalopram	20–60
• Clomipramine	50–250
• Desipramine	100–300
• Duloxetine	40–60
• Escitalopram	10–20
• Fluoxetine	20–60
• Imipramine	75–300
• Mirtazapine	15–60
• Nortriptyline	75–150
• Paroxetine	10–60
• Paroxetine CR	12.5–62.5
• Phenelzine	15–90
• Sertraline	50–200
• Tranylcypromine	30–60
• Venlafaxine	75–300
• Venlafaxine XR	75–225

apparent. Some patients will report a benefit within a matter of days, whereas others will not see any benefit for several weeks, even though in both cases an eventual satisfactory response or remission will occur. Because of this lag, or latency period, patients and clinicians sometimes switch to alternative treatments prematurely, mistakenly concluding that no clinical response will take place. In fact, about one-third of patients who have shown no response at 2 weeks will go on to experience a substantial benefit if the same treatment is continued. When no response is seen after 4 weeks, a full fifth of these patients will still respond to treatment. Of course, as time passes, the odds of response diminish, and at some point alternative treatments become necessary. On average, absent any **sign** of response, it seems prudent to consider modifications to the treatment regime after 3–4 weeks. In the presence of a partial response, this time is commonly extended to about 6 weeks, although a wide range of strategies is utilized by physicians.

Once it has been determined that treatment response is unlikely, physicians have at their disposal a number of choices. These strategies— optimization (push the dose of the current drug to the maximum tolerable), substitution (change from one drug to another) and **augmentation** (keep the first drug but add another so that the combination is often more effective than the first drug alone). Most of these decisions are based on clinical experience and case reports. Presently, the field has no proven, systematic approach to applying these techniques in treating refractory patients. The STAR★D project (Sequential Treatment Alternatives to Relieve Depression) will attempt to provide an answer to this most important and common clinical problem—that is, what is the clinician to do after the patient did not benefit from the first antidepressant course? Do we go to psychotherapy? Do we try a different medication? Or do we combine psychotherapy with medication? The main objective of this study was to develop an evidence-based set of steps to guide the physician in making sequential treatment selections likely to increase the odds of response and remission. The study, which set out to include about 4,000 patients nationwide, tested the benefits and limitations, both from the patient's and the clinician's perspective, of a sequential order of treatment strategies. The sequence design in the study was derived from accepted clinical standards and supported by the practices of physicians considered experts in the field. Patients who did not respond to initial SSRI treatment (in the study design, citalopram was the SSRI used initially in all subjects) progressed to level 2, where they were assigned to one of a number of treatment options. The options available at level 2 included the addition of or the substitution for cognitive-behavioral therapy. If no response occurred at this level, patients then progressed to level 3 and, as necessary, to level 4, where more options were available (see Figure 3.2). The STAR★D protocol also provided for a minimum duration and dosages of each of the treatments utilized in order to avoid failures derived from insufficiency in these areas.

Initial results for the STAR★D study were published early in 2006, providing useful insights for the clinician (Rush et al., 2006; Trivedi, Fava, et al., 2006; Trivedi, Rush, et al., 2006). The Level I patients were all treated with the antidepressant citalopram, and only about 30% of the patients reached remission (that is, their symptoms essentially disappeared). However, about half of the patients experienced a response (a less demanding outcome measure that is commonly used in clinical drug trials and that reflects the rate of patients who experienced at least a 50% reduction in the severity of symptoms). These results are congruent with efficacy trials and with clinical experience. The results from Level I also showed that, in general, responders to treatment have a higher education, have fewer medical problems or psychiatric comorbidities, and are currently employed white women.

Level II results showed that patients who failed to benefit from SSRI treatment (citalopram) are good candidates for augmentation (with sustained-release bupropion or with buspirone) or switching (to sustained-release bupropion or sertraline or sustained-release venlafaxine—three

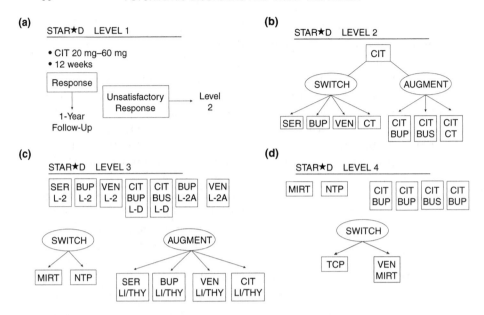

FIGURE 3.2. Protocol for thr STAR★D project. (a) Level 1; (b) level 2; (c) level 3; (d) level 4. CIT, citalopram; SER, sertraline; BUP, bupropion; VEN, venlafaxine; CT, cognitive-behavioral therapy; BUS, buspirone; MIRT, mirtazpine; NTP, nortriptyline; LI, lithium; THY, thyroid hormone; TCP, tranylcypromine.

antidepressants with different mechanisms of action). One third of the patients in each group reached remission. Thus, overall, after two well-delivered (robust doses and sufficient duration) medication treatment courses (results for the group who received CBT were not published yet) about 50% of the patients achieved full remission of symptoms. Level III results showed modest gains and comparable efficacy for lithium and thyroid augmentation, although tolerability was slightly better with the latter. Level IV results also showed very modest treatment improvement in nonresponders (about 10%) and suggested that the venlafaxine XR/mirtazapine combination may be a better choice than MAO inhibitors, based on ease of use. The field is at this time trying to discern the clinical implications of these findings (McGrath et al., 2006; Nierenberg et al., 2006). We will also learn of the percentage of patients who, in spite of these systematic efforts, are still unresponsive to antidepressant treatment and require more drastic or unconventional treatment approaches.

In spite of all the conventional medication and treatments available, there is a subgroup of patients who will not benefit from adequate use of these tools. Several new antidepressant medications are under development that may not only provide results similar to those obtained with the ones currently in use—with a lower side-effect burden—but also offer benefits to those individuals who do not respond to current treatments. And, of course, the search continues for medications that will shorten the latency for onset of response/remission and which will be more effective and better tolerated in a larger number of patients. In addition, some nonmedication alternatives, rTMS (repetitive transcranial magnetic stimulation) and VNS (vagal nerve stimulation) are now approved by the Food and Drug Administration for the treatment of certain types of depression, although many clinicians are skeptical about their place in the antidepressant armamentarium. You can find more information on these treatments in Appendix B, "Future Trends."

Electroconvulsive Therapy

As an alternative form of treatment for depression, a physician may also consider **electroconvulsive therapy (ECT)**. ECT was the first effective antidepressant treatment. More than 65 years after its introduction, it is still considered by many physicians to be the most effective therapeutic tool for moderate to severe depression. Although the relatively benign side-effect profile of the current generation of antidepressants has reduced the need for ECT, more than 100,000 patients currently receive this treatment in the United States each year. This will probably surprise some readers, as ECT is not often talked about in general mental health circles. The very nature of ECT—direct electrical stimulation of the brain—evokes myriad emotional responses among clinicians and the general public. For most people, the dramatic scenes in the classic novel and film *One Flew over the Cuckoo's Nest* have created an indelibly negative—albeit highly inaccurate—impression of ECT. And yet, it is a highly effective and safe form of treatment. It is not without some irony that society can regard direct electrical stimulation of an organ as one of the most dramatic and admired of medical interventions—as is the case of cardiac defibrillation, where the electrical stimulus is applied to the heart—or as a maligned, even barbaric, procedure, as with ECT, where the stimulus is applied to the brain.

Although a number of theories have been proposed, the mechanism of action of this form of treatment is essentially unknown. The main indication for ECT is major depressive disorder, particularly in the presence of certain clinical characteristics. Mania and schizophrenia in some situations also constitute indications for ECT (see Tables 3.18 and 3.19).

The technique used today for the administration of ECT differs considerably from that prevalent during the first 20 years or so following its

TABLE 3.18. Diagnostic Indications for ECT

Major depression
- Unipolar
- Bipolar

Mania

Schizophrenia (acute exacerbations)
- Abrupt or recent onset
- Catatonic subtype
- History of favorable response to ECT

Schizoaffective disorder

Schizophreniform disorder

Medical disorders (efficacy data only suggestive)
- Parkinson's disease ("on–off" phenomenon)
- Neuroleptic malignant syndrome
- Intractable seizure disorder

Note. Data from American Psychiatric Association (2001).

TABLE 3.19. Primary and Secondary Uses of ECT

Primary
- In most cases, ECT is used after treatment failure with psychotropic medications (although there are exceptions).
- Need for rapid, definitive response because of severity of psychiatric/medical condition.
- Risks of other treatments outweigh risks of ECT.
- Past history of poor response medications or of good response to ECT.
- Patient's preference.

Secondary
- Treatment resistance.
- Intolerance to or adverse effects with pharmacotherapy.
- Deterioration of psychiatric or medical condition creating a need for rapid, definitive response.

Note. Data from American Psychiatric Association (2001).

introduction. The modern use includes careful selection of patients who meet the criteria in Tables 3.18 and 3.19. Informed consent is obtained from the patient and, in many cases, from his or her significant others as well. The treatment is given by a trained psychiatrist in a facility where modern equipment and monitoring devices, operated by trained personnel, are readily available. Contrary to popular belief, ECT is a painless procedure. Anesthesia, provided by a physician anesthesiologist or a nurse anesthetist, is necessary so that the patient can be given muscle relaxants only, which will prevent the electrical stimulus of the brain from affecting muscles in the rest of the body. This temporary muscle relaxation includes full paralysis of the diaphragm, rendering the patient unable to breathe on his or her own. During the procedure, the patient will require assisted ventilation. Although this could be done while the patient is conscious, the loss of control over respiratory function can be quite anxiety-provoking for most people, so the procedure is more comfortable under general anesthesia. Once under the effects of anesthesia, the patient is given a very brief electrical stimulus generated by the ECT device, using especially designed electrodes that are applied to specific areas on the skull.

The main, though certainly not the only, challenge of ECT is its effect on memory. Typically, ECT-treated patients will experience various degrees of amnesia. In most, full memory is restored within several weeks after treatment. However, a small minority of patients will continue to have memory problems for months or even years. Two important techniques have reduced, but not eliminated, this problem. One is the use of devices that deliver electrical waves in a form and intensity less likely to induce amnestic complications. The other is electrode placement. Traditionally, the electrodes are positioned bilaterally, one on each side of the skull. Research has shown that placing both electrodes on one side of the brain—usually the nondominant hemisphere, which for most people is the right hemisphere—can substantially reduce the incidence of amnesia. In a number of cases, however, some loss of efficacy may result when unilateral placement is used. Thus the physician and the patient need to make the appropriate risk–benefit analysis in selecting a technique.

Once the electrical stimulus is delivered, a generalized brain seizure follows, of a variable duration of 30–90 seconds. Scientists believe that this seizure activity is the variable responsible for ECT's therapeutic benefits. The patient gradually awakens from anesthesia a few minutes later. There is some cognitive confusion, which usually clears over the next 30–60 minutes. On average, depressed patients need 7–10 such treatments, usually given three times per week. A successful acute course of ECT will induce response and remission but it will not prevent relapse or recurrences. Thus, once a response has occurred, the patient is started on antidepressant medications. In some cases, medications are ineffective in preventing relapses and/or recurrences, and thus ECT may be given as a continuation and/or maintenance treatment at weekly or monthly intervals, depending on the circumstances. Overall, the response rates for ECT in moderate to severe depression are quite good, exceeding 80% of cases, a performance that is superior to that obtained with antidepressant medications and/or psychotherapy.

BIPOLAR DISORDER

> Those affected with melancholia are not every one of them affected according to one particular form; they are either suspicious of poisoning or flee to the desert from misanthropy, or turn superstitious, or contract a hatred of life. If at any time a relaxation takes place, in most cases a hilarity supervenes . . . the patients are dull or stern, dejected or unreasonably torpid, without any manifest cause . . . they also become peevish, dispirited, sleepless, and start up from a disturbed sleep. Unreasonable fear also seizes them; if the disease tends to increase . . . they complain of life, and desire to die.
> —ARETAEUS DE CAPADOCCIA (2nd century A.D.)

This is perhaps the earliest documented clinical description of bipolar disorder. Keen observers noticed not only that certain individuals suffered from depression but also that, seemingly inexplicably, their mood would suddenly switch into the polar opposite: from dejection to unbridled excitement, from profound despair to limitless optimism, or from paralyzing fatigue to superhuman levels of activity and energy. Bipolar disorder, as it is presently termed, historically has been called manic–depressive insanity (as it was called in Kraepelin's [1919/1971, 1976] time) or manic–depressive illness. The term "bipolar" was coined several decades ago in an effort to reflect the hallmark of the disorder: two opposite poles of the affective continuum.

Bipolar disorder affects about 0.5–1.5% of the U.S. population in any given year. These figures cross cultural, economic, and ethnic boundaries. If broader criteria (i.e., the inclusion of subtypes thought to be variants of bipolar disorder) are applied, its prevalence can reach as high as 5%. Bipolar I disorder (defined below) appears to be equally common among females and males, whereas bipolar II disorder is apparently more common in females.

Bipolar disorder is a lifetime disorder for which there is treatment but no cure. It has a profound impact on the patient and his or her family, coworkers, and friends and on society as a whole. Bipolar individuals have a high incidence of broken marriages and remarriages; to illustrate this point, some clinicians anecdotally suggest that a history of four or more marriages strongly suggests the presence of bipolar disorder. Patients often find themselves unemployed, not infrequently having been fired from their jobs. Their friendships end, having been shallow and brief. Bipolar disorder imposes severe disability, and it is a deadly affliction, perhaps one of the most lethal among psychiatric disorders. The lifetime risk of suicide among bipolars is 8–20%. This figure is much higher than the suicide risk in the general population (Goodwin & Jamison, 1990).

Although traditionally thought to be an illness of early adulthood onset, research has demonstrated that bipolar disorder can often begin in childhood, sometimes mistakenly diagnosed as attention-deficit/hyperactivity disorder, oppositional defiant disorder, or **unipolar depression**. In rare instances, bipolar disorder can also first appear late in life, after the age of 50. In such cases, the onset is usually thought to be the result of brain injury or insult (physical, metabolic, pharmacological, or infectious, among others). Of particular importance for our discussion is the well-documented potential that antidepressant medications have for inducing hypomanic (similar to manic but of milder severity) or manic episodes in biologically vulnerable individuals.

The natural course of bipolar disorder is episodic and highly recurrent. Initially, it can present with one or more episodes of depression before the first frankly hypomanic or manic episode occurs. In many cases, manic and hypomanic episodes may precede or follow a depressive episode. Episodes usually last several months and may resolve spontaneously, without treatment. Recurrences every 2 years or so are not uncommon, and over time the frequency and intensity of episodes may actually worsen. In general, there is great variability in its course from patient to patient. A graphic rendition of the median life course of affective illness (based on the life course of 82 patients), including episodes of mania and depression, treatments, and hospitalizations, is illustrated in Figure 3.3.

As much as one-third of the life of a person with bipolar disorder is spent under the cloud of depression. The disorder occurs in cycles. A

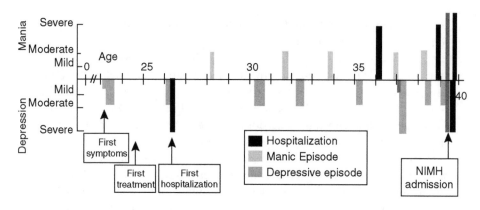

FIGURE 3.3. Median course of affective illness in 82 bipolar patients. Data from Post, Roy-Byrne, and Uhde (1988).

cycle is measured from the beginning of one episode until the beginning of the next one. It includes both the symptomatic period (the "episode") and the intervening **asymptomatic** period that precedes the onset of the next episode. Some patients suffer from a rapidly cycling form of the disorder, with frequent, sometimes ultrabrief episodes that last a few days or even hours. Arbitrarily, a rapid cycler is an individual who suffers four or more episodes (mania, hypomania, depressed, mixed, or a combination thereof) in the course of 1 year. The psychological and social scars resulting from episodes of mania and depression, which often require hospitalization, make it all but impossible for patients to approach a modicum of stability and predictability in their daily activities. Mid- and long-term planning are a constant gamble.

Bipolar disorder is thought to have a strong heritable component. Family, twin, and adoption studies all point at a genetic contribution to vulnerability to developing the illness. First-degree biological relatives of bipolar individuals have, in comparison to the general population, a much higher incidence of bipolar disorder types I and II, as well as of major depression. For example, the **monozygotic twin** (identical twin) of an individual with bipolar disorder has up to an 80% risk of developing the illness him- or herself. For a **dizygotic twin** (fraternal twin) the risk is considerably less, the same as any sibling, in the vicinity of 10–15%. A relationship, possibly genetically determined, has also been recognized among bipolar patients and some individuals suffering from alcoholism. Currently, genetic researchers are vigilantly searching for the specific genes responsible for the biological risk of bipolar disorder.

Contemporary mental health standards recognize several types and subtypes of this disorder, and work on categorizing it for accurate diagnoses is ongoing. DSM-IV-TR (American Psychiatric Association, 2000) includes bipolar type I (episodes of mania, hypomania, and depression), bipolar type II (episodes of hypomania and depression but no mania), cyclothymic disorder (hypomania and minor depressive episodes), and bipolar disorder not otherwise specified (atypical, difficult to categorize presentations). Some episodes may be mixed, wherein both depressive and hypomanic/manic symptoms occur contemporaneously. You can find out more about these diagnostic categories in the DSM and in various psychopathology texts.

Treatment of Bipolar Disorder

> Untreated manic–depressive illness is, by any measure, gravely serious—complex in its origins, diverse in its expression, unpredictable in its course, severe in its recurrences, and often fatal in its outcome.
> —GOODWIN AND JAMISON (1990)

Like many other psychiatric and medical disorders, bipolar disorder is not curable, but it is certainly treatable. Its clinical symptoms can be controlled, modified, and even silenced. Successful treatment must combine drug therapy, psychotherapy, and psychoeducation. More and more frequently, treatment is provided by a team that, at a minimum, includes a physician—usually a psychiatrist—and a therapist. Whenever possible, treatment should involve the patient's immediate family (spouse, parents, and children). Although medication is the core intervention, it is widely recognized that a number of psychological variables can influence the course of the disorder and the patient's adherence to treatment.

During acute episodes, especially mania, hospitalization is almost always unavoidable. The turmoil and disruption resulting from mania, and its profound impact on judgment and behavior, may make it impossible to treat the patient on an outpatient basis. Furthermore, there are significant risks of aggravating existing medical illnesses, of physical injury to self or others, of dehydration, of physical exhaustion, and of suicide. In fact, it is not rare that these patients are hospitalized against their will because of the danger to themselves or others or the severe disability resulting from the mania. Likewise, when depression is severe, the same setting is necessary for successful initiation of treatment. Once the most severe symptoms are controlled, the rest of the treatment takes place initially in a partial hospitalization setting and later in an outpatient setting.

Medical or Somatic Treatment

ACUTE MANIA/HYPOMANIA

Although presently only lithium, valproic acid/divalproex, and several atypical antipsychotics have been approved by the FDA as treatments for acute mania, clinicians prescribe a number of other medications as well for patients in the manic phase (Table 3.20). The strength of the data justifying their use varies, with the strongest evidence occurring with lithium and followed by atypical antipsychotics (aripiprazole, olanzapine, etc.).

Since first reported by Cade in 1949, lithium has been the most frequently studied and used drug for the treatment of bipolar disorder. Recent trends in the United States have shifted to the use of anticonvulsants—mostly divalproex and valproic acid—although the rationale for this switch in emphasis arguably stands on tenuous scientific grounds.

Although lithium is a very powerful antimanic medication and an effective **prophylactic** agent in the prevention of recurrences, its mechanism is unknown. Some hypotheses have suggested that its action occurs intracellularly, in the so-called second messenger system (chemical reactions going on inside the cytoplasm of the neuron), beyond the neurotransmitter receptors. Lithium is given orally. Sustained release preparations enable giving doses twice or even once a day. In mania, its benefits

TABLE 3.20. Some Common Treatments for Acute Mania

Medication	Starting dose	Target dose/level
Lithium	600–1,200 mg/day	600–2,700 mg/day (0.6–1.3 mEq/L)
Olanzapine	5–10 mg/day	10–20 mg/day
Divalproex or valproate	500–1,000 mg/day	500–3,750 mg/day (20 ± 3 mg/kg/day)
Carbamazepine	300–500 mg/day	400–1,800 mg/day (6–16 µg/ml)
Aripiprazole	15 mg/day	10–30 mg/day
Quetiapine XR	300 mg/day	600 mg/day
Lamotrigine[a]	12.5–25 mg/day	50–400 mg/day
Tiagabine[a]	2–6 mg/day	4–48 mg/day
Topiramate[a]	25–75 mg/day	75–600 mg/day

[a]At the present time, there is only very sparse evidence on the benefit of these agents for acute mania.

do not become apparent for several days, so initially additional medications are needed for tranquilization and, if necessary, to control psychotic symptoms. Commonly, lithium has been used in conjunction with conventional or atypical antipsychotics (in the past few years, because of their more favorable side-effect profile, atypical antipsychotics have all but replaced the use of conventional antipsychotics) and/or benzodiazepines (such as lorazepam and clonazepam). Lithium has been found to have antisuicidal properties that are superior to those of divalproex and possibly to carbamazepine, another antiepileptic drug often used for mania. Considering the high prevalence of suicide risk among bipolar patients, this is a key advantage of lithium.

Because of the potential effect it may have on other body systems and the risk of **toxicity**, a baseline medical workup is *de rigueur* in every patient who is a candidate for lithium therapy. This workup includes laboratory tests aimed at evaluating kidney function, thyroid status, complete blood count, cardiac function, and so on.

Lithium is effective within a certain range of concentration in the blood. Therefore, dosing must be tailored to the individual patient to reach levels that fall within the therapeutic range, usually between 0.6 and 1.3 mEq/L (milliequivalents per liter, the units used to express the concentration of lithium in the bloodstream). In general, levels for acute manic episodes fall in the higher end of the range, whereas for maintenance treatment the target level is lower. Exceeding the therapeutic level may result in severe and eventually lethal side effects. A properly managed patient receiving lithium must have periodic blood tests to ensure that the level is neither too low (ineffective) nor too high (potentially dangerous). Typically, blood levels are initially checked at least once a week. Once treatment is established and the individual dosing needs of the patient are better known, lithium level tests are done every 2 to 3 months. A word of caution: lithium blood levels are guideline references, only meaningful in conjunction with an ongoing clinical assessment of the patient. Variations among individuals are common, and although some patients may develop significant, even potentially dangerous side effects at "therapeutic levels," others will tolerate supratherapeutic levels with little or even no discomfort.

Lithium produces a number of side effects, even within the therapeutic range, and they will occur in a large majority of patients (Table 3.21). These effects may lead to treatment nonadherence and an increased risk of relapse. Sometimes, the side effects can be managed with blood-level adjustments and/or modifications in the daily dosage.

TABLE 3.21. Lithium Side Effects

- Decreased renal ability to concentrate urine, leading to polyuria (increased urination) and polydipsia (increased thirst)
- Hand tremors
- Weight gain
- Sedation, lethargy
- Cognitive effects (slow thinking, dulling, impaired memory, confusion, decreased concentration)
- Motor coordination problems
- Gastrointestinal symptoms (nausea, vomiting, diarrhea)
- Hair loss
- Acne, psoriasis
- Water retention
- **Hypothyroidism** (may occur in up to 25%, more frequently in females)

Note. Data from Goodwin and Jamison (1990).

Lithium Toxicity. Lithium toxicity is a life-threatening complication. The blood levels required for a therapeutic effect are very close to those leading to toxicity. Typically, doses of lithium are aimed at reaching blood levels of 0.6–1.2 mEq/L. Early signs of toxicity may appear at levels above 1.5 mEq/L and become quite serious above 2.0 mEq/L. If not recognized and treated on a timely basis, lithium toxicity can lead to serious central nervous system injury and even death. The elderly are particularly sensitive to even therapeutic levels of lithium, and their levels tend to fluctuate more unpredictably, thus requiring closer monitoring.

Lithium toxicity results from any situation that causes either excessive ingestion of the drug or insufficient **clearance** of it from the body (lithium is excreted via the kidneys). For example, patients who misunderstand the physician's directions or who otherwise take higher than prescribed doses can very quickly elevate their blood levels to a dangerous range. Dehydration, interactions with several other medications (e.g., nonsteroidal anti-inflammatory drugs, such as ibuprofen, which are commonly used and obtainable over the counter, and certain diuretics), certain medical illnesses, diarrhea, vomiting, anorexia, crash dieting, strenuous exercise, very hot climate, and pregnancy and delivery can all alter lithium levels and increase the risk of lithium toxicity.

Lithium toxicity constitutes a medical emergency. Because the need for early recognition and treatment are essential, its manifestations are included in Table 3.22 for reference.

TABLE 3.22. Lithium Intoxication

Mild
- Recurrence and/or intensification of a previously transient or mild side effect
- Difficulty concentrating, cognitive impairment
- Muscle weakness, heaviness of the limbs
- Irritability
- Nausea

Moderate
- Drowsiness, lassitude
- Dullness, disorientation, confusion
- Slurred or indistinct speech
- Blurred vision
- Unsteady gait
- Coarse hand tremor
- Restlessness
- Muscle twitches
- Lower jaw tremor
- Giddiness
- Vomiting

Severe
- Intensification of any of the above
- Marked apathy, impaired consciousness, may progress to coma
- Ataxia
- Irregular hand tremor
- Prominent generalized muscle twitches
- Choreiform/parkinsonian movements

Note. Data from Goodwin and Jamison (1990).

Since the observation made in Japan in the 1970s that carbamazepine, an anticonvulsant used for the treatment of epilepsy, was a promising antimanic agent, considerable research has been done on the use of this class of medications for the treatment of bipolar disorder. In fact, several of the medications listed in Table 3.20 are anticonvulsants (carbamazepine, divalproex, lamotrigine, tiagabine, topiramate, and gabapentin), and all of them have been used in the treatment of bipolar disorder, although there is no evidence to support the use of some of them. At the present time, the only one that has received FDA approval as an antimanic agent is divalproex, and it is presently the most commonly used drug for the treatment of mania. It also requires doses to be adjusted to a blood-level range thought to be associated with optimal therapeutic benefit (50–100 μg/mL [micrograms per milliliter, the units used to express its concentration in the bloodstream]), but its therapeutic blood level is well below its toxicity level, making it, in this respect, an easier drug to use. Also, when given in a rapid-loading fashion, with the dose based on the patient's weight, it appears to have an onset of antimanic action that is faster than lithium. Side effects may occur as well (see Table 3.23). Many patients will initially experience these effects more markedly, but habituation to side effects tends to develop (the side effects tend to lessen or become less noticeable with time) after several weeks of treatment.

A new class of medications has been recently introduced for the treatment of mania: the atypical antipsychotics. These medications, commonly used for the treatment of schizophrenia and other psychoses, have been found to have powerful antimanic effects. Olanzapine was the first atypical antipsychotic approved for this purpose by the FDA, and others in this class soon followed.

Lamotrigine is an anticonvulsant agent approved for maintenance in bipolar disorder. Lamotrigine, with ambiguous evidence as an antimanic agent, has been found to be useful in the adjunct treatment and in the prevention of the depressive phase of bipolar disorder. This is a particularly useful tool, considering the high prevalence of depression among bipolar patients. Lamotrigine use has been associated with skin rash in about 10% of patients. Rarely, this rash can be severe enough to require hospitalization and can be life-threatening. Gradual escalation in the dose over a period of several weeks is thought to significantly decrease the risk of a rash.

Not infrequently, treatment (for maintenance or acute mania) with a single agent proves ineffective, and combinations are necessary. Some of them are based on controlled studies, mostly of patients who suffered

TABLE 3.23. Some Side Effects of Divalproex

- Stomach discomfort, nausea, and vomiting
- Dullness and sedation
- Hand tremors, unsteady gait
- Headache
- Alopecia (hair loss)
- Thrombocytopenia (decreased platelet count) and risk of bleeding

Note. Data from Goodwin and Jamison (1990).

from breakthrough episodes of hypomania or mania while receiving treatment with **monotherapy**. Some are based on case reports only. Common combinations include lithium + divalproex, lithium + atypical antipsychotics, and olanzapine + divalproex with or without lithium. ECT is an excellent antimanic treatment and, in fact, has been found to be more effective than the combination of lithium and haloperidol, a conventional antipsychotic. (ECT is reviewed in detail earlier in this chapter.)

Evaluation of potentially useful antimanic agents continues. Studies are in progress to determine whether other novel antipsychotics and anticonvulsants are effective. Omega-3 fatty acids, contained in large amounts in certain fish oils, have been reported in several publications as effective agents as well. Further research on these compounds is needed before determining their true value in antimanic therapy.

DEPRESSION

As mentioned earlier, bipolar patients struggle frequently and for long periods of time with the depressive phase of the illness. In general, from a phenomenological perspective, depressive episodes in bipolar patients are often indistinguishable from those in individuals with unipolar depression. Since bipolar disorder tends to manifest itself first with one or more depressive episodes before the first hypomania or mania occurs, an initial diagnosis of major depressive disorder, unipolar type, is often made and later changed to bipolar only when the first episode of abnormally elevated mood and **psychomotor** function manifests itself. However, the more astute clinician will inquire about family history and the presence of atypical depressive symptoms, which are more common in bipolar disorder than in unipolar depression. It has been suggested that certain clinical characteristics—for example, hypersomnia and profound psychomotor retardation—can distinguish the two types of depression. However, there is considerable overlap of symptoms among unipolar and bipolar depression, making reliance on phenomenology alone an uncertain method. Nevertheless, the presence of a positive family history of bipolar disorder and/or the antecedent of cyclothymic-like episodes should raise the index of suspicion for bipolar disorder in a patient with a depressive episode and no prior history of mania or hypomania.

The goal of treatment for bipolar depressive episodes is, of course, to achieve remission and mood stabilization. As opposed to unipolar depression, a specific risk must be considered: antidepressant treatment may, in some cases, precipitate a hypomanic or manic episode, a phenomenon commonly known as a "switch to mania" or "switching." It is unclear how many patients actually suffer from an antidepressant-induced switch to hypomania or mania, and figures vary roughly between 5 and 15%. The risk is significant enough to require specific management adjustments. Choices for the treatment of bipolar depression include the combination of either lithium or divalproex + lamotrigine, or the use of quetiapine or the olanzapine/fluoxetine combination. The field is at this time trying to discern the clinical applications of these findings. In fact, considering the high suicide risk among bipolar patients, primary consideration should be given to lithium, in spite of its bothersome side effects, since it has been shown to significantly decrease suicide risk more effectively than divalproex.

When no response occurs to a mood stabilizer alone, an antidepressant is *added* to the treatment regimen. SSRIs and non-SSRI antidepressants have been found to be effective for this purpose. The concern of inducing a switch must always be kept in mind, and thus there is a need to continue the use of the mood stabilizer in the presence of antidepressant treatment. Because it has been suggested, and the evidence is inconclusive at best, that bupropion may pose a lesser risk than other antidepressants in inducing hypomania or mania, some physicians prefer this drug over others.

The risk of switching into mania, once the patient has emerged from depression, continues to be a factor in treatment considerations. Physicians often choose to discontinue the antidepressant relatively soon after recovery and to continue treatment with the mood stabilizer alone, in order to diminish this risk. This approach is diametrically opposed to the strategies for unipolar depression, where antidepressant treatment must continue at least for 1 year and often longer.

Lamotrigine is approved for the treatment of bipolar depression. This anticonvulsant has been shown to have antidepressant properties that are apparently unique among other anticonvulsants currently used for the treatment of bipolar disorder. Although lamotrigine's antimanic properties may be modest, because of its contribution to the often difficult-to-treat bipolar depressive episodes, we are likely to see its use increase.

As with mania and unipolar depression, ECT is a very effective treatment for the depressive phase of bipolar disorder, especially in cases with psychotic symptoms. It is at least as effective as antidepressant medications and probably more effective. Curiously, in spite of its proven antimanic properties, when ECT is administered to depressive bipolars, it may precipitate a switch into mania in some cases. Several other treatments have been tried for bipolar depression, especially in refractory cases, with variable success but in generally small patient samples. Continuous sleep deprivation for a full night is well documented as a very effective antidepressant. Patients can dramatically convert from profound depression into euthymia from one evening to the next morning. In fact, sleep deprivation, like other effective antidepressant treatments, is also capable of inducing switches into hypomania or mania. The antidepressant effects of sleep deprivation (which have also been documented in unipolar depression) are very short-lived, and typically, depression returns after the first night of recovery sleep. This has made it difficult to incorporate the technique of sleep deprivation into a comprehensive treatment program. (Sleep deprivation is used quite frequently at the University of California San Diego Medical Center as a treatment to jump start euthymia, with medications and light therapy used to sustain it.) However, it remains a valuable research tool to further the understanding of the different mechanisms at play in bipolar disorder.

Other interventions used for refractory bipolar depressed patients include atypical antipsychotics, thyroid hormones, stimulants (often used in the treatment of attention-deficit/hyperactivity disorder), and phototherapy. Repetitive transcraneal magnetic stimulation (rTMS) and vagal nerve stimulation (VNS) are techniques currently being researched.

As mentioned earlier, some bipolar patients are prone to rapid cycling episodes. This subtype is particularly difficult to treat and seems to be less amenable to treatment with lithium and carbamazepine. Divalproex appears to be more effective and, in some cases, lamotrigine as well, the latter especially in rapidly cycling patients in whom depression predominates. High doses of thyroid hormone can also be effective in some cases. In general, the management of rapid cycling requires a combination of different agents coupled with patience and persistence until the appropriate regimen is found for each particular patient.

MAINTENANCE TREATMENT

Bipolar disorder is a lifetime condition, and accordingly, treatment must be given for the duration of the patient's life. The purpose of maintenance treatment includes full and partial breakthrough episode relapse prevention, suicide prevention, mood stability, and improved functioning. In particular, low-grade symptoms, like mild to moderate depressive symptoms and unpredictable mood fluctuations, can have noticeable effects on functioning.

Many studies have confirmed the efficacy of lithium as an effective prophylactic agent in the prevention of mania and depression. During long-term treatment with lithium, it is necessary to periodically monitor lithium levels, thyroid function, renal function, other functions. Perhaps the most challenging issue at this stage is treatment adherence. Evidence is solid in showing that discontinuation of lithium is often followed by a high risk of relapse. In some cases, abrupt discontinuation has been associated with increased suicidal risk, when compared to gradual tapering and discontinuation. Often, side effects tend to erode the patient's motivation to take the medication regularly, perhaps especially because it tends to be more effective in preventing the ego-syntonic hypomanic episodes than the depressive breakthroughs.

Divalproex has also been shown to be an effective maintenance treatment, although the evidence is less conclusive than in the case of lithium. Recently, quetiapine XR has gained approval by the Food and Drug Administration for use as adjunct to lithium or divalproex for maintenance treatment in bipolar disorder.

Psychotherapeutic Interventions

Medications are the core feature in the treatment of bipolar disorder. Without their skillful application, there is little hope for a good result. However, the illness and its course, coupled with the current imperfections of medication, make the use of psychotherapy and other psychosocial interventions essential tools. Bipolar patients are faced with myriad issues and obstacles that have a profound impact on how they perceive themselves and their future (Table 3.24).

TABLE 3.24. Issues for Psychotherapy in Bipolar Patients

- Patient education
- Family education
- Medication compliance
- Dealing with anger, denial, and ambivalence
- Dealing with reaction to partial treatment response
- Dealing with impact of side effects, including the "loss" of hypomanic mood
- Fears of recurrence
- Learning to discriminate normal from abnormal moods
- Concerns about spouse, family, other relationships
- Concerns about genetics
- Support groups

Note. Data from Goodwin and Jamison (1990).

The chronic, unpredictable, and recurrent nature of the illness creates fear and uncertainty in the patients, their families, and their friends. Tremendous strain is put on marital relationships; frequent divorces and impulsive marriages are a common feature in the history of some of these patients. It is a complex and difficult process for most patients to come to terms with the reality and permanence of their illness, the need for long-term medications, and the inevitable side effects that accompany their use. Treatment adherence is often an ongoing challenge, especially when the patient is doing well or during hypomanic states. The fear of transmitting the illness to one's children is ever present. All these issues form the core of the psychotherapeutic intervention, one that must be ongoing and long term, with variable degrees of frequency, as the issues dictate. As for the symptomatic manifestations of the disease itself, hypomania and mania are basically immune to psychotherapy. Cognitive therapy can be effective in the depressive phase of the illness but usually as an adjunct to medication.

The clinical management of bipolar disorder and its challenges make it a particularly appropriate condition for the collaborative model of care. There will be no successful medication treatment without psychotherapeutic intervention and no psychotherapeutic hope without medication. The prescribing physician—ideally a psychiatrist, given the need for specialized and often complex treatment—and the psychotherapist must work closely together to ensure the best possible results. The therapist must be knowledgeable about the course of the illness, its variability, the limitations and side effects of medication, and the need for different medication regimens imposed by the varying clinical manifestations. The physician must be keenly aware of the many psychosocial issues that arise in the course of treatment and the impact they have on the patient's day-to-day life and the adherence to treatment. An excellent and detailed review of all these issues may be found in several texts specifically devoted to bipolar disorder, most notably the psychotherapy chapter in Goodwin and Jamison (1990).

In utilizing the collaborative model in the management of bipolar disorder, as well as depression, the psychotherapist supports the inherent coping skills of the patient, assesses progress and resistance, and tracks medication compliance. The psychotherapist can then inform the psychiatrist of any changes that have occurred and/or are required, and vice versa, thereby resulting in a more comprehensive and quality-driven level of care.

In summary, mood disorders are common in the general population. Depressive disorders are occasionally referred to as "the common cold" of psychiatry. During the past half century, we have greatly enhanced our understanding of these disorders and now we know what we have long suspected: both genetics and the psychosocial environment play critical roles in the expression of major depression and manic–depressive illness.

We have also gained substantial understanding—alas, much is still unknown—on the pharmacology and molecular biology of these illnesses, and in parallel, we have developed medications that can substantially alter, for the better, their natural course. These medications must be used skillfully by well-trained physicians in a constant effort to achieve the best cost–benefit ratio, that is, the most efficacy with the least possible adverse effects. Moreover, we are beginning to understand how to select medications for mood disorders, how to start them, how long to use them and on whom and when, and how to stop them. We have also reviewed the endemic problem of lack of adherence to treatment and its consequences and the vital role that the treatment team—the medication "manager" and the therapist—plays in educating the patient and sustaining adherence to treatment. Experienced clinicians know that when treatment collaboration is meaningful, frequent, and goal-directed, treatment outcomes are maximized.

CHAPTER 4

Anxiety Disorders

Anxiety is a normal part of life. Our brains are "wired," as a result of thousands of years of evolution, to react to external threats or hazards with a protective and highly tuned set of psychological and physical alarm responses known as the fight-or-flight response. We share this survival and escape reaction with most other species. In humans, it includes rapid heartbeat and respiration, diversion of blood to the muscles, enlarged pupils, increased muscle tone, fear, and increased alertness and awareness. This carefully modulated response occurs in a continuum and is generally proportional to the gravity of the threat. In fact, within limits, it is quite beneficial. A little anxiety and alertness improves our performance when we take a test or give a speech. A reasonable fear that her children may be injured prompts a mother to insist that they wear helmets when biking. When this array of psychological and physical manifestations exceeds the point where it helps us adapt and becomes an impediment to functioning in daily life, it becomes a disorder: the bright college student flunks out because he panics when faced with an exam, or a mother's pervasive fear of harm to her children prevents them from engaging in normal developmental activities. So when the response occurs in the absence of a threat or with disproportionate intensity, or when a malfunctioning processing system makes a situation be perceived as falsely ominous, then the fight-or-flight response becomes a maladaptive mechanism. It is, in a sense, a false alarm, not unlike an automobile alarm going off when no one is attempting to break into the vehicle. These are the patients who seek our help, and medication can often be very useful for them.

Before we discuss treatment issues unique to some of the most prevalent anxiety disorders, it is important to review some concepts common to all of them.

The brain mechanisms involved in the regulation of anxiety are quite complex and still insufficiently understood. Several areas in the brain have been implicated, and some of them are thought to be particularly relevant to specific anxiety disorders, as summarized by Anderson and Reid (2002). The brainstem area has been linked to the fight-or-flight response and is probably the origin of spontaneous panic attacks; the hypothalamus controls the autonomic (rapid heartbeat and respirations) and **endocrine system** components (cortisol levels) of the anxiety response; the amygdala plays a role in classical conditioning and in the coordination and integration of fear responses, and it is possibly involved in phobias and posttraumatic stress disorder (PTSD); the septohippocampal system has been linked to anticipatory anxiety and avoidance behavior; and the temporal and prefrontal cortex, which process higher order functions like social situations, are likely to be involved in socially induced anxiety.

Several neurochemical hypotheses have been set forth to explain the mechanisms leading to the clinical manifestations of anxiety disorders. Although a detailed account goes beyond the scope of this book, it is enough to state that norepinephrine, serotonin, and **GABA (gamma-aminobutyric acid)** are three of the neurotransmitters most often implicated. The medications found to be most useful for the treatment of anxiety disorders—SSRIs, TCAs, MAOIs, and benzodiazepines—have profound effects on these neurotransmitters and their respective neuroreceptors.

Anxiety disorders include a range of diagnoses in which panic or disabling anxiety is a prominent feature. These include panic disorder with and without agoraphobia, specific phobias, PTSD, social phobia, OCD, and generalized anxiety disorder (GAD) (Table 4.1).

Also, several other psychiatric disorders have anxiety as a prominent feature. For example, approximately two-thirds of depressed patients suffer from anxiety as a significant part of their symptomatology. Because there is considerable overlap in symptoms, diagnosis can be tricky, but a correct diagnosis can make a big difference in whether a patient is referred for medication and which medication

TABLE 4.1. DSM-IV-TR Anxiety Disorders

Generalized anxiety disorder

Panic disorder
- With agoraphobia
- Without agoraphobia

Phobic disorders
- Specific phobia
- Social phobia

Posttraumatic stress disorder

Obsessive–compulsive disorder

Adjustment disorder with anxious features

Acute stress disorder

Anxiety disorder due to a general medical condition

Substance-induced anxiety disorder

Anxiety disorder not otherwise specified

---

regimen a physician might choose. Consider, for example, a 27-year-old woman who has had panic attacks and is now unable to leave her house without considerable fear and anxiety. We would certainly think about panic disorder with agoraphobia, and we know medication can be very effective in blocking panic attacks. But as we probe further, we discover that her two panic attacks occurred in automobiles and she stays at home because she is afraid of cars (**ubiquitous** in her urban environment), not because she fears an unprovoked panic attack. Now it begins to look as if she has developed a specific phobia. The distinction is important because there is no evidence that any currently available medication works for specific phobias. But if we inquire even further and find out that her fear of cars began when she was badly injured in a car accident, and she fears them because they prompt extremely distressing memories of the accident we would be inclined to consider PTSD, for which there is some evidence that SSRIs are effective.

Making these distinctions may well be up to the clinician, especially if he or she is planning to refer the patient to a primary care physician. In addition to the different diagnoses listed above, the physician will also explore many other causes of anxiety, including those induced by substances (excessive caffeine intake, known as "caffeinism"—usually seen in individuals who consume large amounts of coffee, tea, and/or cola drinks—is surprisingly common and overlooked in clinical practice).

Also, a number of medications, and withdrawal from some of them, may be associated with anxiety symptoms.

Finally, it is important for the clinician to keep in mind that there are myriad medical disorders capable of producing anxiety symptoms, not in response to the perception that one is suffering from a disabling or even lethal condition, but as part of one's own symptomatological picture. These disorders may involve one or more bodily systems and require a proper clinical workup by a physician so that the clinician is not treating an "anxiety disorder" when in fact treatment for a medical disorder is needed. Some examples of medical conditions that may present with anxiety are listed in Table 4.2.

Anxiety disorders are quite prevalent in the general population and, of course, more so among patients in primary and specialty care. Also, some affect one gender more than the other (see Table 4.3). It is also common in clinical practice to see patients with symptoms that overlap two or more anxiety disorders or an anxiety disorder and another psychiatric condition; for example, there is a high degree of **comorbidity** for depression and anxiety.

GENERAL TREATMENT CONSIDERATIONS

Both pharmacological and psychotherapeutic interventions have proven effective, to various degrees, in the treatment of anxiety disorders. Usually, a combination of both techniques seems to yield the best results. A number of factors (e.g., patient preference, availability of specially trained therapists, cost, and prior results) will determine whether medications, psychotherapy, or both are selected. Among the psychotherapies, the evidence shows cognitive-behavioral techniques as the preferred approach.

The treatment strategies are implemented in a stepwise fashion, with single treatments first and then, depending on response and

TABLE 4.2. Some Medical Conditions with Associated Anxiety

• Anemia	• Chronic obstructive pulmonary disease
• Asthma	• Pheochromocytoma
• Hyperparathyroidism	• Irritable bowel syndrome
• Hyperthyroidism	• Vestibular dysfunction
• Cardiac arrhythmias	• Certain seizure disorders
• Mitral valve prolapse	• Hypoglycemia

TABLE 4.3. Prevalence of Anxiety Disorders in Men and Women

Anxiety disorder	% women	% men
Specific phobia	15.7	6.7
Social phobia	15.5	11.1
Agoraphobia without panic disorder	7.0	3.5
Generalized anxiety disorder	6.6	3.6
Panic disorder	5.0	2.0
Posttraumatic stress disorder	10.4	5.0

Note. Data from Kessler et al. (1994, 1995).

tolerability, combination and/or substitution treatments. Since anxiety disorders tend to relapse, the long-term effects of treatment are paramount. In general, with some exceptions, medication treatments, when successful, tend to maintain their benefit while treatment is ongoing. However, following discontinuation, even after months or years of treatment, patients will commonly experience a relapse. Conversely, appropriately instituted cognitive-behavioral treatments tend to have much longer beneficial effects, often lasting well after formal treatment has concluded.

When medications are used, treatment is typically started with an SSRI. Responses may take weeks or months to occur. For example, OCD tends to have a rather large latency period before a benefit is observed. Panic disorder and social phobia tend to respond sooner, although, like depression, the lag period is measured in weeks, not days. A notable exception is the group of benzodiazepines, which have an almost instantaneous antianxiety effect. However, their use is limited because of possible cognitive side effects and the potential for addiction in susceptible individuals.

When the initial SSRI fails to produce the desirable response or if it is poorly tolerated, a second SSRI can then be tried. Partial responders are candidates for agents that augment or enhance the action of the original medication or for the addition of cognitive-behavioral techniques, whereas nonresponders should be tried on a non-SSRI class of antidepressants (e.g., clomipramine, venlafaxine, or duloxetine) or switched altogether to cognitive-behavioral therapy. In fully refractory cases, clinicians try different kinds of medication permutations and combinations, as well as intensive cognitive-behavioral techniques. These approaches are mostly predicated on published case reports and uncontrolled studies. Very little evidence exists to conclusively prefer one specific combination over another. It is also useful to reassess refractory cases to ensure that all possible contributing factors have been addressed. Comorbid substance abuse, situational and family stressors, and medical problems can sometimes be easily overlooked as perpetuating elements. The case below exemplifies some of the complexities.

CASE: COMORBID ANXIETY DISORDERS

Case Description

Mr. K is a 24-year-old man who is coming to see his primary care physician about a sinus infection he's had for the last year. Dr. W is the fourth doctor Mr. K has seen for this complaint, and this is the third time he has seen her in the last 2 months. As she examines him, he tells her the same story about spending the night at his cousin's house, sleeping on his cousin's pillow, only to find out a few days later that his cousin had a sinus infection. Since then he's been obsessed with the idea that he became infected with a horrible bacteria, and he visits doctors monthly to try to find a cure. Dr. W finds no signs of infection; refers him to an ear, nose, and throat specialist; and also refers him to an in-house therapist to help him work through "all the stress this congestion has caused."

Beginning Collaboration

Upon receiving the referral, Ms. J contacts Dr. W to find out more about Mr. K's medical concerns. Dr. W says that Mr. K does appear to have some congestion but no clear signs of infection. He has been treated with several courses of antibiotics, yet still complains of the same symptoms and fears. She says that Mr. K does not complain of any other symptoms or illnesses but consistently tells the exact same story about his cousin's house, displaying a significant amount of anxiety each time he tells it.

Ms. J schedules an appointment with Mr. K. When he comes in, he tells her the same story about his sinus infection and spending the night at his cousin's house; he says that he thinks about that night *all* the time and that he thinks about that pillow every morning when he feels the sinus congestion and "just can't seem to get over it." Ms. J probes for other obsessive thoughts, and Mr. K starts describing his obsession with germs and cleanliness. Mr. K buys only canned food from the grocery store, and he leaves no open containers in his refrigerator or cupboard for fear of contamination. When he buys lunch at work, he usually buys packaged cookies or chips. When he goes to a restaurant to eat, he frequently throws away the food uneaten because he can't get it out of his head that someone contaminated it. He describes feeling anxious and "uptight" almost all of the time, finding it hard to remember the last time he felt relaxed.

As Ms. J hears his story, she begins to think that Mr. K may benefit from a consultation with a psychiatrist, to clarify a diagnosis and to consider medication. Ms. J brings this up by asking Mr. K if he'd ever been given any medication to help deal with all this stress. Mr. K gets a fearful look in his eyes and says, "Oh no, I'm not taking that kind of medication." He explains that once, in high school, he had gone to the doctor after his father died because he was depressed. His doctor gave him an antidepressant medication. After taking it a few times, he began to have difficulty sleeping and one night woke up with his heart pounding, feeling as if he was "losing it." Since then he has developed a fear of all psychotropic medication and refused to consider even a trial of a different medication. He has also had panic attacks, with no particular trigger, intermittently since that time. After the session, Ms. J confers with Dr. W, who agrees that a medication consultation would be very helpful in treating Mr. K. She decides to work with Mr. K to help allay his fears about medication and encourage him to consider a consultation with a psychiatrist.

Ongoing Collaboration

Over the next 2 months, Ms. J and Dr. W work with Mr. K to help him decrease his anxiety in general and, specifically, his anxiety about medication. Having no success, they decide to consider another option. Twice a month, a collaborative team of therapists, primary care physicians, and psychiatrists meet in Dr. W's clinic to interview patients and discuss complex cases. Dr. W and Ms. J decide that maybe Mr. K will consider being interviewed by this team. At this point, he's starting to trust Ms. J, and when she asks him to join her for this interview, he agrees. He's particularly interested in having some new doctors hear about his sinus condition, which he still thinks about daily despite a CT scan of his sinuses, indicating that no infection is present.

During the interview, Mr. K reveals his various struggles to the team who ask questions for clarification as he goes along. The team members then send Mr. K to the waiting room for a few minutes while they consult about his treatment plan. Unfortunately, the collaboration process was not as fruitful as Dr. W and Ms. J had hoped. The team begins to consider various diagnoses, from OCD, to delusional disorder, to bipolar disorder. By the end of the meeting, there is no agreement on diagnosis and no agreement on treatment. The psychiatrist, who is considered the head of the team, agrees to address treatment with Mr. K. Mr. K is brought back into the room; addressed by the psychiatrist, who tries to convince him he has bipolar disorder; and leaves feeling misunderstood and frustrated.

At his next session with Ms. J, he says that he didn't connect with the psychiatrist and didn't like how "she kept pushing the bipolar thing." Although Dr. W and Ms. J both disagree with the bipolar diagnosis, they respect their psychiatrist colleague enough to be hesitant about how to proceed with treatment until Mr. K receives a more thorough psychiatric evaluation.

Despite continual reassurances from Dr. W, Mr. K still refuses to consider psychotropic medication or a psychiatric consultation. Ms. J works with Mr. K over the next month, trying to help him find ways to deal with his various fears. He appears to be making some mild progress until, one day, he calls Ms. J to cancel their appointment because he broke his foot. He explains that he is afraid to ride in elevators and usually takes the stairs to attend his appointments with her on the fourth floor. He is now unable to use stairs and refuses to consider the elevator for fear of "losing it." Unable to accommodate him on a lower floor, Ms. J agrees to some phone therapy during his recovery. Mr. K finds it difficult to keep the phone appointments and gradually loses touch with both Ms. J and Dr. W.

Two months later, Mr. K comes back to see Dr. W about his sinus infection. As he's getting ready to leave the appointment, he asks for the number of a psychiatrist and for Ms. J's number, which he had lost in the last few months. He never contacts Ms. J, but she and Dr. W are hopeful that he will follow through on his desire to see a psychiatrist.

Questions for Consideration

• *Why did Ms. J think a psychiatric evaluation for Mr. K was so important after meeting him only once?* First, Ms. J saw that his symptoms could be indicative of at least a couple of different disorders. As for Mr. K's sinus complaints, she was having trouble distinguishing between an obsessional thought and a delusion. In addition to wanting more information from Mr. K himself, she also wanted the opinion of another mental health professional. Second, Ms. J knew that OCD can be very difficult to treat without medication. She knew that for Mr. K to experience optimal relief from his symptoms, medication should at least be considered as part of the treatment plan.

• *Why did the team have so much difficulty agreeing on a diagnosis and treatment plan for Mr. K?* Mr. K had an interesting combination of symptoms that could be viewed from a variety of perspectives. Ms. J and Dr. W saw his symptoms as indicating comorbid anxiety disorders of OCD, panic disorder, and specific phobia. Dr. H, a psychiatrist, thought his reaction to the antidepressant medication in high school and his constant feelings of being "uptight" were both indicative of mania and thus believed he had bipolar disorder. Other colleagues focused on his ongoing concern about his sinuses (which he spent a large portion of the interview discussing) and saw his primary diagnosis as delusional disorder, somatic type. Because of these differing perspectives, the team found it difficult to identify a clear plan for treatment as each diagnosis would warrant a different treatment protocol. Clearly, a more thorough evaluation was needed.

• *One possible risk of having a collaborative team is that team members don't agree on the diagnosis or treatment plan. How should these issues be resolved?* Although there is a chance that team members will never reach consensus, often more information and the opportunity to follow the patient over time can clarify diagnostic quandaries. Unfortunately, many patients don't have the patience for this process and lose confidence in their providers. Therapists have a certain amount of "relationship capital"—the trust, patience, and hope that patients have because of their relationships with their therapists. An expert, giving a one-time consultation, may have no "relationship capital," or the therapist might lend some of her "capital" to the psychiatrist if more time is needed. For example, the therapist may use her relationship with the patient to explain the diagnostic process and ask the patient to wait while the issues are resolved.

PANIC DISORDER

Panic disorder typically starts in the third decade of life, although it may start in childhood or late in life as well. It is a recurrent, chronic, and disabling condition, in which relapses after remission are common. Panic disorder affects females twice as often as males, and after remission, women are more likely to relapse than men. The long duration of illness and the presence of agoraphobia portend a less favorable **prognosis**. Suicide risk is comparable to that seen among patients with major depression.

Panic attacks are the common symptom for many of the anxiety disorders. A panic attack is a brief and intense experience of fear or distress accompanied by some of the symptoms listed in Table 4.4 (DSM-IV-TR requires four or more symptoms for this diagnosis but acknowledges that patients can be severely anxious with fewer than four different symptoms). A panic attack—or even several panic attacks—is not by itself a disorder. Many people have a panic attack at some point in their lives. However, about 4% of individuals develop recurrent panic attacks, and 3.5% actually meet DSM-IV-TR criteria for panic disorder.

TABLE 4.4. Symptoms of a Panic Attack

- Palpitations, racing or pounding heart
- Sweating
- Trembling or shaking
- Chest pain
- Nausea or abdominal pain
- Numbness or tingling sensations
- Chills or hot flushes
- Shortness of breath
- A feeling of choking
- Feeling dizzy, lightheaded, or faint
- Feelings of unreality (derealization) or of being detached from oneself (depersonalization)
- Fear of losing control, of "going crazy"
- Fear of dying

Panic disorder is diagnosed when a patient has recurrent, unexpected panic attacks and one of the attacks has been followed by a month or more of persistent concern about future attacks, worry about the implications of the attacks (e.g., having a heart attack or losing control), or a significant behavior change as a result of the attacks or worry about them. If the attacks are always or frequently triggered by identifiable objects or situations, a specific phobia or social phobia may be a more likely diagnosis, although patients with panic disorder may also have some triggered panic attacks or may have both panic disorder and a phobia. Panic disorder may or may not be accompanied by agoraphobia—literally, "fear of the marketplace," once the most crowded public setting that most people would typically encounter—now defined as anxiety about being in places where escape would be difficult or help might not be available if panic symptoms were to occur. In agoraphobia, which occurs in roughly one-third of patients with panic disorder, those situations are typically avoided, though a patient may be able to tolerate them with a companion or may suffer through them with considerable anxiety. Agoraphobia develops in panic disorder as a very crude kind of "self-help," that is, the patient's only perceived way of controlling what seem to be uncontrollable and intolerable symptoms. Typically, agoraphobia develops over time (most often during the first year after the onset of panic attacks) when initial efforts to seek help from medical or other resources don't produce a solution. As panic attacks recur, they provoke more and more anticipatory anxiety (worry about when the next one will happen). At the same time, patients give up on the sources of help they have tried and increasingly resort to avoiding any situation that might provoke an attack or be a frightening or embarrassing place to have an unexpected attack.

Treatment

Treatment of panic disorder aims at stopping the panic attacks, treating any comorbid disorders (including agoraphobia and, if present, depression), and achieving and maintaining remission (see Table 4.5). In most cases, treatment options include two classes of medications—benzodiazepines and antidepressants—and one form of psychotherapy that has been proven effective for panic disorder: cognitive-behavioral therapy. Many patients see even greater benefits from some combination of these treatments. As with other disorders, treatment here includes psychoeducational interventions and an invitation to the patient to become an active partner in the treatment effort. An example is the patient who, well informed of the mechanisms leading to the symptoms of a panic attack, is trained to recognize and rate the intensity and frequency of panic attacks.

Several different classes of medications have been used in the treatment of panic disorder, some much more effective than others (Table 4.6). SSRIs, the same class of medication used in the treatment of depression, are the current medications of choice. Many studies have conclusively shown that these medications (paroxetine, escitalopram, sertraline, fluoxetine, etc.) are usually very effective in blocking panic attacks after a few weeks of treatment. Tricyclic antidepressants also work—also following a lag period—but their side effects generally make them the second choice. This period of waiting for the medication to begin working can be difficult for patients. A significant disadvantage of these agents is the appearance of side effects well before any benefit becomes

---

TABLE 4.5. Goals of Pharmacotherapy for Panic Disorder

- Block panic attacks
- Treat comorbid conditions (e.g., depression, substance abuse, or dependence)
- Achieve remission
- Maintain remission

**TABLE 4.6. Medications Used
in the Treatment of Panic Disorder**

- Selective serotonin reuptake inhibitors
- Tricyclic antidepressants
- High-potency benzodiazepines
- Monoamine oxidase inhibitors
- Other agents
- Combination treatments

apparent. If this were a commercial transaction, it would be akin to paying first and receiving the service later. This can be quite frustrating to patients, who in the short term actually feel worse than when they started treatment: Now, not only do they suffer from anxiety, but they also have to put up with side effects like nausea, insomnia, diarrhea, dry mouth, headaches, blurred vision, and others, depending on the medication being used. Patients need to be prepared for and supported through this initial period of treatment so that the discouraging experience of taking pills daily with no immediate improvement in their anxiety and panic doesn't undermine their faith in the treatment and willingness to stick with it. In general, patients will develop habituation to side effects, which means that their intensity will gradually diminish after several weeks of treatment.

Usually, anxious patients tend to be more sensitive to and less tolerant of side effects of all kinds, particularly those associated with the stimulation effects of SSRI treatment. In the short term, the medication may actually make the anxiety worse rather than better. The physician will usually select a less stimulating SSRI and typically will begin treatment with a very low dose, increasing it gradually.

Certain patients with panic disorder and substantial anticipatory anxiety have actually almost persistent and free-floating anxiety, symptoms that for all practical purposes have rendered them fully disabled. In these cases, in which acute anxiety is so prominent, immediate or quick relief is necessary, and it is useful to begin treatment not only with SSRIs but, concomitantly, with benzodiazapines (e.g., diazepam [trade name Valium], clonazepam [trade name Klonopin], alprazolam [trade name Xanax], and lorazepam [trade name Ativan]). These medications have the advantage of producing antianxiety effects very quickly. Patients feel their effects shortly after taking them, and the drugs are very effective in blocking panic attacks and diminishing anticipatory anxiety. There are problems with this class of medications, making them a less attractive choice as a long-term treatment (see Table 4.7).

Used short term, the benzodiazepine will provide immediate partial or complete relief and will "buy time" until the full effect of the SSRI becomes apparent several weeks later. Once the disorder is stabilized with the SSRI, the physician can then proceed with a gradual discontinuation of the benzodiazepine. Long-term use of benzodiazepines should generally be avoided as they can cause excessive sedation or drowsiness and slow down thinking and reaction times. Sometimes, memory function can be impaired since they can interfere with neural learning processes.

In some cases, there can also be significant problems with drug **dependence** and difficulty in withdrawal (the clinician will certainly want to include in the referral letter to the physician any known history of substance abuse or dependence). After daily use for more than a few weeks, sudden discontinuation of any benzodiazepine is very uncomfortable and can be potentially dangerous or even fatal. Patients should be strongly discouraged from ever discontinuing these drugs without proper medical supervision (Table 4.8). It is also important to remember that some patients—those who metabolize the drug much faster than the average person and who therefore have rapid drops in benzodiazepine blood levels—may occasionally have "mini withdrawals" between doses, characterized by anxiety symptoms that can easily be misinterpreted as a relapse of the primary anxiety disorder. This phenomenon is seen more frequently with those benzodiazepines that have an ultrashort half-life, like lorazepam and alprazolam, than with clonazepam or alprazolam XR (extended release).

TABLE 4.7. Side Effects of Benzodiazepine Medications

- Drowsiness
- Dizziness
- Psychomotor dysfunction or incoordination
- Headaches
- Blurred vision
- Memory deficits
- Disinhibition and/or excitability (in children and the elderly)

TABLE 4.8. Manifestations of Benzodiazepine Withdrawal

- Psychological
  Anxiety, difficulty concentrating, dysphoria,
  insomnia, irritability, depersonalization,
  dizziness, visual misperceptions, sensorial
  hypersensitivity

- Physical
  Tremors, headaches, sweating, ataxia, loss of
  appetite, nausea, vomiting, seizures

For a limited number of patients, a benzodiazapine may be all they need. For example, a patient who functions well between rare but unexpected panic attacks may prefer to have a diazepam or alprazolam handy for those infrequent occasions, rather than take a daily medication. Bear in mind that using benzodiazepines in this fashion for patients with panic attacks will have no effect in blocking the panic attack itself because the drug's action will not be apparent for 30–60 minutes. However, it may alleviate the lingering symptoms of a panic attack. Clinical experience suggests that for some patients, just knowing that a pill is available in their pocket or purse for immediate use if necessary can have a powerful **placebo** effect in preventing panic attacks or in assisting patients to better cope with them.

Overall, benzodiazepines are excellent agents when used in carefully selected patients, when use is preferably limited to short term (with some exceptions), and when use is systematically avoided in individuals with a documented history of substance abuse.

The third option for treatment of panic attacks is cognitive-behavioral therapy (CBT). There is some evidence that CBT alone can be effective in stopping panic attacks, especially when the therapist is specifically trained and experienced in its use, but generally studies show that fewer patients respond to CBT alone than to medication alone. For many patients, especially those with agoraphobia, a combination of medication and CBT is the preferred treatment. The medication will block the panic attacks but will not always treat the agoraphobia because, to the extent in which we can make these distinctions, agoraphobia is a learned response to the biological event of repeated panic attacks. So although the medication can address the biological event, the anticipatory anxiety and behaviors such as avoidance are not directly treated by the medication. In some patients, agoraphobia does resolve "spontaneously" (i.e., without the need for formal CBT) when the panic attacks are effectively being blocked and anticipatory anxiety is thus less intense. What's really happening in these cases is that the patients are doing their own informal version of CBT. As the panic attacks lessen or stop, the patients cautiously venture out, try something previously avoided, and discover that no panic attack occurs (because of the medication). Then they try something else, perhaps more "daring." Success leads to success, and the agoraphobia gradually fades away. Other patients will need the structure and support of a more formal program of CBT. In addition, patients with panic disorder may also have other disorders, although these may not be as apparent while the panic attacks are prominent. Specific phobias, social phobia, and depression are common problems comorbid with panic disorder that may need to be addressed directly. In fact, one of the advantages of using SSRIs over benzodiazepines is that the medication will not only block panic attacks but will also directly address the depressive symptoms.

Long-term follow-up of patients with panic disorder has shown that this condition tends to be chronic and recurrent in a significant number of cases. Medications have great benefits, but their effect is likely to be lost after discontinuation. Medication treatment should continue for at least 1 year, preferably 2. Then an attempt can be made to very slowly and gently taper off the medication over an extended period of time, perhaps several months. Should a relapse occur, treatment must be restarted. Some patients relapse quite quickly after discontinuation of medication, whereas others are asymptomatic for a year or longer before the panic attacks return. In this regard, CBT appears to be more effective in that its benefit is much longer lasting, at least up to several years following discontinuation of formal CBT.

SOCIAL PHOBIA

Social phobia has a lifetime prevalence of about 13% and a 1-year prevalence of about 8% (Kessler et al., 1994), making it the third most common psychiatric disorder, after depression and alcoholism. It is estimated that approximately 30 million Americans suffer from social phobia, affecting women twice as often as men. The disorder typically starts in the midteens, and some of the patients have a history of shyness or inhibited behavior dating back to childhood. Social phobia may start acutely, for example, following a particularly humiliating social experience, or it may develop insidiously, with no apparent precipitating event.

Without treatment, symptoms tend to be continuous and become especially worse in certain particularly stressful situations. Once the individual reaches adulthood, some adaptation occurs, resulting in ameliorating manifestations or outright remission. Although it is more common among relatives, overall it appears to have low heritability. Further research is ongoing to clarify the possible contribution of genetic factors.

Comorbidity in social phobia is quite common as it may overlap with other anxiety disorders and with depression. Suicide risk is increased, and substance abuse—interpreted by clinicians as an effort to self-medicate—is commonly seen among these patients.

The hallmark of social phobia is an excessive and ongoing fear of being embarrassed or scrutinized in social or performance situations (including fear of being embarrassed by the physical symptoms of social phobia—trembling, blushing, sweating, etc.). It can present in generalized form; that is, the fears are present in most social settings, including interactional and performance situations. In almost all of these patients, it will overlap with avoidant personality disorder. Generalized social phobia is the most disabling of the social phobias. It tends to run in families and generally has a chronic course. In other cases, the phobia may be restricted to a single or to very few situations, usually of a performance nature. Fearful situations include those in which the patient must speak to or before others, as well as other contexts in which the patient may be observed (urinating in public bathrooms, eating in public, or writing checks at the checkout line). See Tables 4.9 and 4.10.

Exposure to these social and performance situations consistently causes anxiety, which may or may not amount to a full-blown panic attack. Although patients recognize that the fear is out of proportion to the actual risk, their severe anxiety generally causes them to avoid the activities they fear or otherwise endure the situation at the cost of great discomfort and suffering (Table 4.11). It is easy to imagine the impact

TABLE 4.9. Typical Social Phobic Situations: Performance

- Speaking in public
- Performing in public (e.g., musical instrument)
- Eating in public
- Writing in public
- Urinating in a public bathroom
- Entering a room where people are already seated

Note. Data from Kessler et al. (1998); Stein et al. (1996, 2000).

**TABLE 4.10. Typical Social Phobic Situations:
Social Interactions**

- Conversing on the telephone
- Meeting someone for the first time
- Attending social gatherings (e.g., parties)
- Asking someone for a date
- Dealing with people in authority (e.g., boss, teacher)
- Returning items to a store
- Making eye contact with unfamiliar people

Note. Data from Kessler et al. (1998); Stein et al. (1996, 2000).

these symptoms can have on the social and occupational life of such an individual. For example, patients who are unable to use a public restroom may fear going to any place from which they could not immediately return home if necessary; as a result, they might be homebound to the extent that they appear (erroneously) to be suffering from agoraphobia.

Treatment

The goals of treatment for social phobia have been summarized by Davidson (2003), as seen in Table 4.12.

A patient whose phobia is limited to relatively infrequent performance situations can sometimes be successfully treated with **beta-blockers** (a class of medications normally used in the treatment of high blood pressure and other cardiovascular conditions). Beta-blockers work on a short-term basis by reducing the peripheral and physical man-

TABLE 4.11. Concerns in Social Phobic Situations

- Doing or saying something embarrassing or humiliating in front of others
- Making a poor impression or being negatively evaluated by others
- Having hand tremble when writing in front of others
- Mind going blank when speaking to others
- Saying foolish things
- Blushing or showing other signs of anxiety that will be noticeable to others

Note. Data from Kessler et al. (1998); Stein et al. (1996, 2000).

TABLE 4.12. Treatment Goals for Social Phobia

- Eliminate anxiety/phobic avoidance
- Eliminate functional disability
- Remission of social anxiety and comorbidities
- Choose therapy that is tolerable for long-term

Note. Data from Davidson (2003).

ifestations of arousal and anxiety (e.g., heart palpitations, hyperventilation, and sweating) and can be used to treat performance-based phobias, for example, before giving a speech or otherwise performing in front of an audience.

Patients with generalized social phobia, when the phobia interferes with their lives in many ways or on many occasions, need ongoing treatment. Both CBT and certain antidepressants work well with social phobia, and as in other anxiety disorders, CBT can have a long-lasting effect. Among the antidepressants, SSRIs are the current medication of choice. Their characteristics have already been discussed in this chapter, and their use in social phobia is essentially quite similar to that in panic disorder. Other antidepressants (MAOIs, but not tricyclic antidepressants) and the benzodiazepines are also effective, but as with treatment for panic disorder, these medications can have more problematic side effects or risks. Beta-blockers and the antianxiety drug buspirone have not been effective in the treatment of generalized social phobia. Some patients who are successfully treated with medication expand their social horizons on their own, but others may benefit from training in social skills they missed developing.

POSTTRAUMATIC STRESS DISORDER

Since the appearance of PTSD is directly associated to the occurrence of specific traumatic events, its prevalence will vary significantly in different countries and even within countries. Exposure to war, torture, crime, natural disasters, traumatic social situations, motor vehicle accidents, and other traumatic events will all determine the rate of PTSD. Although the risk of experiencing a traumatic event sometime in one's lifetime is over 50%, only one-fifth of those who do so will develop the disorder. Overall, in the United States it is estimated that its lifetime prevalence is about 8% (Kessler et al., 1995). We would typically look for PTSD in survivors of military combat and sexual assault, but it can also result from other events, such as being robbed or physically attacked; being kidnapped, tortured, or the victim of a terrorist attack; being diagnosed with a life-threatening illness; and experiencing natural disasters. Witnessing others being harmed or threatened in these ways and even hearing about them happening to people close to you can also lead to PTSD (see Table 4.13). Of course, it may affect individuals of any age and of both genders, although women are affected twice as often as men. Not all individuals exposed to traumatic events develop PTSD; in fact, only a minority do. Most victims of trauma fully recover a few weeks or months after exposure, with only a small proportion developing the full-blown picture of PTSD, one that tends to be chronic—in many cases, lasting for years—and considerably disabling. Comorbidity is also common among patients with PTSD. Many suffer comorbid depression, panic disorder, and an increased risk of suicide comparable to that seen in major depression.

Both therapists and patients sometimes have the sense that medication is not needed or not helpful in situations like PTSD, where the precipitant of the disorder is obviously environmental. It's one of the legacies of the mind–body split that we may assume that a disorder that stems so directly from a traumatic event is not "biological." But, of course, although we may not yet understand the specific mechanisms, a neurochemical reaction occurred in the patient's brain when he or she experienced the trauma—as, indeed, every mental experience is mediated by some kind of neurochemical event in the brain, the patient's ongoing symptoms included.

The diagnosis of PTSD requires both a certain kind of external traumatic experience—one causing or threatening injury or death to oneself or others—and a specific emotional response to the experience: intense fear, horror, or helplessness. The disorder develops when the patient continues (for more than a month) to reexperience the trauma through intrusive memories, recurrent dreams, flashbacks (which feel as though the event were occurring in the present), and/or intense physical and

---

TABLE 4.13. Common Traumatic Events

- Witnessing injury/death
- Sexual molestation/rape
- Natural disaster/fire
- Physical attack or abuse/threatened with a weapon
- Life-threatening accident
- Combat

Note. Data from Kessler et al. (1995).

emotional responses to reminders of the event. Patients actively avoid any reminders or recollections of the event, sometimes even "forgetting" important elements of the event itself. They experience a general blunting of feeling and detachment from others and from their normal interests. They develop new symptoms of increased, ongoing arousal, such as insomnia, irritability, difficulty in concentrating, hypervigilance, or an exaggerated startle response (Table 4.14). Symptoms can be especially intense and long lasting when the trauma was intentionally inflicted by another person, such as in torture or rape.

Treatment

The treatment of PTSD is best accomplished with careful integration of both medications and CBT. Medication use is aimed at reducing the symptomatology of depression and hyperarousal, including sleep disturbances, whereas CBT will help in reintegrating and processing the trauma. Psychotherapy is almost always necessary to deal with the trauma's profound effects on self-concept, understanding of and faith in other people and the world in general, and ability to imagine and plan a future. In witnesses of trauma to others, survivor guilt is also an issue.

Several studies have shown that SSRIs are effective in reducing the symptoms of PTSD, although there are insufficient long-term data to reliably guide therapeutic practices. When SSRIs are used, initial doses must be low, with a gradual increase dictated by the clinical response. Combination with benzodiazepines is often necessary, although preferably this should be only on a short-term basis (see previous comments in this chapter). Some physicians are exploring the benefits of using atypical antipsychotics (e.g., olanzapine and aripiprazole). Other promising pharmacological approaches include the use of propanolol (a β-adrenergic blocker sometimes used in the treatment of certain forms of social phobia), ketamine (an intravenous anesthetic, which has been used with some success in the short-term relief of refractory depression), and prazosin (an α-1 adrenergic blocker used primarily for the treatment of nightmares associated with PTSD). d-cycloserine, a broad-spectrum

---

TABLE 4.14. Core Symptoms of PTSD

- Intrusive symptoms, reexperiencing
- Avoidance behavior
- Numbing
- Hyperarousal symptoms

---

antibiotic with cognitive-enhancement properties, is being tested as an adjunct to prolonged exposure treatment (Cukor et al., 2009). In general, further carefully controlled studies are needed to clarify the role of medications in PTSD. As for the duration of treatment, these decisions are made empirically at the present time as no well-established data exist. Clinicians tend to treat for at least 1 year and then discontinue the medication very cautiously and gradually. Individual clinical results essentially dictate pharmacotherapeutic behavior.

GENERALIZED ANXIETY DISORDER

Like other anxiety disorders, GAD is also relatively common, with a lifetime prevalence of about 5% and a 12-month prevalence of about 3% (Kessler et al., 1994). GAD occurs rarely in children, and although it may start early, it tends to increase in prevalence in the 30s and 40s, making it the most diagnosed anxiety disorder after midlife. It also tends to be chronic, with exacerbation and amelioration of symptoms over time, even with periods of remission. Women are affected twice as much as men, and the rates appear to increase very substantially in women once they reach their 40s. Psychiatric comorbidity is common, especially with depression and other anxiety disorders. GAD can be seriously disabling and can lead to substantial impairment in familial, social, and occupational functioning. As with other anxiety disorders, a partial genetic transmission model is suspected.

Unlike the disorders we have discussed so far, in GAD anxiety is not focused on a specific event, situation, or object. People with GAD worry and feel anxious about many aspects of their lives, such as the demands of their work or school, finances, the safety of loved ones, and even the minor challenges of everyday life (e.g., getting the car repaired or being on time to an appointment). Of course, from time to time, we all have problems we worry about, but in GAD the worry is far out of proportion to the actual likelihood of danger or risk and so persistent that patients cannot control their worries, which, along with the associated symptoms (e.g., tension, anxiety), interfere with their lives. This pervasive anxiety also results in various physical symptoms: restlessness, easy fatigability, difficulty in concentrating, irritability, muscle tension, and sleep problems.

Treatment

Benzodiazepines, which have a GABA-enhancing effect, have long been the standard treatment for GAD, but as discussed earlier, there are the problems of side effects and addictive potential. An antianxiety medication, buspirone, has been effective in some studies and is FDA-approved for the treatment of GAD (but not for other anxiety disorders such as panic disorder). Although overall study results for buspirone support its use in these patients, in the reality of clinical practice the results have been mixed, and many clinicians have abandoned its use. However, it may work well for some patients, especially those who have not previously taken benzodiazepines. It seems less effective in people who have previously taken benzodiazepines for anxiety, although perhaps this perception results from the fact that, unlike benzodiazepines, buspirone does not have an immediate onset of action; like antidepressants, it can take several weeks to reach full effectiveness. Buspirone does have the advantages of safety, good tolerability, the absence of a withdrawal syndrome, and no apparent addictive potential. For patients with substance abuse problems, it may be preferable to a benzodiazepine.

The mainstay of medication treatment for GAD is, once again, antidepressants. Their success in alleviating or eliminating anxiety is comparable to that of benzodiazepines but with many of the advantages discussed earlier. Both SSRIs and dual-action antidepressants (like venlafaxine and, sometimes, some of the older TCAs) are drugs commonly used. Overall, treatment discontinuation often leads to the relapse of symptoms, although the actual rates are poorly understood at this time.

Current research is also exploring the possible benefit of certain antiepileptic medications (pregabalin and tiagabine) for the treatment of GAD, but conclusive results are still pending. CBT, alone or in combination with medications, is effective for GAD as well, and its benefits tend to extend beyond the completion of formal treatment and exceed the protective effect conferred by medication.

OBSESSIVE–COMPULSIVE DISORDER

OCD affects about 2–3% of the U.S. population. It can have a major impact on the quality of life, including the marital, familial, social, and occupational realms. It, too, is thought to follow a partial genetic form of transmission, can be highly comorbid with other anxiety disorders and depression, and is associated with substance abuse at rates higher than those seen in the general population. In OCD, as in other disorders in this section, anxiety is a core phenomenon. However, the anxiety itself may be much less apparent because of the compensating role that compulsions play in temporarily relieving it. OCD symptoms focus on thoughts and behaviors. Obsessions are recurrent distressing thoughts, images, or impulses that feel unwanted, intrusive, inappropriate, and uncontrollable. Some common themes include obsessions about contamination by dirt or germs; repeated doubts about safety (is the door really locked?; is the stove really turned off?); a need for objects to be in a specific order or symmetrical arrangement; impulses to harm others or to behave in grossly inappropriate ways; and intrusive, distressing sexual imagery (see Table 4.15). As would be expected, these unwanted thoughts and impulses are capable of inducing considerable anxiety and distress.

Patients respond to the anxiety thus provoked by trying to ignore or suppress their obsessions or to counteract them with some other thoughts or behavior. These attempts to control obsessive thoughts may become compulsions, repetitive acts designed to decrease anxiety or ward off some impending embarrassment and doom. So, someone with an obsessive fear of contamination may feel driven to wash repeatedly, and someone with intrusive impulses to shout obscenities in the midst of a religious service or a funeral may develop a compulsive mental ritual such as counting or repeating a pattern of words. In some cases, patients will have developed compulsive behaviors without a clear connection to an underlying obsession, but they still feel driven to perform the behaviors to avoid a nameless dread or satisfy a rigid set of arbitrary rules (Table 4.16).

How the patient experiences these thoughts and behaviors is an important diagnostic feature. In OCD, they feel alien, unwanted, and ego-dystonic, not a thought or behavior the patient would normally want to have. They are distressing and time consuming to the point of interfering with daily life. Although the degree of insight may vary, most patients with OCD recognize that the thoughts are the products of their own minds (in contrast, e.g., to a delusion that their thoughts are being implanted by others) and that they are excessive and unreasonable. Ritualized behavior per se is not necessarily OCD. To take an extreme example, a professional baseball player may eat the identical meal before every game, line up his equipment in a specific order every day, wear the

TABLE 4.15. Common Obsessions

- Contamination
- Aggression
- Safety/harm
- Sex
- Religion (scrupulosity)
- Somatic fears
- Need for symmetry or exactness

TABLE 4.16. Common Compulsions

- Cleaning/washing
- Checking
- Ordering/arranging
- Counting
- Repeating
- Hoarding/collecting

same (sometimes unwashed) socks or underwear as long as a hitting streak continues, and cross himself and tap his bat three times against his right shoe every time he enters the batter's box. He feels a strong need to do all this and would probably feel some distress if his lucky socks were accidentally washed. Although none of these behaviors are rationally connected to his ability to hit the baseball (and he would admit that, at least in the off-season), the ritual probably isn't OCD. The behaviors aren't distressing to him; he feels in control of them, and they are acceptable behaviors in the subculture of professional baseball. Thus, it can be important to consider cultural context in diagnosing OCD. Many cultural and religious groups prescribe rituals that may seem irrational or compulsive to outsiders but perfectly ego-syntonic and appropriate to members of the culture. On the other hand, people can develop obsessions and compulsions related to the content of their cultural rituals. A man whose religion forbids certain foods may develop an obsessive fear of accidentally ingesting a forbidden food and a compulsion to repeatedly check his kitchen for hidden traces of it. If a clinician does not know this man's culture, it might be helpful to find out whether his wife and his religious leader think his behavior is excessive to help the clinician distinguish between an unfamiliar ritual and a compulsive behavior of clinical significance.

Treatment

Treatment of OCD naturally lends itself to collaboration because it is dual-focused, utilizing both psychotherapy and medication. For the receptive patient, the combination can be quite effective in symptom reduction and/or alleviation. Psychotherapeutic intervention incorporates two fundamental elements designed to elicit anxiety and then cope with it: exposure and response prevention. However, it is important to note that between 20 and 25% of patients with OCD will flatly refuse this method of treatment out of considerable fear of exposing themselves to unacceptable levels of anxiety.

As with many of the other anxiety disorders, SSRIs and other powerful serotonergic drugs, notably the tricyclic clomipramine, are effective for OCD. The course of response for patients with OCD differs from that observed among depressed or other anxious patients. In OCD, doses often have to be greater than for other disorders, and response time is much slower. It may take up to 30 weeks of treatment for the maximum response to become apparent (Table 4.17). Unfortunately, the maximum response is often less than full remission, but that failing should not discourage anyone from trying medication. Even when symptoms cannot be completely eliminated, a partial response—a significant drop in obsessive thoughts and compulsive behaviors—can amount to a major improvement in the patients' quality of life, in both their functioning and their subjective experience.

Many patients relapse when medication is discontinued, even after long-term use. However, the additional implementation of CBT in conjunction with medication has been shown to be effective with OCD, with a much lower risk of relapse after treatment; in effect, the therapist educates the patients in how to treat themselves on an ongoing basis. So we could expect that combined therapy and medication might maximize effects and perhaps allow medication to be discontinued without relapse at some point.

Anxiety disorders are ubiquitous, and like affective disorders, they appear to be expressed clinically only when the combination of genetic vulnerability and psychosocial forces are critically combined in a given individual. Included in this phenomenon, of course, is the fact that medi-

---

TABLE 4.17. Medication Considerations in the Treatment of OCD

- Duration and dose
  - Response may take 8–12 weeks.
  - Medication doses are higher than those used for depression.
  - Full benefit may not be apparent for 3–6 months.
- Full remission is rare.
  - Most patients exhibit only 20–40% improvement.
  - 25% of patients experience no response at all.
- Medication treatment must be long term.
- If attempted, medication tapering must be slow and closely scrutinized.
- About 90% of patients relapse quickly after medication discontinuation.

---

cations used for unrelated medical conditions and over-the-counter drugs (even coffee) can induce anxiety disorders in susceptible individuals. The same is true for some illegal substances.

Although anxiety disorders, when untreated, can be the cause of substantial personal suffering, disability, and marital and family disruption, the progress made in the therapeutic area for conditions like panic disorder, OCD, and GAD, among other anxiety disorders, makes these conditions very gratifying to treat. Indeed, the skillful use of psychotherapies—cognitive-behavioral therapies appear to be most effective—and medications can produce dramatic and lasting improvement in many patients.

Most of the medications used in the treatment of anxiety disorders are those used in treating depressive disorders, and many of the comments made in the previous chapter are applicable here, including the rational selection of mediation, initiation, and duration of treatment, as well as the identification and management of side effects. An important observation to remember is that patients with anxiety disorders have a tendency to relapse relatively quickly once medications are discontinued, whereas the impact of behavioral therapies appears to be longer lasting. Once again, a close collaborative effort between the therapist and the physician can guide the selection of the most appropriate form of treatment and/or combination of treatments, as well as their duration.

CHAPTER 5

Schizophrenia and Other Psychoses

Perhaps only few other disorders are as cruel as schizophrenia. Recent discoveries suggest that certain deficits, of a "soft" nature and usually not regarded as ominous by parents and close relations, are present during the developmental years of an individual marked to manifest schizophrenia later in life. But the illness takes its real bite just when the patient reaches late adolescence or early adulthood, as he or she prepares to enter the central stage of life, the years of productivity, independence, family building, and personal creativity. It destroys all dreams, and it truncates the development of new ones for the rest of the patient's existence.

For the rest of their lives, schizophrenic patients, with a few painfully rare exceptions, will be unable to lead a truly independent existence, will be unable to support themselves, will not raise a family, and will spend frequent periods of time in a hospital, in outpatient programs, and even in jail. All the while, they will be besieged by auditory hallucinations, persecutory delusions, confused thinking, and mood swings. And this existence will be shrouded by discrimination or, at the very least, indifference on the part of a society that by and large acts as if this illness does not exist.

Most of this chapter focuses on schizophrenia—its **epidemiology, pathophysiology**, and treatment. Schizophrenia, however, is not the only disorder in which psychosis is a primary feature. Many other illnesses have this characteristic. In some, like mood disorders, psychosis is present only in the most severe forms. In others, like paranoid disorder, the main psychotic feature—the delusion—is an isolated feature, and the rest of the patient's mental functioning is generally preserved (Table 5.1). The use of a number of substances, some prescribed for medical disorders and some used illegally for mind-altering purposes, can also result in psychotic symptoms (Table 5.2). It is estimated that about 5–6 million people in the United States suffer from psychotic symptoms at any given time.

Schizoaffective disorder, given the frequency with which it is diagnosed, and delusional disorder merit a few comments. Schizoaffective disorder is, depending on one's perspective, a kind of "better prognosis" schizophrenia or a "worse prognosis" type of bipolar disorder. The psychiatric field is divided on the validity of this diagnosis, although it is listed in DSM-IV-TR (American Psychiatric Association, 2000). Roughly, schizoaffective disorder incorporates elements of thought disorder, hallucinations, and other psychotic symptoms typically observed in schizophrenia, with significant mood symptoms (depression, hypo-

---

TABLE 5.1. Disorders That Manifest Psychotic Symptoms

- Schizophrenia
- Schizophreniform disorder
- Schizoaffective disorder
- Delusional disorder
- Brief psychotic disorder
- Shared psychotic disorder
- Mood disorders (e.g., mania, psychotic depression)
- Brain tumors
- Stroke
- Head trauma
- Endocrine/metabolic abnormalities (e.g., severe hypothyroidism)
- Substance-induced psychoses
- Dementia (e.g., Alzheimer's disease)
- Delirium
- Neurological conditions (e.g., Huntington's chorea, Tourette's syndrome)
- Infections
- Other psychoses

TABLE 5.2. Some Drugs Known to Induce Psychosis

• Amphetamines	• Indomethacin
• Marijuana	• Corticosteroids
• Hallucinogens	• Procainamide
• Cocaine	• Phenytoin
• Beta-blockers	• Carbamazepine
• Bupropion	

mania, and mania) classically associated with bipolar disorder. Delusional disorder is characterized by the presence of a single (although there can be more than one), unshakeable, nonbizarre delusion. Several subtypes of delusional disorder are recognized, emanating from the main delusional concern (erotomanic, grandiose, jealous, persecutory, somatic, and mixed). In addition to interventions called for by the specific syndrome, treatment for all these psychotic conditions includes the use of antipsychotic medications of the same classes used in the treatment of schizophrenia. The case below illustrates the myriad considerations in the assessment and treatment of delusional disorder.

CASE: SCHIZOPHRENIA

Case Description

Ms. P, a 53-year-old Caucasian woman, visits her primary care physician, Dr. K, because she feels pain in her arms and pressure around her eyes, and she senses some changes in her vision. Dr. K examines her, finding no medical cause for her complaints. He adds them to the long list of symptoms she has reported over several visits that have no clear medical etiology. She also tells him that she's been feeling very "nervous and stressed out" over the past several weeks.

Ms. P currently lives alone in a government-subsidized apartment complex. She has been married and divorced twice, maintains close contact with her mother, has an adult daughter who refuses to speak to her, and has an adult son who was recently released from an inpatient substance-dependence treatment facility.

Beginning Collaboration

Dr. K refers Ms. P to an eye specialist and asks her if she would like a referral to an in-house therapist for some extra support. She agrees, and Dr. K fills out a referral for one of the clinic therapists, Ms. L.

Ms. L contacts Ms. P, who agrees to come in for an initial therapy session. She reveals several of her worries, including concerns about her health, her family, and her neighbors. She denies any symptoms of depression, mania, or psychosis and is given a diagnosis of anxiety disorder not otherwise specified. Over the next several sessions, Ms. L starts to wonder if these anxieties are based in reality or are symptoms of a psychotic disorder. Ms. P starts to describe a discoloration of her skin that is not at all visible to Ms. L. She later describes an ability to smell food she sees on television and an incident in which she saw her whole living room turn purple. In subsequent sessions, Ms. P describes several phone calls to the police and landlord about a neighbor stalking her, which were investigated and then dismissed as unfounded. She also tells Ms. L about her special ability to know the thoughts of people she talks to on the phone, and to even hear special voices, as if she "has a satellite dish attached to her head." Throughout this time, Ms. P holds strong to her belief that she is "not mentally ill" but that she has several undiagnosed physical ailments, a very bothersome neighbor, and some special abilities that most people don't have.

As Ms. L gathers this information, she and Dr. K decide that it is time to involve a psychiatrist in the treatment process. Ms. L suggests on several occasions that Ms. P may benefit from having the "additional support of an extra doctor added to her treatment team," but as soon as Ms. P hears the word "psychiatrist," she insists she is not mentally ill and has no need for "one of those kinds of doctors." One day, Ms. P comes to therapy particularly agitated. She describes herself as feeling very stressed, unable to sleep well, and unable to shut off her mind. Ms. L again mentions the idea of seeing a doctor who specializes in "dealing with stress," and this time Ms. P agrees to the offer.

Ongoing Collaboration and Outcome

Ms. L contacts Dr. M, a psychiatrist in her healthcare network whom she knows to be warm, tactful, and very experienced. Ms. L knows how important it is for the psychiatrist to establish a good rapport with Ms. P right from the beginning because Ms. P is so hesitant about seeing a psychiatrist, and she appears to greatly need one. Dr. M agrees to see Ms. P, and Ms. L helps Ms. P schedule an appointment.

Ms. L decides to attend the psychiatric appointment with Ms. P. Dr. M does a thorough evaluation and decides to prescribe for Ms. P an "atypical" antipsychotic medication that will help "calm down her mind, reduce her stress, and help her sleep." Ms. P is thankful for the medication and agrees to take it as prescribed. But by her next session with Ms. L, she has read more information about her medication, found out it is used to treat "people who are crazy," and has stopped taking it.

Ms. L assures her that taking medication does not mean she is "crazy" and reminds her that Dr. M prescribed that medication to help with her "stress" and "calm down her mind." Ms. L encourages Ms. P to contact Dr. M to discuss her concerns, and Ms. L calls Dr. M to update her.

Over the next several months, Dr. M and Ms. L work closely with Ms. P, who has decided to take her medication as prescribed. She likes that it helps her sleep and brings "a sense of peace to her mind." Unfortunately, when she starts to feel better, she frequently discontinues her medication until she starts to feel "stressed" again, despite Dr. M's and Ms. L's encouragement to take her medication as prescribed.

Questions for Consideration

• *Why did Ms. L continue to see Ms. P even though she clearly needed psychiatric care more than therapy?* Ms. L saw fairly quickly that therapy was not particularly helpful to Ms. P while she was actively psychotic. She continued to see her so that she could serve as a bridge into the psychiatric care she saw as crucial to Ms. P's treatment. Because Ms. L was located in the same office as Dr. K (Ms. P's primary care physician), Ms. P found it very natural to come in to see her. She often made medical appointments or had her blood pressure checked while she was at the clinic. This comforted her by keeping her symptoms in the category of "physical illness" rather than "mental illness," and it ultimately enabled her to trust Ms. L enough to follow her advice to see a psychiatrist.

• *Why did Ms. L attend the psychiatry appointment with Ms. P?* Although Ms. L knew and trusted Dr. M enough to feel confident in her ability to establish a good rapport with Ms. P, she wanted to be at the appointment for several reasons. First, she wanted to support Ms. P and help her muster up the courage even to go to the appointment. Second, she wanted to be able to encourage Ms. P to give information to Dr. M that she might not disclose unless asked directly. Second, she knew that if Ms. P disliked anything about the appointment, she would be quick to disregard everything Dr. M said. Ms. L wanted to have the opportunity to debrief the session with Ms. P and highlight the good parts rather than allowing her to focus on her concerns.

• *How much should Ms. L talk with Ms. P about her psychotropic medications?* Ms. L is limited in what she can say to Ms. P about her medications. First, Ms. L always prefaces her statements about medications by reminding Ms. P that she is not a doctor, nor is she an expert on medication. She then chooses to make only general statements about medications as a whole (e.g., "taking medication doesn't mean you're crazy") and always recommends to Ms. P that she discuss any medication concerns with Dr. M. Instead of encouraging Ms. P to "take her medicine every day," she simply encourages Ms. P to take her medication as prescribed by her doctor and to stay in close contact with Dr. M about any side effects or concerns.

- *Research suggests that many patients who are prescribed psychotropic medication fail to complete an adequate trial, that is, to take enough medication for enough time to see if it treats the symptoms. How did Ms. L's presence influence the patient's adherence to the medication trial?* During the critical first weeks, when Ms. P was skeptical about the medication and what it meant if she took it, Ms. L was able to help her address her worries. She could help her address her self-image problems—whether taking medication meant that she was crazy—and she was able to help her get answers to the questions about the medication that emerged as she started taking it. Without Ms. L's helpful encouragement, there is a good chance that Ms. P would have simply stopped the medication and not returned to Dr. M.

EPIDEMIOLOGY

Schizophrenia, among the leading causes of disability, affects approximately 1% of the U.S. population. It affects men and women equally, although its average age of onset appears to be earlier in men (15–25 years old) than in women (25–35 years old). Many cases of schizophrenia have begun much earlier in life, during childhood. Although we are discovering that many deficits are present in many schizophrenia patients during their early years, the age of onset is often referred to as the time when the major symptoms appear. Also, recent research has established the notion of late-onset schizophrenia for those individuals who develop the illness in their 50s or later.

Schizophrenia accounts for about 40% of mental health hospital beds and about 15% of all hospital beds. The costs to society are staggering: $19 billion per year in the United States for direct costs (hospitalization, physician and therapist services, and medications) and $46 billion in indirect costs (disability, lost productivity, etc.). It accounts for 2.5% of all U.S. health costs and about 20% of the total days of Social Security benefits.

The course of schizophrenia is chronic and relentless, with periods of exacerbation marked by prominent psychotic symptoms interspersed between long periods with lesser psychotic symptoms but disabling cognitive, mood, interpersonal, and thought process deficits. Although they have been reported, **spontaneous remissions** are very rare. It is felt that women have a somewhat better prognosis than men. Other prognostic features have been identified (see Table 5.3).

Schizophrenic patients are also at a great disadvantage in other health concerns and in life expectancy. Their mortality rates are between 1.6 and 2.6 times higher than those for the rest of the population, and their life expectancy is about 20% shorter (61 years vs. 76 years). Patients with schizophrenia have smoking rates much higher than the general population and are therefore exposed to all the cardiovascular and pulmonary risks, among others, inherent to long-term tobacco use. They are also more likely to be obese (some of this is medication-induced) and suffer from diabetes, heart disease, and other conditions. Finally, the schizophrenic patient is at great risk for suicide. About half of patients with schizophrenia will attempt suicide sometime in their lives, as a result of either command hallucinations, delusions, or severe depression, and 10–15% of patients with schizophrenia will die as a result of suicide.

ETIOLOGY AND PATHOPHYSIOLOGY

Studies conducted several decades ago confirmed suspicions that the illness occurs more often among relatives of schizophrenic patients than in the general population. Clever research designs, utilizing adoption records, separated the familial environmental influences from the genetic determinism. However, genetics (the number and location of the genes is still unclear) is merely part of the story since only about 50% of monozygotic (identical) twins are concordant for the disorder (Table 5.4).

TABLE 5.3. Some Prognostic Features of Schizophrenia

Feature	Prognosis
• Early age of onset	Worse
• Presence of precipitating factors	Better
• Slow, protracted onset	Worse
• Good premorbid functioning	Better
• Presence of mood symptoms	Better
• Single marital status	Worse
• Available support system(s)	Better
• Positive family history	Worse

TABLE 5.4. Genes and Schizophrenia

• General population prevalence	1%
• Parent of individual with schizophrenia	5–10%
• Sibling of individual with schizophrenia	8–14%
• Offspring of individual with schizophrenia	9–16%
• Offspring of two parents with schizophrenia	46%
• Uncle or aunt of individual with schizophrenia	2%
• Nephew or niece of individual with schizophrenia	1–4%
• Grandchildren of individual with schizophrenia	2–8%
• Half-sibling of individual with schizophrenia	4%
• First cousin of individual with schizophrenia	2–6%
• Monozygotic twin concordance	40–60%
• Dizygotic twin concordance	10–16%
• Heritability	~80%

Note. Early age at onset and more severe illness may indicate higher risk to relatives. Data from National Coalition for Health Professional Education in Genetics (2004).

Further study has suggested that environmental factors must play a very important role. These factors and their impact are poorly understood at the present time, but they include the possibility of maternal **intrauterine** viral infections during the **gestational period**, obstetrical complications during delivery, and **perinatal** conditions during the early days or months of the patient's life. Essentially, it would appear that schizophrenic patients have a genetic vulnerability to develop the disorder, which is manifested later in life if and when certain environmental conditions occur.

Although the nature of the brain abnormalities seen in schizophrenia is not clearly known at present, certain pieces of the puzzle are being identified. Overall, schizophrenic patients appear to have some degree of cerebral atrophy (about 5% loss of cerebral mass), enlarged cerebral ventricles, and decreased size of certain other brain structures. From a functional perspective, the prefrontal and medial temporal brain appear to be particularly affected. Several neurochemical abnormalities are also associated with the disorder, and several neurotransmitter systems have been implicated (Table 5.5).

The dopamine system is the most studied in relation to schizophrenia, and the so-called dopamine hypothesis can be reasonably argued as the basis for several of the cardinal symptoms (e.g., hallucinations). The dopamine hypothesis posits that certain dopaminergic pathways in the

TABLE 5.5. Neurotransmitter Systems Postulated to Be Involved in Schizophrenia

- Dopamine
- Acetylcholine
- Norepinephrine
- Serotonin
- Glutamate
- GABA
- **Neuropeptides** (e.g., cholecystokinin)

brain are dysregulated. A brief review of these neural pathways will be helpful in understanding the targets of antipsychotic medications and some of their more prominent side effects. There are at least four dopamine-mediated pathways in the brain, projecting to different areas of the brain, thus controlling different functions (Table 5.6).

The dopamine hypothesis postulates that there is an *increased* dopamine drive in the mesolimbic system, leading to the causation of positive symptoms and a *decreased* dopamine drive in the mesocortical system, leading to the causation of negative symptoms. Antipsychotic drugs tar-

TABLE 5.6. Dopamine Pathways in the Brain

Pathway	Projections	Function
Mesolimbic tract	From the midbrain ventral tegmental area to the nucleus accumbens, olfactory tubercle, and parts of the limbic system.	Arousal, memory, stimulus processing, locomotor activity, motivational behavior. Hyperactivity implicated in positive symptoms.
Mesocortical tract	From the midbrain ventral tegmental area to the frontal cortex. It has been implicated in aspects of learning and memory.	Cognition, communication, social activity, learning, and memory. Hypoactivity implicated in negative symptoms.
Nigrostriatal tract	Substantia nigra and striatum.	Motor control. Hypoactivity implicated in parkinsonian-like side effects of antipsychotics.
Tuberoinfundibular tract	Projects from the hypothalamus to the anterior pituitary gland.	Controls prolactin secretion. Hypoactivity implicated in breast enlargement, milk production, and other side effects caused by many antipsychotic medications.

get these two dopamine pathways. The other two dopamine pathways are also prone to be affected by many of these drugs, resulting in some of the familiar side effects associated with medication.

PSYCHOPATHOLOGY

Psychotic symptoms, the most prominent and recognized manifestations of schizophrenia, are not the exclusive domain of the illness. From a psychopathological perspective, the disorder is much more complex and overreaching, leading to the profound deficits displayed by these patients in interpersonal, social, and occupational functioning. Four symptom clusters are recognized: positive symptoms, negative symptoms, cognitive deficits, and mood symptoms and their associated manifestations (Table 5.7).

MEDICATION

The most effective treatment for schizophrenia incorporates a multidisciplinary approach in which antipsychotic medications are a necessary but insufficient component. Medication must be complemented by specific psychotherapy modalities, including family therapy, skills training, psychoeducation, supportive intervention, vocational training, and self-help groups.

Prior to the introduction of antipsychotic medications in the 1950s, the main treatments, all with very paltry results, included ECT, insulin coma, nonspecific sedating medications (e.g., **barbiturates**), psycho-

TABLE 5.7. Clinical Clusters of Schizophrenia

Cluster	Examples
Positive symptoms	Hallucinations, delusions, conceptual disorganization, disorganized speech, excitement, grandiosity, paranoia
Negative symptoms	Alogia, affective flattening, avolition, social withdrawal, anhedonia
Cognitive deficits	Attentional impairment, memory dysfunction, impaired executive functions
Mood abnormalities	Depression, excitement, aggression, anxiety, hostility, associated substance abuse

surgery, liberal use of physical restraint, and psychosocial interventions. Since the introduction of chlorpromazine—the first antipsychotic medication discovered—treatment has progressed significantly. However, compared to other psychiatric conditions (i.e., depressive and anxiety disorders), the benefits of medication for schizophrenia are still quite modest. As an illustration, consider that in order to gain FDA approval for marketing an antipsychotic medication, the candidate drug must show that, compared to a placebo, it causes a 20–30% improvement in symptoms. For antidepressants, the bar is considerably higher, at 50%. These figures reflect the current status of research development and knowledge about these disorders.

Antipsychotic medications constitute the backbone of pharmacological agents for these patients. Other categories of medications are used when specific clinical features so require, and they include antidepressants, anticonvulsants, benzodiazepines, and for the management of certain side effects, anticholinergic medications. In practice, clinicians are likely to find that many of the patients suffering from schizophrenia will indeed be on a complex multimedication regime. This reflects both the unique characteristics of the patient and our rather limited understanding of the disorder and its treatment.

First-Generation or "Conventional" Antipsychotics

The first generation of antipsychotics has been used in the United States since the 1950s, and although gradually replaced by newer agents, they are still seen as part of the medication regimen for many patients. Examples of conventional antipsychotics appear in Table 5.8.

All these antipsychotic medications have a common mechanism of action: they block the dopamine receptor (at the same time, they unfortunately affect a number of other neurotransmitter systems—e.g., cholinergic, alpha-adrenergic, and histaminergic—and thus cause myriad undesirable and unintended side effects). In blocking the dopamine receptor, they fulfill an important goal of antipsychotic therapy, the reduction of drive in the hyperactive mesolimbic dopamine pathway (see earlier in this chapter). The result is a noticeable improvement in positive symptoms, like hallucinations and delusions. Since medications are essentially distributed throughout the brain, the blockade of the dopamine receptor will occur wherever such receptors exist, including the three other pathways reviewed earlier. As expected, this will result in detectable clinical effects on the functions regulated by the respective pathways. Typically, therefore, antipsychotic therapy with conventional

TABLE 5.8. Some Conventional Antipsychotics

- Chlorpromazine (Thorazine)
- Haloperidol (Haldol)[a]
- Thioridazine (Mellaril)
- Trifluoperazine (Stelazine)
- Fluphenazine (Prolixin)[a]
- Perphenazine (Trilafon)
- Thiothixene (Navane)
- Loxapine (Loxitane)
- Molindone (Moban)

Note. Trade names are in parentheses.
[a]Available in injectable depot (long-term) formulation.

antipsychotics will result in minimal improvement of "negative symptoms" since the dysregulation in this pathway, it will be recalled, is characterized by a decreased dopamine drive. If anything, the medication is likely to make negative symptoms worse. Likewise, blocking the dopamine receptors in the nigrostriatal pathway causes several motor symptoms like muscle rigidity, inexpressive facial features, and tremors, reminiscent of the manifestations of Parkinson's disease. Consequently, this category of side effects is commonly referred to as **parkinsonian** and **extrapyramidal symptoms** (after the name of the neural tracts involved). Table 5.9 lists the common side effects associated with conventional antipsychotic therapy.

Blockade of the dopamine receptors in the tuberoinfundibular pathway will increase the production and release of a hormone called prolactin. Prolactin is normally elevated in pregnancy and is responsible for breast enlargement and milk production. Sometimes, patients—including males—treated with these medications will develop gynecomastia (breast enlargement) and lactation. There are several other consequences to abnormally elevated prolactin levels, and they can be quite distressing to the patients (Table 5.10). Other side effects, related to effects in other areas, include photosensitivity (which can lead to severe skin burns when overexposed to sunlight), electrocardiogram abnormalities, jaundice, and decreased white blood cell count.

Motor side effects deserve particular mention. Some can occur as early as a few hours after administration of the first dose (acute **dystonia**), whereas others (like **tardive dyskinesia**, a usually irreversible condition) may not appear until after many years of treatment (although

TABLE 5.9. Neurological Side Effects of Conventional Antipsychotics

Side effect	Clinical manifestations	Chronology of onset
Acute dystonia	Spasm of tongue, throat, face, jaw, eyes, neck, or back muscles (torticollis, facial grimacing, oculogyric crises)	24 hours to <1 week
Akathisia	Restlessness, inability to sit still, strong urge to move about	<1 week to 2 weeks
Pseudoparkin-sonism	Bradykinesia, rigidity, sialorrhea, mask-like facies, resting tremor, "pill rolling," shuffling gait	~1 week
Tardive dyskinesia	Protrusion of tongue, puffing of cheeks, chewing movements, involuntary movements of extremities and trunk	3 months to years

elderly patients are at risk for a much earlier onset, sometimes months, of this adverse effect). These extrapyramidal symptoms are easily observable and are extremely distressing and bothersome to patients, contributing to the high rate of treatment nonadherence in this population (approximately 50% of patients with schizophrenia will discontinue medications after 4–6 months of treatment, mostly because of side effects). It is important for therapists to develop some familiarity with this constellation of adverse effects, although their prevalence has diminished somewhat since the introduction of the atypical antipsychotics (see Table 5.11). Management of this class of side effects includes dose modifications (of limited value since dose reduction may aggravate the pri-

TABLE 5.10. Clinical Effects of Hyperprolactinemia

Menstrual function	Sexual function
• Anovulation	• Decreased libido
• Shortened luteal phase	• Orgasmic dysfunction
• Oligomenorrhea	
• Amenorrhea	
Breast	Bones
• Engorgement	• Decreased bone density mediated
• Nonpuerperal lactation	by estrogen deficiency

TABLE 5.11. Neurotransmitter Effects of Conventional Antipsychotics and Their Associated Side Effects

Neurotransmitter	Side effect
Histamine	Sedation, weight gain, hypotension
Acetylcholine (muscarinic)	Urinary retention, increased heart rate, memory deficits, confusion, dry mouth, blurred vision, constipation
Norepinephrine (alpha-adrenergic)	Low blood pressure, constricted pupils, increased heart rate
Dopamine	Parkinsonian symptoms, other motor symptoms, increased prolactin

mary symptoms of the disorder) and the addition of agents specifically aimed at reducing or eliminating the movement disorder (see Table 5.12). Of course, these so-called anticholinergic medications, although effective in reducing movement abnormalities, have side effects of their own.

Conventional antipsychotics were the only class of antipsychotics available for about 35 years. There are several advantages to these medications, and they still have a place in the contemporary treatment of schizophrenia: they are remarkably effective against positive symptoms, prescribers have had many years of experience in their use, and they are inexpensive. Until recently, they were the only antipsychotics available in depot long-term formulation, a strategy aimed at simplifying treatment

TABLE 5.12. Drugs Used in the Treatment of Extrapyramidal Symptoms

Antimuscarinics
    Benztropine (Cogentin)
    Biperiden (Akineton)
    Ethopropazine (Parsidol)
    Orphenadrine
    Procyclidine (Kemadrin)
    Trihexyphenidyl (Artane)

Antihistaminic
    Diphenhydramine (Benadryl)

Dopamine agonist
    Amantadine (Symmetrel)

Note. Trade names are in parentheses.

by administering the medication by injection once every 2–4 weeks and thereby improving treatment adherence. On the other hand, conventionals fall short in efficacy—only about 30% of patients will respond—and they have little or no impact on negative and cognitive symptoms. Relapses and troublesome side effects are common. A rare but potentially fatal condition, **neuroleptic malignant syndrome**, can also develop in patients treated with conventional antipsychotics.

Atypical Antipsychotics

An important leap in the treatment of schizophrenia occurred in the late 1980s with the introduction of the first of a number of medications that offered a wider spectrum of action and relatively improved tolerability. Some of these atypical antipsychotics, also called second-generation antipsychotics, are listed in Table 5.13.

The first of the atypicals, clozapine (trade name Clozaril), produced results that raised expectations of antipsychotic therapy. For the first time, negative symptoms were amenable to treatment. This effect is thought to be mediated by certain serotonin receptors. This capability, along with the ability to block the dopamine receptor, has led some to call this new generation the "atypical" antipsychotics. Further clinical study showed that clozapine was able to induce noticeable improvement

TABLE 5.13. Atypical (Second Generation) Antipsychotics

- Clozapine (Clozaril)
- Risperidone (Risperdal)
- Olanzapine (Zyprexa)
- Quetiapine (Seroquel)
- Ziprasidone (Geodon)
- Aripiprazole (Abilify)[a]
- Paliperidone (Invega, Invega Sustenna)
- Iloperidone (Fanapt)
- Asenapine (Saphris)

Note. Trade names are in parentheses.
[a]Aripiprazole is sometimes called a third-generation antipsychotic because of its unique mechanism of action (see text).

in patients hitherto unresponsive to other antipsychotics (efficacy in particularly refractory cases is not necessarily shared by the other atypicals, and it appears to be a particular advantage of Clozaril). Also, a worldwide study has shown that clozapine—in a distinct advantage over other antipsychotics, both conventional and atypical—appears to have a specific antisuicidal effect in patients with schizophrenia. Finally, clozapine (and the atypicals that followed it into the market) displayed a much lower incidence of extrapyramidal symptoms and the dreaded tardive dyskinesia.

In spite of these advantages, clozapine use was accompanied by many disturbing side effects and dangerous adverse reactions, notably an increased risk of potentially fatal **agranulocytosis** (a severe drop in white blood cell count). This potential risk (which occurs in 1–1.5% of cases) requires patients to take weekly blood tests for the first 6 months of treatment, with a decreased frequency thereafter, for as long as they are on clozapine; it is easy to understand why so few patients were willing to continue long-term treatment, in spite of the benefits obtained. Other side effects of clozapine that further limit its use are listed in Table 5.14.

In spite of its limitations, clozapine brought renewed impetus in the quest for improved antipsychotic medications. For the first time, negative symptoms, so disabling to patients in the interpersonal, social, and occupational spheres, were seen as amenable to treatment. Other atypicals followed, all with important contributions to the treatment of positive, negative, and cognitive symptoms. These properties, as in the case of clozapine, are thought to result from a balanced effect on dopamine and serotonin receptors. These compounds also have a broader spectrum of action, leading to their proven use in the treatment of manic episodes and efficacy in the management of agitation associated with other conditions (e.g., Alzheimer's disease).

TABLE 5.14. Some Potential Side Effects of Clozapine (Clozaril)

- Risk of agranulocytosis
- Drowsiness and sedation
- Marked weight gain
- Orthostatic hypotension
- Hypersalivation
- Dizziness and vertigo
- Seizures
- Increased heart rate

From the perspective of tolerability, these new atypicals are clearly superior to conventionals. The rates of extrapyramidal symptoms, tardive dyskinesia, and anticholinergic effects are much lower. However, as their use has become more commonplace, these drugs appear to have their own adverse effects, some of which have raised substantial concerns. They include increased rates of extrapyramidal symptoms at higher than usual doses, prolactin elevations, and electrocardiogram changes.

Weight gain and metabolic side effects, in particular, merit special attention. It will be remembered that individuals with schizophrenia are at a higher risk for developing several chronic medical conditions, including heart disease and diabetes (Consensus Development Conference on Antipsychotic Drugs and Obesity and Diabetes, 2004). They tend to be more overweight and to have higher rates of obesity, and compared to the general population, they also have a shorter life expectancy. This is true also for bipolar patients, another diagnostic category in which atypical antipsychotics are being used with increased frequency (Kupfer, 2005).

Treatment with atypical antipsychotics—some more than others—has been associated with increased risks by promoting weight gain, **hyperglycemia** (elevated blood sugar), diabetes, and **hyperlipidemia** (elevated blood fats). The effect is significant enough to warrant recommendations for proper monitoring of patients in order to improve the chances of early detection (Consensus Development Conference on Antipsychotic Drugs and Obesity and Diabetes, 2004). All mental health providers should ensure that patients adhere to a program of monitoring as recommended by their primary care physician or psychiatrist (Marder et al., 2004). The program should include periodic monitoring of several parameters, including weight measurements and baseline and follow-up blood sugar and lipid levels. Furthermore, given that the evidence shows that not all atypical antipsychotics currently available are equal offenders in increasing the risk for **metabolic syndrome** (see Table 5.15), clinicians must give consideration to this, among other factors, when selecting antipsychotic medications. Note that data regarding metabolic risks for the new atypicals (paliperidone, iloperidone, and asenapine) are at this time insufficient to provide a meaningful clinical assessment. Additionally, a large population study by Yood et al. (2009) concluded that, relative to conventional antipsychotics, among atypical antipsychotics, only clozapine and olanzapine use are associated with an increased risk (paliperidone, iloperidone, and asenapine were not studied). Although the exact nature of these risks is still being researched, given the fact that, at the present time, schizophrenia treatment is essentially needed for the lifetime of the patient, the long-term impact of these side effects may be considerable.

TABLE 5.15. Atypical Antipsychotics and Metabolic Abnormalities

Drug	Weight gain	Risk for diabetes	Worsening lipid profile
Clozapine	+++	+	+
Olanzapine	+++	+	+
Risperidone	++	D	D
Quetiapine	++	D	D
Aripiprazole[a]	+/–	–	–
Ziprasidone[a]	+/–	–	–

Note. D, discrepant results. Data from Consensus Development Conference on Antipsychotic Drugs and Obesity and Diabetes (2004).
[a]Newer drugs with limited long-term data.

CASE: DELUSIONAL DISORDER, SOMATIC TYPE

Case Description

Mr. F, a 42-year-old Caucasian male, visits his family physician, Dr. T, with myriad health concerns, including aches, pains, rashes, numbness, fatigue, sadness, memory disturbance, and weight loss. He says the symptoms began after an extramarital affair, which occurred 2 weeks before this meeting. Mr. F is particularly concerned that he might "have AIDS," since this is his only explanation for his health problems. He explains that he had seen another physician near his mother's house in a neighboring community and reported similar complaints. He had an HIV test during this previous medical exam, which he said was negative. Despite this reassuring news, he still firmly believes that he has AIDS, which scares him to the point of considering suicide.

Beginning Collaboration

Dr. T evaluates Mr. F for suicidality and implements a crisis intervention plan to ensure his safety. He meets with him for extended visits over the next 2 months, starts him on an SSRI, and refers him to Dr. E, a therapist who works in Dr. T's office. A general medical and cardiac evaluation is started as well. Over the course of 3 months, Mr. F requests and receives two more HIV tests, both of which are negative. Unfortunately, these negative results do little to weaken his belief that he has AIDS. On a scale of 0–100, Mr. F says he is 90% sure he has AIDS.

Ongoing Collaboration

Over the course of several months, Mr. F has an extensive medical evaluation, including specialty evaluation by a neurologist, cardiac stress testing, podiatry evaluation, and laboratory testing including eight HIV tests. All evaluations are negative. Dr. T and Dr. E also recommend a psychiatric evaluation. Mr. F sees a psychiatrist but finds it unhelpful and refuses to return. The psychiatrist who performed the evaluation recommended an antipsychotic, prescribed by Dr. T, to address Mr. F's delusional thinking.

Outcome

Mr. F's certainty and worry about AIDS infection follows a predictable pattern: After a negative result, he feels relief and gratitude for the work of the health care team but gets increasingly anxious and irritable the further he gets from the most recent test. When Mr. F becomes highly distressed about AIDS, he often questions the intent and honesty of Dr. T: "Maybe the AIDS test is positive but he's not telling me because he's afraid that I'll kill myself." He also questions whether Dr. T is doing enough to find the cause of his symptoms. Dr. E reassures Mr. F that everyone is being honest and trying to provide the best possible care. In a joint meeting, Dr. T and Dr. E restate their commitment to helping Mr. F and offer a referral to another primary care physician for a second opinion. Mr. F declines this suggestion.

Questions for Consideration

• *What role did collaboration play in Mr. F's treatment?* First, success with Mr. F would have been much less likely without close collaboration. Mr. F demonstrated reluctance to follow through with referrals to a variety of specialists. When he did follow through with an initial appointment, rarely did he continue contact with these providers, such as the psychiatrist. The reason he attended the first and subsequent mental health appointments was due to the strong relationship between Dr. E and Dr. T., which was facilitated by the colocation of their practices.

Second, the medical clinic where Mr. F received his medical care was a second home for Mr. F. As his extended family, which included his medical providers and front desk staff, the clinic became a holding environment for his suffering. When he arrived for his appointments, the staff greeted him with a familiar kindness and respect. Furthermore, multiple needs could be met at one time and in one place. For example, Mr. F arrived for one appointment feeling particularly anxious and distraught because he was waiting to hear the results of his latest HIV test.

Dr. E interrupted the session and invited Dr. T to join them. After finishing the care of another patient, Dr. T entered the mental health meeting and was able to give Mr. F the test result. This one-stop shopping was convenient and secure.

Finally, Dr. E and Dr. T were a united front, frequently reassuring Mr. F with a more hopeful reality than the one he frequently described. Furthermore, when his distortions convinced him that they were hiding information, such as a positive test result, they provided consistent information because of their frequent communication and shared charting and could vouch for each other's noble intentions. Mr. F was appreciative of their communication about him, which delivered a message that he was an important patient and that the doctors were working as a team devoted to giving him the best possible care.

• *What are some risks and possible strengths of the close collaborative relationships that Dr. T and Dr. E had?* The close physical proximity, strong historical relationship (built by sharing multiple cases over time), mutual respect, and frequent communication between Dr. T and Dr. E helped them create a holding environment for Mr. F. Without these qualities, Mr. F could have easily triangulated Dr. E and Dr. T. For example, Mr. F might try to convince Dr. E that Dr. T wasn't taking his concerns seriously enough. Dr. E might feel the need to pressure Dr. T into doing more evaluation, and this could become frustrating for Dr. T. Clearly, the strength of the bond and communication between Dr. T and Dr. E facilitated Mr. F's treatment.

In addition, because Dr. E was working in Dr. T's office, he did not feel rushed in treating Mr. F. He knew that Mr. F would be a long-term patient, coming in for many needs. Dr. E could take his time, build his relationship with Mr. F, and wait for the most opportune times to encourage him to consider multiple explanations for his fears.

The Dopamine Partial Agonists

A new, so-called third generation of antipsychotics has recently been introduced, and at this time one drug, aripiprazole, is available and others are in the late stages of development. This new class of medications has a novel mechanism of action that, at least in theory, should deal with several of the limitations of other atypicals. It will be remembered that all antipsychotics preceding this class had the ability to block the dopamine receptor, and they did so in all four dopamine pathways. As discussed, this had both benefits and drawbacks: dopamine blockade resulted in the improvement of positive symptoms (mesolimbic pathway) but had a limited benefit in negative symptom reduction (mesocortical pathway), as well as extrapyramidal symptom (nigrostriatal pathway) and prolactin elevations (tuberoinfundibular pathway). The dopamine blockade occurred as an "all or nothing proposition" wherever dopamine activity was present.

Dopamine partial agonists have a unique mechanism of action. Their net effect on each dopamine pathway is influenced by the level of dopamine activity in that specific pathway: it will reduce dopamine drive where it is too high, it will increase dopamine drive where it is too low, and it will have little effect where the drive is normal. In the case of schizophrenia, these drugs are expected to improve positive symptoms by *reducing* excessive dopamine drive in the mesolimbic pathway while improving negative symptoms by *increasing* reduced dopamine drive in the mesocortical pathway. They should also cause much fewer changes (or none at all) in the other two dopamine pathways, thus avoiding extrapyramidal symptom and prolactin elevations. In addition to its partial dopamine agonism, aripiprazole has serotonin receptor effects that have been associated with mood and cognitive improvements, both desirable features in treating schizophrenia.

GENERAL TREATMENT CONSIDERATIONS IN ANTIPSYCHOTIC THERAPY

It is unquestionable that current antipsychotic therapy is comparatively effective and at the same time disappointingly insufficient. These drugs can treat the symptoms of the disorder but certainly do not provide a cure. The great majority of patients will have between 20 and 50% reduction in symptom severity. Some will have marked improvement beyond these figures, although this is rare, and a small minority of patients will be entirely refractory to all forms of treatment currently available. Full results from antipsychotic therapy take considerable time (although initial effects on some positive symptoms can be seen in a few days). Whereas the effect of benzodiazepines on anxiety and sleep can be measured in hours, and that of antidepressants in weeks, the full impact of antipsychotic therapy is measured in months. A study by Robinson et al. (1999) showed that only 20% of patients responded after 4 weeks of treatment with conventional antipsychotics, whereas after 26 weeks the number of responders had grown to about 70%. Similar results were reported with clozapine treatment, where a response was observed in 40% of subjects after 4 weeks and in 60% of subjects by week 17 (Kane et al., 2001). Clinical observations clearly show that improvement in schizophrenia is not synchronous along the main symptom clusters. Typically, antipsychotic medication therapy will result in noticeable improvement in positive symptoms (e.g., hallucinations and delusions) within a few days of initiating treatment, whereas negative symptoms (e.g., social withdrawal and affective flattening) will lag behind for weeks or months. Similarly, mood and cognitive symptoms will take longer to improve than positive symptoms. It is critical to keep this asynchronic pattern of response in mind to avoid premature judgments about the efficacy of a particular antipsychotic medication.

The time necessary for remission appears to be a function, among other factors, of the episode number being treated. It has been demonstrated that the average patient being treated for a first acute episode of schizophrenia reaches remission of symptoms in about 4–6 weeks, whereas the same average patient, now in the third episode, will take 4 months to reach the same benefit level.

The duration of treatment is also a function of episode number. Experts recommend at least 1 year of treatment for the first episode (and many find this approach rather unrealistic), 5 years after a second episode, and lifetime after three episodes. And when treatment adherence figures are factored in, it has been suggested that if one could double the rate of adherence to neuroleptic maintenance programs, the relapse rate could be cut in half (Kissling, 1991).

Given the relatively modest results currently seen with antipsychotic therapy, clinicians are often searching for medication combinations or dose increases in order to maximize benefits. Mostly, this is done on a fully empirical basis and, in some cases, with little published evidence to justify these approaches. In general, the following techniques are used:

- Monotherapy—replacing one antipsychotic with a different antipsychotic (either conventional or atypical).
- Increasing the dose beyond that supported by placebo-controlled studies.
- Polypharmacy—adding a second antipsychotic (conventional or atypical) to the first antipsychotic.
- Augmentation—adding a non-antipsychotic medication to an antipsychotic.

The rationale and evidence for the use of these strategies are not very well substantiated. Generally there is more evidence to support the use of monotherapy and augmentation and less for higher doses and **polypharmacy.**

The management of schizophrenia poses unique challenges, depending on the stage of the illness being treated. In an emergency room, where one may find psychotic patients with aggressive, hostile, and violent behavior, immediate symptom control is essential. During outpatient follow-up care, where the most severe symptoms are essentially controlled, adherence to treatment becomes a major issue, and simplicity of dosing and the ability to confirm compliance are preferable. In the interest of addressing the latter, pharmaceutical companies have developed different modes of administration for some of their products (Table 5.16).

Such is the current status of antipsychotic medication: probably minor efficacy improvements (the debate still goes on), substantial reduction of medication-induced involuntary movements, and increased risk of metabolic syndrome. It would seem plausible to speculate that, with the current advances in molecular biology, genetics, and genomics, a substantially better understanding of schizophrenia and other psychoses is perhaps not more than a decade or two away. Once the pathological processes leading to the clinical manifestations are elucidated, more specific treatments may then be possible. Given the protean nature of schizophrenia, it is likely that many different neural circuits are involved in multiple permutations, essentially moving us beyond the concept of one disorder with a few subtypes to the discovery of multiple conditions that will probably require medications or other interventions with more than just one mechanism of action, including interventions aimed at modifying genetic function.

TABLE 5.16. Routes of Administration for Antipsychotic Medications

Route	Examples	Comments
Intramuscular injection[a]	Haloperidol, ziprasidone, olanzapine	Maximum blood levels achieved in a short period of time
Dissolvable tablets	Olanzapine, risperidone, aripiprazole	Quicker absorption, provides alternative to injection
Liquid concentrate	Haloperidol, risperidone	Same as above
Tablets or capsules	All	Standard route
Injectable depot	Fluphenazine, haloperidol, risperidone, paliperidone	Slow release; allows for dosing every 2–4 weeks

[a]Intravenous route, which delivers quasi-instantaneous blood levels, is sometimes used. This constitutes an off-label use.

CHAPTER 6

Cognitive Disorders

An advertisement shows a picture of an elderly woman and a very lovely child of about 6 years of age, and it reads: "70 years ago she learned to tie her shoes . . . yesterday she forgot how." The pain of dementia is shared by millions of families.

When evaluating a new patient, all therapists must be aware of the disorders that often present with cognitive impairment or behavioral symptoms as their first sign of illness. A person may consult a therapist about relationship problems, stress at work, depression symptoms, or impulse control problems, and all of these could be symptoms of a dementing process at the early—and most treatable—stages. It is critical that therapists consider the differential diagnosis of cognitive impairment when deciding on a course of therapy and whether or not to recommend a medical evaluation specifically targeted to these symptoms.

DEFINITION OF DEMENTIA

Before focusing on dementia, let us consider what dementia is *not*. Dementia is not *amnestic disorder*, in which there is impairment of memory but other functions are quite intact. Amnestic disorders may be due to general medical conditions (e.g., head trauma and cerebrovascular problems); they may be substance induced (by alcohol or other depressants); and they may be related to dissociative disorders, but the only symptom is the memory disorder and the patients do not have any other features of dementia.

Dementia is also not *delirium,* which is a disorder of consciousness, a disorder of perception, and an inability to keep one's attention on a given task. Delirium develops quickly, over minutes or hours, and it fluctuates over the course of minutes, hours, or days. There may be slurred speech, language disturbance, or no speech at all. A person with delirium may have memory impairment as one symptom, but it is the difficulty in maintaining attention that is the hallmark symptom. The person may become incoherent, see an electric cord on the floor and perceive it to be a snake, or see spots on a sheet or bedspread and perceive them to be insects; the person may be irritable and agitated in the night and hypoactive and apathetic in the daytime. Delirium is due to some physical cause, and time is critical in finding that cause and remedying it. Often the cause is the primary medical condition of the patient, such as head injury, insufficient oxygen delivery to the brain, heart failure, respiratory failure, kidney disease, liver disease, brain tumors, infections such as pneumonia, urinary tract infection, dehydration, and many other medical conditions. Delirium may also be due to the side effects of medications. This is such a common and readily treatable cause of delirium that the first question a physician asks when meeting a patient with delirium is this: "What are *we* giving to, or doing to, this person to cause this delirium?" If a therapist feels that the patient may have a delirium, the person must be sent for medical evaluation for the specific symptoms of delirium that day, often in the emergency department of a hospital, since failure to treat the underlying cause may result in death. It is also important to recognize that delirium and dementia may coexist. If a patient who has dementia suffers an acute worsening of function, then a delirium may have developed in addition to the dementia, and the underlying cause may represent a potentially life-threatening emergency.

Dementia is also not the mild decline in cognitive ability that is a normal process of aging, sometimes called age-related cognitive decline or benign senescent forgetfulness. People with age-related cognitive decline may have some trouble remembering names or may misplace objects, but they fully compensate by using notes, calendars, and other prompts. They take the small memory challenges in stride, and there is minimal or no impact on life functioning. Sometimes patients and their families worry about whether the mild symptoms that they observe are the precursor to dementia. Studies of those who suffer mild cognitive impairment (MCI), which is more significant than age-related cognitive decline, have shown that many of those with MCI, especially those who have significant impairment in executive function, will develop dementia (Petersen et al., 2001). Executive function refers to the ability to plan and think abstractly, to do things that require sequencing, such as gathering clothes for the laundry, starting the appropriate cycle on a washing machine, adding the soap, moving the clothes to the dryer, and removing and hanging them in the right closet. This is a simple task, yet it requires one to follow a sequence of planned actions. Other examples of executive functioning include making financial and other life decisions. Mild memory symptoms without difficulties in executive functioning may be just benign forgetfulness, but mild memory symptoms with significant disturbance in executive functioning could mean that the patient has MCI and may be a candidate for screening for dementia, with a particular focus on finding treatable, reversible causes.

TYPES OF DEMENTIAS

Dementia is an illness characterized by memory impairment, plus at least one additional cognitive deficit, which might include *aphasia* (a defect or loss of the power of communication by, or comprehension of, speech, writing, and signs), *apraxia* (inability to perform purposeful movements or to use objects correctly), *agnosia* (inability to recognize the nature of sensory input; e.g., not being able to tell the difference between a coin and a key placed in one's hand without looking is tactile agnosia), or a disturbance in *executive functioning* (described above). The cognitive deficits must be severe enough to cause problems in occupational or social functioning, and they must represent a decline in function from the patient's previous level. The impairment must not occur exclusively during a delirium (American Psychiatric Association, 2000). Dementia is a clinical diagnosis, and there is no definitive test or screening procedure. In clinical practice, the Folstein Mini-Mental State Examination (MMSE; Table 6.1) is often used as a screening tool for dementia.

The MMSE has been widely used and standardized, but it does have some limitations. A person who has had limited education may not do well, and a person who is very bright and well educated may have suffered a great deal of cognitive impairment and yet still score well; moreover, the MMSE is culture-bound. For example, when an elderly woman was asked what date it was, she answered, "Early in the season when the

TABLE 6.1. The Mini-Mental State Examination

	Points
Orientation	
• "Name the season, day, date, month, year."	5 (1 for each correct)
• "Name our location (what building are we in, what floor of the building, what town, what state, what country?)."	5 (1 for each correct)
Registration of information	
• Identify three objects by name and ask the patient to repeat them immediately (e.g., cat, book, door).	3 (1 for each correct)
Attention and calculation	
• Serial 7s (subtract 7 from 100, then 7 from that) or spell "world" backward (D-L-R-O-W).	5 (1 for each correct)
Recall	
• "Tell me the three objects I named earlier."	3 (1 for each correct)
Language	
• "What is this?" (point to pencil, then watch).	2 (1 for each correct)
• "Repeat this phrase: 'No ifs, ands, or buts.' "	1
• "Do this exactly as I tell you: Take this paper, fold it in half, and place it on the table."	3 (1 for each step)
• "Do what I have written on this paper" (write CLOSE YOUR EYES on the paper and show it to the patient).	1
• Tell the patient to write a sentence on a paper (it does not matter what it says, but it must have at least a subject and a verb and make sense).	1
• Draw intersecting pentagons on a paper, and ask the patient to copy the drawing.	1
Total score	30

Note. Data from Folstein, Folstein, and McHugh (1975).

thunder sleeps." This was completely appropriate in her Navajo culture for a date in the middle of October. Many clinicians track serial MMSE scores, although some studies suggest that this is not a reliable tool for tracking dementia (Clark et al., 1999). The diagnosis and tracking of dementia is a clinical skill. There are many different types of dementia, sorted by differences that are known in their cause and/or in their symptomatic presentation.

CASE: COGNITIVE DISORDER

Case Description

The M family (Hector, 9-year-old son; Sara, mother; Maria, aunt/sister) arrives for counseling services at an urban free clinic with the following concerns: Maria states that Sara has significant problems with memory and is hitting Hector for no apparent reason. For example, when Hector tried to take a piece of food from the table, she immediately reacted by slapping him in the face. Maria also reports that Sara has pulled Hector's hair when he sought food or water. Maria states that Sara's behavior has been a concern for several months, following an incident of domestic violence involving her ex-husband, which resulted in a 2-week hospitalization for head injury and a coma. Prior to this incident, Sara had been hospitalized for overdosing on pills and alcohol. Sara states that she is here to apply for a job and does not think there is anything wrong with her or her family.

Beginning Collaboration

Because of Sara's previous cognitive impairment and violent behavior toward her son, the therapist refers her to a physician at the free clinic for immediate attention. The therapist also reports the suspected child abuse to Child Protective Services (CPS).

A family physician/psychiatrist concludes that Sara has a history of hypoxic brain injury with consequent significant cognitive impairment, inability to perform activities of daily living, and impulse control problems (disinhibition because of her frontal lobe injury) in her role as a parent. Sara is given trazodone for her impulse-control problems. The therapist continues to work with Maria, Hector, and Sara to develop coping strategies for the family of this brain-injured woman.

Questions for Consideration

• *What are some of the legal issues inherent in this case? How can the collaborative team deal with them?* There are two key legal issues in this case—child protection and confidentiality. The therapist, Dr. E, addressed the first key issue by immediately reporting the situation to CPS. He set the tone for this referral by talking to the sisters about the need for outside support and help since Sara was a single mother with no health insurance. He framed the call to CPS as a call for help and resources and told CPS about this framing.

Dr. E also had both Sara and Maria sign releases so that he could talk with either of them at any time about clinical concerns. He did this to ensure that if he ever saw Sara alone and found out about dangerous or high-risk behaviors, he could immediately get Maria involved. At the same time, he talked to Maria about using the clinic and the team as a resource to help Sara be the best parent possible for Hector. Dr. E made sure that he reviewed these issues with the psychiatrist and that they planned together the ways in which they would help this family.

• *The therapist doesn't know much about hypoxic brain injury. How can collaboration help him address his concerns about his unfamiliarity with the diagnosis?* Dr. E has never treated someone with hypoxic brain injury. While he feels confident in his abilities to help set boundaries, establish a safety net for Hector, and encourage frequent communication between the clinic and the family, he is unsure about the course and prognosis of Sara's illness. He meets with the psychiatrist to learn some basic information. The psychiatrist is pleased to tell him what he knows and even has a few articles on brain injury for Dr. E to read. Together, they decide to do a quick literature review and share their findings with each other.

Dementias That Are Reversible or Partially Reversible

There is no blood test or X-ray to diagnose Alzheimer's-type dementia per se, but there are tests for causes of dementia syndromes that may at first look like Alzheimer's disease, and often those causes are treatable.

A 47-year-old woman came to the therapist's office, stating that she felt depressed, and she attributed this to her excessive work schedule. The therapist, who elicited a history of fatigue, difficulty concentrating, and sleep problems, as well as a subjective sense of depression, referred her patient to a physician for a medication evaluation, with a presumptive diagnosis of major depression. On the first visit with the physician, the patient gave the same history as she gave to the therapist, but the physician noted that the patient had no prior history of depression and that most of her distress was related to her "memory problems." The patient owned her own business, and she prided herself in getting the orders filled for her customers "just exactly right—the right goods delivered to the right customer on the right day at the right time." But in recent weeks, she found herself making lots of mistakes, delivering goods to customers on the wrong day or delivering the wrong goods to a customer on the right day, and she was distraught: "I just can't think straight anymore!" The patient also complained of fatigue, crying about her deteriorating business, and feeling very grim about her future. An MMSE (Table 6.1) was administered to the patient, and she scored 29 out of 30 points, missing the date by a few days. (She was very bright and well educated.) Mild cognitive impairment was suspected, and laboratory tests were ordered. This patient had no measurable vitamin B$_{12}$ in her blood, and she did not have anemia, which is sometimes used as a screening test for vitamin B$_{12}$ deficiency. (In our vitamin-taking society, many vitamins contain folate, which will prevent the anemia of B$_{12}$ deficiency, but it will not prevent the neurological damage.) This patient had an excellent diet; she did not become deficient in vitamin B$_{12}$ because of lack of intake, and vitamin supplements would not have helped her. She and others like her become deficient because of lack of absorption of vitamin B$_{12}$ from her food. Lifelong injections of vitamin B$_{12}$ restored her memory, resolved her "depression," and restored health to both the patient and her business.

This clinical case involves cognitive impairment and mood changes due to vitamin B$_{12}$ deficiency, sometimes called pernicious anemia. This is one of many illnesses that must be considered and tested for when a patient presents with cognitive symptoms. Other causes of cognitive impairment that are treatable are found in Table 6.2. It is critical that patients be examined and tested for these conditions as soon as symptoms are identified since the passage of time may lessen the probability of cure or improvement in function.

The Degenerative Dementias

The most common types of degenerative dementias are listed in Table 6.3. Although Alzheimer's disease is the presumed diagnosis for the majority of patients who suffer from dementia, it is important for the therapist to be familiar with the clinical features of other types because some of those discerning features are behavioral in nature. In the early stages of Alzheimer's disease, the symptoms may be subtle and attributed to forgetfulness. Alzheimer's disease is progressive, and as the symptoms become more severe, they interfere with daily activities. Language skills deteriorate, as does comprehension and ability to perform the basic tasks of living and self-care. Hallucinations and delusions often

TABLE 6.2. Causes of Dementias That Are Reversible or Treatable

Disorder	Management
Vitamin deficiencies, including B_{12}, nicotinic acid, thiamine	Therapeutic dose replacement
Endocrine disorders • Hypothyroidism • Parathyroid disorders • Adrenal disorders	Therapeutic dose replacement or adjustment
Infectious disorders • Chronic meningitis • Tuberculosis, fungal, parasitic • HIV disease • Tertiary syphilis • Slow virus (Creutzfeldt–Jakob disease)	Treatment of infection
Disorders with space-occupying effect • Primary brain tumor • Metastatic brain tumor • Subdural hematoma (posttrauma) • Normal-pressure hydrocephalus	Neurosurgical management
Toxic disorders • Drug, narcotic, heavy metals • Organic toxins • Medications (prescription) • Alcohol consumption • Dialysis dementia (aluminum)	Removal of offending toxin
Vascular dementia • Multi-infarct • Diffuse white matter disease (Binswanger's dementia)	Control of blood pressure
Miscellaneous • Vasculitis/inflammatory • Sarcoidosis/porphyria • Dementia pugilistica (recurrent head trauma) • Parkinson's disease/Huntington's disease • "Pseudodementia of depression"	Diagnosis and treatment varies

TABLE 6.3. Types and Features of the Most Common Dementias

Type	Selected features
Alzheimer's disease	Most common type; first symptoms often memory problems and word-finding difficulty, but behavior is socially correct in early stages. Progressive, with survival time 5–10 years after definitive symptoms. Diagnosis is presumptive in a living person and can only be certain at autopsy, with the finding of senile plaques, neurofibrillary tangles, gliosis, and amyloid angiopathy seen in neurons.
Pick's disease	Difficult to distinguish clinically from Alzheimer's disease at times; slowly progressive dementia; hyperoral behavior; disinhibition; irritability; persistent aimless wandering; memory loss; language difficulties; frontal lobe atrophy seen on brain imaging; diagnosed at autopsy by "Pick bodies" in neurons.
Frontotemporal dementia	Approximately 10% of dementias. Initial complaint is often personality changes. Disinhibition; withdrawal; apathy; hyperoral behavior (including weight gain); compulsions; memory problems; speech and language difficulty. Familial cases have approximately 40% autosomal dominant inheritance and may develop signs of Parkinson's disease.
Lewy body disease	Difficult to clinically distinguish from Alzheimer's disease at times and may coexist with Alzheimer's disease; frequent fluctuations in cognition and behavior (can look like delirium but persists); tremor and rigidity similar to Parkinson's disease; repeated unexplained falls; unusual sensitivity to neuroleptic medications (more side effects). Lewy bodies are found in neurons at autopsy.
Vascular dementia	Brain imaging (CT or MRI) reveals brain lesions, examination reveals neurological signs, usually there is a long history of hypertension

develop, sleeping patterns deteriorate, and agitation puts tremendous stress on caregivers. At end-stage Alzheimer's disease, the patient is often bed-ridden, not eating or drinking, incontinent of stool and bladder, not recognizing family members, and showing primitive movements like sucking and snout reflex. Some patients have a continuously downhill course over 5–10 years, and others have plateau periods between times of deterioration, but the typical time course is similar. When there is an exacerbation in Alzheimer's disease symptoms, the patient should be examined to be sure that he or she has not developed an infection or other illness that is causing the acute change.

EPIDEMIOLOGY, COSTS AND RISK FACTORS

Alois Alzheimer first described Alzheimer's disease in Germany in 1907. There are approximately 3–4 million people in the United States with Alzheimer's disease, about 10% of all those over 70 years of age. The health care cost of treatment is more than $80 billion per year, and the cost of caring for one patient with Alzheimer's disease is more than $50,000 per year when the disease is advanced. Alzheimer's disease is one of the most common reasons that a person is placed in a nursing home. Several genetic factors have been tied to Alzheimer's disease and other dementias, but very often there seems to be no family history, and the cause of Alzheimer's disease is unknown at this time.

BIOLOGY AND BIOCHEMISTRY OF COGNITIVE DISORDERS

A great deal of research is in progress to learn the cause of Alzheimer's disease and to understand its disease mechanisms and molecular biology. A full review of these exciting studies is beyond the scope of this book, but a few indicate the kinds of findings that may become clinically important in the future: Luukinen, Viramo, Koski, Laippala, and Kivela (1999) found that major head injuries caused in falls of those over 70 years of age were associated with increased risk of cognitive decline. And Petersen et al. (2001) found that mild cognitive impairment was associated with increased risk of developing dementia. These studies, along with the genetic and molecular biology studies, are only a sampling of the work in progress to understand, diagnose, and prevent Alzheimer's disease. Some research focuses on the acetylcholine (ACH) receptors and the amount of ACH present in brain synapses because the cognitive deficits of Alzheimer's disease have been associated with a decrease of ACH activity in the brain, and some of the medications that are helpful for patients with Alzheimer's disease work in that area.

TREATMENT PLAN FOR ALZHEIMER'S DISEASE

Medication Treatment

There is no cure for Alzheimer's disease. Historically, management has been aimed at enabling the patient to have the best life function for as long as possible, minimizing the distressing symptoms for the patient and family, and supporting family members and other caregivers through this very stressful time. In recent years, several medications have been developed that slow the progression of Alzheimer's disease, working best when they are started early. The comparative features of the most commonly used medications for cognitive impairment and dementia are listed in Table 6.4. None of them represents a cure; all of them are expensive; and when they are stopped, the patient is in about the same stage of disease as controls who did not take medication. Nevertheless, any medication that can slow the progress of disease somewhat, and allow a person to remain in his or her own home longer because the symptoms are manageable, is definitely worth trying. The savings from avoiding a nursing home may more than compensate for the expense of the medication in many cases.

A new class of medication, N-methyl-D-aspartate (NMDA)-receptor **antagonist** called memantine, was approved by the U.S. FDA and released in early 2004 under the brand name Namenda. It has been approved for the treatment of moderate to severe Alzheimer's disease and has been used in Germany for over 20 years. Clinical studies in the United States have shown modest effectiveness, with the main benefit being delayed deterioration of basic functions, such as the ability to go to the bathroom independently, feed oneself in a less messy fashion, be less easily distracted, and perhaps have less agitation. There is no evidence that it has any effect in the early stages of Alzheimer's disease or that it alters the ultimate course. Although these are modest benefits, they may allow a person to remain at home with family care and delay nursing-home placement for some period of time (Abramowicz, 2003).

Medications commonly used for the treatment of several target symptoms often seen in Alzheimer's disease are listed in Table 6.5. The goal for the use of each medication is to assist the family and the patient by making the patient as comfortable and functional as possible, for as long as possible, with minimal side effects.

Side Effects

The most common side effects of the Alzheimer's disease drugs are listed with each drug in Table 6.4. The most common side effects of the other drugs are listed when they are discussed in detail (e.g., the SSRIs). The point here is that any drug can cause anything, and the therapist can encourage the patient and family to tolerate minor reactions and talk to their physician about the important side effects. A comprehensive list is beyond the scope of this text.

TABLE 6.4. Comparison of the Medications Most Commonly Used for Dementia in the United States

Tacrine (Cognex)

- The first medication demonstrated to have any effectiveness in slowing the progression of moderate Alzheimer's disease.
- 30–40% of patients who completed the drug trials showed modest improvement, compared to 10% of those receiving a placebo.
- Response is dose related (as is hepatocellular injury), and both response and increased liver function tests (LFTs) resolve with stopping the drug.
- Less commonly used now that several other medications are available that have fewer side effects.
- Side effects
  - 30% develop three times the upper limit of normal LFTs, and 5–10% must stop the drug because of increases of 10 times or more—this resolves with stopping the drug.
  - More common in women.
  - Tend to occur at about 6–8 weeks of treatment.
  - Spectrum of cholinergic side effects: nausea, vomiting, bradycardia, increased stomach acid.

Donepezil (Aricept)

- Improvement in cognitive function or no change (as compared to decline in controls) is seen in 80% of patients with Alzheimer's disease: improvement in 35–60%, stabilization in 20–45%.
- Benefits seen in up to 2 years of treatment.
- Return to controls 3–6 weeks after stopping the drug.
- Well tolerated, with no increased LFTs.
- Dosing/side effects
  - 5 mg/day to start: increase to 10 mg/day after 1 week, as tolerated.
  - Dose-related side effects: nausea, insomnia, diarrhea.
  - Incidence of treatment-emergent adverse events (68–78%) with both dosages was similar to incidence in group receiving a placebo (69%).

Rivastigmine (Exelon)

- Improvement in 25–30% of patients at 6–12 mg/day.
- Improvement maintained for about 40 weeks before declining.
- No liver toxicity.
- Fewer adverse drug interactions (not metabolized by CYP450).
- Dosing/side effects
  - 1.5 mg twice a day, which can be increased to 3, 4, 5, and up to 6 mg twice a day.
  - Should be taken with food.
  - Approximately 20% of patients were unable to tolerate because of side effects; most common were gastrointestinal in nature: nausea, vomiting, diarrhea, abdominal pain, loss of appetite.

Galantamine (Razadyne)

- Superior to placebo at 16–32 mg/day.
- Improvement was sustained 6 months in some studies, 24 months in others.

(continued)

TABLE 6.4. *(continued)*

Galantamine (Razadyne) *(continued)*

- Liver metabolized by CYP2D6 and3A4, and high plasma levels may develop in the 7% of the population who lack CPY2D6 enzymes.
- Adverse drug interactions may occur if concurrent medications also metabolized by CYP2D6 and 3A4.
- Dosing/side effects
  - Start with 4 mg, twice a day; increased after 4 weeks to maintenance dose of 8 mg, twice a day.
  - Should be taken with food.
  - Avoid if liver or kidney impairment.
  - Most common side effects are nausea, vomiting, diarrhea, loss of appetite, weight loss, dizziness. Very slow heart rate may occur.

Memantine (Namenda)

- Approved for use in the United States in early 2004; used in Germany for more than 20 years.
- Main benefit is delayed deterioration of basic functions, such as self-feeding, toileting, decreased agitation.
- Only drug available that may work at more advanced stages of Alzheimer's disease.
- Dosing/side effects
  - Start with 5 mg/day; increase by 5 mg/day at weekly intervals to a maximum of 20 mg/day. Divide total daily amount into two doses per day when over 5 mg/day.
  - Most common side effects are headache, constipation, elevated blood pressure, confusion, and fatigue.

Note. All of these medications are used for the target symptom of cognitive impairment. Most are cholinesterase inhibitors, which result in an increase in ACH in the brain, and they are indicated for treatment of mild to moderate Alzheimer's disease.
Data from Abramowicz (2000, 2001, 2003).

The Therapist's Role in Treatment

A patient may come to a therapist with many complaints that are early symptoms of Alzheimer's disease or other types of cognitive impairment, and the therapist's first responsibility is to recognize the importance of prompt medical evaluation and treatment. The therapist may also be assisting a patient with mild cognitive impairment and depression, a common co-occurrence. Because medications are likely to be indicated for major depression in Alzheimer's disease, the patient may benefit from the therapist's assistance in learning to cope with mild symptoms. Most likely, the therapist will work with the family members and care-givers of those who suffer from Alzheimer's disease and other dementias.

TABLE 6.5. Medications Used for Specific Target Symptoms in Alzheimer's Disease

Psychosis and agitation

- Assess why now—new medical problem, change in environment, depression, constipation—try all nondrug approaches first.
- When drugs are used, "start low–go slow" on the dose, and reevaluate need often.
- Antipsychotics, such as risperidone, haloperidol (0.5–2.0 mg/day), olanzapine.
- Non-FDA approved but commonly used: trazodone, buspirone, SSRIs.
- Anticonvulsants in treatment-resistant cases (carbamazepine, valproate).
- Avoid high-potency drugs (e.g., haloperidol) in Lewy body disease.

Benzodiazepines/sedation

- Save them for special needs (dental procedures, CT scans, etc.).
- Regular use results in habituation and ineffectiveness as a sedative; risks disinhibition and worsening cognitive impairment.
- Use only drugs with no active metabolites (lorazepam, oxazepam).
- Do not use flurazepam (too long a half-life) or triazolam (worsening dementia).

Depression

- First choice, SSRIs
  - Sertraline 25 mg/day to start (150 mg maximum)
  - Paroxetine 5–10 mg/day to start (40 mg maximum)
- Nortriptyline; low doses (often 10–50 mg/day) with drug level monitoring.
- Absolutely avoid amitriptyline.

Insomnia

- Sleep hygiene comes first—treat underlying problem (depression, agitation, etc.).
- Avoid benzodiazepines and others that exacerbate sleep apnea and cause rebound insomnia and worsening cognition.
- Avoid diphenhydramine (anticholinergic).
- Avoid amitriptyline (number one cause of anticholinergic delirium in the elderly).
- Trazodone 25–100 mg as needed for sleep.
- Zolpidem 5–10 mg nightly sleep.

Note. None of these medications have FDA indication for the treatment of Alzheimer's disease. The literature and practice guidelines support the use of these medications for specific target symptoms. The FDA has issued a "black box" warning regarding the use of certain antipsychotic medications in the elderly, especially haloperidol, olanzapine, and risperidone. The warning notes that the use of these drugs is associated with an increase in death rates when used by the elderly patients with dementia.

There are no FDA-approved drugs for the treatment of these symptoms in persons with dementia. All antipsychotics, when used in patients with dementia, carry a small but measurable increased risk of death.

Assisting Families and Caregivers

When a patient and family have learned that the diagnosis is presumptive or probably Alzheimer's disease, there is often widespread dismay, and all the stages of grief may be expressed at one time or another. Because they need a little time to process this dismaying news, the family may have difficulty planning such necessary items as wills, trusts, durable power of attorney for health care, and the patient's wishes for end-of-life care. The therapist should encourage early planning of these matters because once the patient's dementia has progressed to the point that he or she is not considered legally competent, the patient can no longer have input into these critical decisions. The therapist can also help the family by mentioning the need to attend to matters of safety, such as driving and wandering, as well as the patient's type of residence. If a move to a different residence will be needed eventually, it is best to help the patient to settle into the new living situation early in the course of the disease to maintain stability as long as possible. Moves at a later stage in illness will be poorly tolerated. The therapist can be of tremendous help to the family in setting realistic goals and plans and supporting the family through what might be a guilt-provoking time when it becomes necessary to transfer the patient to a nursing facility.

The therapist can also help the family by advising them of educational sources and available support groups, such as the local chapter of the Alzheimer's Disease Association, social service and home health agencies, assistance with home behavioral management, Meals-on-Wheels, transportation and recreational programs, and respite care.

Depression is very common among caregivers of patients with Alzheimer's disease. With the typical course of illness being 10 years—beginning with gradual onset, then progressive memory loss, cognitive decline, and on average, institutionalization for the last 3 years of life—caregivers are vulnerable to mental illness exacerbations (or illness *de novo*) because of the hard work of care. Prevention of caregiver burnout treats two patients and benefits the extended family indirectly. The therapist should be vigilant for signs that the caregivers are overwhelmed because then the patient will be institutionalized. The most common symptoms that acutely precipitate institutionalization of patients with Alzheimer's disease are the following:

- Insomnia, night-time wandering
- Incontinence of urine, feces, or both
- Agitation, aggressive behavior

Many excellent resources teach caregivers how to best assist their family member with Alzheimer's disease. A special report, prepared by Kahn et al. (1998), provides the answers to many critical questions:

- An understanding of the causes of agitation in dementia
- Treatment options for agitation
- Tips on providing the right environment for the patient
- How to supervise activities of the patient
- Tips on how to talk with a person who has dementia
- Getting support and improving coping skills
- A primer on medications used in Alzheimer's disease
- A comprehensive list of resources

The therapist can help the family and caregivers find such essential and concise how-to survival guides as this special report (Kahn et al., 1998) and many other resources available through the Internet. One very helpful website, www.alzheimers.org, is that of the ADEAR (Alzheimer's Disease Education and Referral) Center, a service of the National Institute on Aging of the National Institutes of Health in the U.S. Department of Health and Human Services. The website of the Alzheimer's Disease and Related Disorders Association, Inc., www.alz.org, also provides resources and information for patients, families, and caregivers.

Alzheimer's disease and other dementias rob patients and families of what is arguably their most precious belonging—their very identity and personhood. The therapist can play a key role in helping the patient and family cope with this trying and long illness.

CHAPTER 7

Alcoholism and Substance Abuse

Alcohol has been called the "universal solvent": It dissolves stomachs, livers, brains, jobs, families, bank accounts, credit ratings, drivers' licenses, and the future hopes and dreams of those who suffer from alcoholism.

—ANONYMOUS

Substance use disorders (SUDs) are collectively the most common coexisting condition that therapists will see in their patients who present with relationship problems, depression, or anxiety disorders. SUDs are common and often unrecognized, at least in the initial evaluation of the patient and family. This chapter does not propose to be a comprehensive treatise on the management of SUDs. It focuses on some features germane to the collaboration of physicians and nonphysician therapists in treating SUDs. We discuss alcoholism first, as the most common and the prototype of the SUDs, and then touch on selected features of several other types of SUDs.

ALCOHOLISM

Definition

A person is said to suffer from the medical disorder called alcoholism if he or she continues to drink alcohol in spite of the knowledge that this continued use will lead to dire consequences in health, school, employment, relationships, or the law. That is, the person knows that alcohol use can cost him or her the loss of career, family, friends, liberty, or health, and yet the person has no control over the use of alcohol and continues to drink in spite of the consequences. It is important to note that the *amount*, and the *type* of alcohol consumed (e.g., beer, whiskey, and wine) does not enter into the definition of this disease. DSM-IV-TR (American Psychiatric Association, 2000) defines substance abuse and substance dependence as described in Table 7.1.

TABLE 7.1. DSM-IV-TR Substance Use Disorders

Substance dependence

- Maladaptive pattern of substance use, leading to significant impairment or distress, as evidenced by three or more of the following, occurring any time during the same 12-month period:
  - Tolerance.
  - Withdrawal.
  - Taking larger amounts of the substance or taking the substance over a longer period than expected.
  - Persistent desire for the substance or inability to decrease use or control use of the substance.
  - Spending a great deal of time in substance-related activities (using, obtaining, recovering from use).
  - Giving up important life activities because of the substance use.
  - Continuing in substance use in spite of the knowledge that it is causing harm to life and/or health.
- With physiological dependence: evidence of tolerance and/or withdrawal.
- Without physiological dependence: no evidence of tolerance/withdrawal.

Substance abuse

- Maladaptive pattern of substance use, leading to significant impairment or distress, as evidenced by one or more of the following, occurring any time during the same 12-month period:
  - Recurrent substance use, resulting in failure to perform major obligations at work, school, home.
  - Recurrent substance use in physically hazardous situations.
  - Recurrent legal problems related to substance use.
  - Continued substance use in spite of continued social, relationship, or interpersonal problems related to it.
- The symptoms above are not attributed to substance dependence for this class of substance.

Note. Adapted from American Psychiatric Association (2000). Copyright 2000 by the American Psychiatric Association. Adapted by permission.

Several terms warrant discussion as we talk about alcoholism and other substance use disorders:

- *Tolerance* refers to the need to consume progressively larger quantities of the substance (e.g., alcohol, benzodiazepines, or opiates) to achieve intoxication or the desired effect, or the state of needing a progressively increasing dose in order to maintain a sense of normality.
- *Withdrawal* is a syndrome of very unpleasant cognitive, psychological, and physical symptoms that occurs when the amount of the substance declines in the bloodstream. The onset of withdrawal symptoms generally brings an intense craving for the substance, and use of the substance results in resolution of the withdrawal syndrome.
- *Dependence* refers to any one or the combination of cognitive, behavioral, and physical symptoms that indicate that the individual continues to use the substance in spite of significant harm or life problems. Typically a person who has substance dependence also experiences tolerance and withdrawal, as well as compulsive use and drug-seeking behavior.
- *Abuse* is the maladaptive pattern (over at least a 12-month period) of substance use, leading to impairment or distress, but this does not include substance dependence, tolerance, or withdrawal.

When considering the issues of alcohol tolerance and withdrawal, it is useful to review what is expected for the normal person in response to various blood alcohol levels (BALs):

- At a BAL of 20–30 mg/dl, a person will have slowed motor performance and thinking ability (i.e., after one or two drinks).
- At a BAL of 30–80 mg/dl, there are increases in motor and cognitive problems (80 mg/dl is the legal intoxication limit in California).
- BALs of 80–100 mg/dl denote legal intoxication in most states.
- BALs of 80–200 mg/dl show coordination problems and judgment errors, labile mood, and deterioration in cognition.
- At BALs of 200–300 mg/dl there is nystagmus, marked slurring of speech, and blackouts.
- BALs of > 300 mg/dl may lead to respiratory arrest, impaired vital signs, and death (Schuckit, 1995).

Tolerance may occur to the point that patients can appear to be alert and talking coherently with blood alcohol levels in excess of 400 mg/dl, but these individuals are still at risk of respiratory arrest and death at that level of intoxication. Later, they will not remember what occurred during this time (they are in a blackout), and they may experience alcohol withdrawal symptoms when their BAL drops from 400 to 200, a level that is still indicative of intoxication for most people.

CASE: ALCOHOL ADDICTION AND ABUSE

Case Description

Ms. A, a 25-year-old Caucasian female, presents to her primary care physician, Dr. D, with myriad health concerns, including skin rashes, symptoms of "panic attack" (described by the patient as periods of dizziness, increased heart rate, tingling sensations and extremity numbness, shortness of breath, and feeling trapped), headache, hopelessness, and weight gain. Dr. D assesses Ms. A for depression and anxiety and refers her to an in-clinic therapist for regular individual therapy. She meets with the therapist once per week over the next 2 months and discusses her concerns about her drinking, as well as her concurrent symptoms of depression and anxiety.

Beginning Collaboration

Ms. A reports that her symptoms began after a traumatic experience— her mother's near fatal car accident, which occurred 3 years before this meeting. Ms. A is particularly concerned because she notes that she has become more and more dependent on alcohol as a way to "get through the stress," and she drinks nearly every day. She notes that her mother has been an active alcoholic for 20 years, and even though she was drunk at the time of her accident and almost died as a result of her injuries, she is still an active alcoholic and refuses to address her addiction. Ms. A has moved back home since her mother's accident in order to provide care; she notes that she inherits "addictive personality traits" from her mother, and she is becoming increasingly concerned that she is losing control over her own drinking. She claims that over the course of the last year, she has begun drinking more regularly and more heavily, to the point of intoxication on most occasions. She reports having always known she had the potential to be an alcoholic, but she fears she has truly become one recently and cannot control it on her own. Ms. A claims that she feels herself "losing ground" in battling her drinking.

Over the course of 2 months, Ms. A has an extensive medical evaluation, including evaluation by a dermatologist and a nutritionist. The evaluations conclude that she suffers from a chronic skin condition, Hidradenitis Suppurativa, and that her current state of morbid obesity threatens her general health. The therapist meets weekly with Ms. A in order to address her alcohol abuse and concurrent feelings of anxiety. It is concluded, by both the therapist and Ms. A, that a pattern exists whereby Ms. A alleviates rising stress and feelings of guilt, hopelessness, feeling trapped, etc., by drinking alcohol. Ms. A has been able to identify the emotions and feelings connected to her urge to drink. She identifies familiar feelings of rising tension, worry, and restlessness, which subside very quickly as soon as she begins to imbibe alcohol. She notes that if she tries to stop drinking at some point during this activity, her restlessness and anxiety continue to increase, as if she is afraid of what she will feel like if she does not continue the very act of drinking itself.

The therapist and Ms. A decipher a heretofore unidentified link among the past events in her life: her mother's own alcoholism; the incredible trauma of the accident, with an accompanying 3-month coma; the patient's return from college to become full-time caretaker; the patient's feelings of frustration at giving up her own life to care for her mother; and the concurrent guilt she experiences when she feels angry at her mother for affecting her life in this way, for "trapping her" with the accident, recovery, and care needs. Ms. A's drinking follows a predictable pattern: She feels resentful about being trapped; she then feels guilty yet powerless to change her situation, her anxiety levels rise, and to quell this discomfort she seeks out alcohol, whether at home or elsewhere.

The therapist continues to work collaboratively with Dr. D to address Ms. A's many health concerns: her skin disorder, her symptoms of anxiety and depression, her weight gain, and her continued alcohol abuse. Physician, therapist, and patient make explicit that connection among the various problems she experiences; her inability to identify the source of her stress and her reluctance to express that stress seem to cause her skin disorder to flare up. She seeks alcohol in order to soothe herself, and as the months pass with no improvements in her physical or emotional health, she continues to turn to drink as the only way to combat the anger and frustration she feels about many aspects of her life.

The therapist continues to work with Ms. A to identify, normalize, and express those feelings of frustration and resentment. Recognizing self-destructive patterns in connection with the drinking helps shed light on the reasons she feels she cannot control her behaviors. Seeking alternate methods of soothing stress and addressing troubling emotions is essential. Finally, the therapist recommends that the patient attend Alcoholics Anonymous (AA) meetings in order to gain the support of a group with whom she can meet regularly.

Question for Consideration

• *What role did collaboration play in Ms. F's treatment?* First, a favorable therapeutic outcome with Ms. A would have been more difficult to achieve without close collaboration. Ms. A initially presented to her physician with the physical symptoms of illness. Any emotional and mental component to her physical symptomatology would have been more difficult to identify had the patient's only contact been with her primary care physician. Successful treatment in this case required a number of lengthy, regular, "nonrushed" structured sessions with Ms. A to allow her the time and space to reflect on her past, to begin investigating and identifying possible maladaptive behavioral patterns, and to build the therapeutic trust required to finally express the intense anger and frustration underlying her physical presentation.

Second, the medical clinic where Ms. A received her medical care and attended her regular therapy sessions provided a safe haven for her. It was essential for her to find a place, physically apart from her family and home, where she could begin to express her anger and frustration, feelings that she would have felt guilty to express in front of her already-suffering mother. Without the risk of hurting her mother further, Ms. A was able to release those emotions that seemed to rest at the very heart of her physical ailments, her emotional struggles, and her alcoholic addiction. A collaborative environment—to treat both the physical and the emotional aspects of her current issues—was essential. Having the trust that the therapist and physician would work together to care for her, not let her "slip through" when she lacked the motivation and energy to continue pursuing her own care and health upkeep, aided in Ms. A's continued treatment and improvement, as she herself reported.

• *How was time an important variable in treating Ms. A? By "time" we refer to both having enough time to talk to the patient, often 30–45 minutes weekly, and the passing of weeks and even months when Ms. A felt connected to the clinic team.* Dr. D usually had 10–15 minutes set aside for his appointment with Ms. A. At most, he could schedule a 30-minute visit on rare occasions. Dr. D often felt frustrated by the lack of time he had with Ms. A because they often had only enough time to go through their mutual problem list and no time to explore anything else, including Ms. A's feelings about her family and life.

One resource the therapist, Ms. L, offered was that she could spend more time with Ms. A—45 minutes every week for several months. That time, in turn, gave them the chance to explore the connections among Ms. A's early life, her current life, her physical symptoms, and her alcohol use. Then, Ms. A's understanding of her own behavior helped her initiate changes in her alcohol intake and health-related behaviors.

Epidemiology and Risk Factors

Over 90% of adults in the United States drink alcohol, and nearly half of men and 3–10% of women develop significant alcohol-related problems at some point in their lives (Schuckit, 2001). Many drinkers of alcohol will have an occasional problem during excess drinking, and this does not mean they are alcoholics. Up to 40% of men in their late teens and early 20s have experienced at least one blackout (drinking to the point of amnesia concerning all or part of the time during which they were drinking and awake), but most of them do not go develop alcoholism (Schuckit, 2001). Only 5% of alcoholics are homeless; most alcoholics have a job, marriage, and family and are living in mainstream America. Many studies demonstrate the genetics of alcoholism. There is a fourfold increased risk for children of alcoholics to develop alcoholism themselves, even if adopted at birth and raised without knowledge of the alcoholism in their biological parents (Schuckit, 2001). A 15-year follow-up of 453 men originally studied at age 20 has shown that sons of alcoholic fathers showed a lower level of response to alcohol: they felt less intoxicated, less impaired on cognitive and psychomotor tests, and more willing to drive even though intoxicated than their peers who did not have alcoholic fathers (Schuckit, 1994, 2001; Schuckit & Smith, 1996). This low level of perception and response to intoxication at age 20, when they were alcohol-naive, was a powerful predictor of the development of alcoholism later in life. In short, they seemed genetically vulnerable in that they could not tell when "enough is enough." The genetics of alcoholism is complex, with studies suggesting loci on chromosomes 1, 2, 4, 7, and 11, but the identity of the genes involved is not known (Messing, 2001).

There are also genetic factors that are protective against alcoholism. Approximately half of Asian populations have a gene that interferes with the metabolism of alcohol, and a toxic metabolite of alcohol accumulates in their body. When they drink alcohol, **acetaldehyde** accumulates, and they experience the very unpleasant symptoms of rapid heartbeat, flushing, heat, and dropping blood pressure, and they feel intoxicated with very low levels of alcohol in their blood. These individuals rarely, if ever, abuse alcohol. All the genetic factors combined explain about 60% of the risk of alcoholism, with environmental factors contributing about 40% (Schuckit, 2003).

Approximately 20% of the patients entering a primary care medical office are alcoholic, and alcoholism is a significant factor in at least 25% of all hospitalizations. If the drug "alcohol" was just discovered today, most likely it would not be released by the FDA because it would be regarded as too toxic to bodily organs and too dangerous to release to the public. The prohibition of alcohol in the United States in the 1920s did not work, as alcohol has been around a long time and is an integral part of many cultural celebrations.

Treatment Plan

Establishing the Diagnosis

Most patients who say they are alcoholic are already in recovery. Those with an active disease most often deny that their alcohol use is causing problems in their lives, and collateral historians play an essential role in understanding alcohol's true impact. Very often, the patient will stress that he or she consumes "only a few [usually two] beers a day" and therefore could not possibly have alcoholism. That patient, and possibly the family as well, will need education and support to understand that the amount and the type of alcohol consumed do not by themselves define alcoholism. Rather, it is the impact of the alcohol on the person and the inability to stop its use that define the problem.

Alcoholism is ubiquitous and often occult. All physicians are instructed to screen for SUDs, and this is also an essential component of every mental health assessment. There are many tools to accomplish this, and one of the simplest was advocated by the American Medical Association (AMA). The AMA has suggested the CAGE questions about alcohol use as a routine screening test for every adult and adolescent. The CAGE questionnaire consists of the following four questions:

> Have you ever:
> thought about Cutting down?
> felt Annoyed when others criticize your drinking?
> felt Guilty about your drinking?
> used alcohol as an Eye opener?

Scoring is 1 point for each positive answer, and a score of 2–3 is suggestive of alcohol problems (Kinney 1989). Whether a therapist or physician uses the CAGE questions or any other questionnaire or style of inquiry, it is important to have a regular method for screening every single patient. One should ask adolescents and most adults the alcohol-screening questions when interviewing them alone, and then ask collateral historians the questions again later. Some adolescents, for example, will be more honest when asked alone; others will deny the importance of their substance use, and it will be the family's history that brings it to light.

Sometimes the patient denies alcoholism, yet there are physical signs and symptoms that make the therapist suspect it. The person who suffers from alcoholism for an extended period of time may have any of many physical findings: redness of the palms; disproportionately large abdomen ("beer belly"); elevated blood pressure; frequent trouble with the stomach (gastritis or ulcer disease); hemorrhoids; problems with recurrent abdominal pain (due to pancreatitis); male impotence (due to shrinkage of the testicles and liver dysfunction, leading to the accumulation of estrogen); liver cirrhosis, leading to bleeding problems; and heart problems. In advanced stages of alcoholism, there may be cognitive difficulties and neurologic complications, some of which may improve greatly if the person abstains from alcohol. A CT scan or MRI of the brain of an alcoholic patient may show an increase in the size of brain ventricles and sulci, although this is due to the loss of white matter in the brain, not necessarily to the loss of neurons (Jensen & Pakkenberg, 1993). This loss of white matter may help explain some of the functional impairment in chronic alcoholism. Some of these structural changes are reversible with the restoration of white matter if the patient abstains from all alcohol and replaces certain nutrients often deficient in alcoholics, such as thiamine and other B-vitamins (Jensen & Pakkenberg, 1993; Schuckit, 2001).

Alcohol Dependence and Withdrawal

A person who is addicted to alcohol may begin to show signs and symptoms of physical withdrawal within hours of abstinence. These may include tremors, insomnia, anxiety, craving for alcohol, loss of appetite, nausea, vomiting, sweating, high blood pressure, rapid heartbeat, agitation, and irritability (see Table 7.2). Withdrawal symptoms may start within hours of a decreased intake of alcohol and usually resolve within 2 or 3 days. As mentioned, a person who has very severe alcohol tolerance and dependence may start to have withdrawal symptoms even when his or her BAL is still quite elevated. During alcohol withdrawal, one or two generalized seizures may occur, usually within 24–48 hours after decreased alcohol intake, and some patients may develop a more severe withdrawal syndrome, including hallucinations, with or without delirium tremens. Those who are dependent on other central nervous system (CNS) depressants, such as benzodiazepines, meprobamate, or

TABLE 7.2. Signs and Symptoms of Physical Withdrawal from Alcohol

- Tremor
- Insomnia
- Anxiety
- Craving for alcohol
- Loss of appetite
- Nausea
- Vomiting
- Sweating
- High blood pressure
- Rapid heartbeat
- Agitation
- Irritability

barbiturates, may have a similar withdrawal syndrome. It is critical for the therapist to quickly recognize the patient with a withdrawal syndrome from alcohol or other CNS depressants in order to determine whether he or she can be managed as an outpatient (low risk and mild symptoms) or whether hospitalization will be necessary. If the withdrawal syndrome progresses to full delirium tremens (DTs), there can be up to a 15% mortality rate, even when well managed, so hospitalization is essential when there is a history or probability of DTs.

Many alcohol-dependent patients manage their withdrawal outside of the hospital when they have only mild symptoms and are in generally good health. Very often these patients will visit their primary care physician, seeking a short course of benzodiazepines (such as diazepam or chlordiazepoxide) for a few days, as well as some prescription-strength vitamins and thiamine to assist in their withdrawal and recovery. It is critical that a responsible adult monitors these patients around the clock to be sure that they are not developing confusion, unstable blood pressure, or other vital signs and to provide essential support for the detoxification process.

Treatment Approach to Alcoholism and SUDs

A comprehensive review of the therapist's role in the treatment of patients with SUDs is an entire text in itself and beyond the scope of this book. Here we consider the therapist's role as a collaborator with physicians and others in the health care system in the management of a patient with SUDs. This can generally be organized into six areas of collaboration:

1. Accurately identifying the alcoholism or SUD.
2. Empathically confronting the patient so that he or she can acknowledge the illness; this often involves a specific intervention session with the patient and family.
3. Ensuring that the patient is referred for management of the detoxification process; this may be a "social detox" or a "medical detox" program, depending on the severity of the dependence and the probability of life-threatening withdrawal.
4. Ensuring that the patient is referred for a comprehensive medical history and physical examination in order to obtain treatment for the medical and psychiatric complications of the alcoholism or other SUD.
5. Referring the patient to alcohol and substance abuse rehabilitation programs that will help him or her to:

   a. Maintain the essential motivation for abstinence.
   b. Learn to adjust to life and friends without alcohol.
   c. Prevent relapse.

   AA is one readily available resource that every recovering alcoholic should know about.
6. Providing counseling or therapy to the patient in the inpatient or outpatient setting, as appropriate, with the same long-term goals as listed in number 5. Cognitive therapy may be particularly beneficial to the recovering person, who is learning to reframe many events that have, in the past, been triggers for alcohol use and abuse.

After successful completion of an alcoholic rehabilitation program, at least 60% of middle-class alcoholics will maintain abstinence for at least 1 year, and many for a lifetime (Schuckit, 2001). There is no evidence to support the claims that any one specific recovery approach is any better than others, so it is best to keep the treatment approach simple, to ensure that it is something that the patient can do and that it is something the patient is willing to work with. There is no place for dogmatism in the treatment of SUDs since it is harmful to the patient to be forced into a treatment paradigm that may be the only one in the therapist's belief system but a poor fit for the patient. Twelve-step programs, such as AA, have a strong track record of success, and most patients should be encouraged to incorporate AA into their recovery plan. But some patients cannot work with AA, and they can do well with other approaches. The therapist must help the patient find a good fit that will maximize the probability of successful treatment, regardless of the therapist's own biases.

Medications in Alcoholism Recovery

During the acute withdrawal phase of recovery, benzodiazepines are typically used to lessen symptoms of withdrawal and decrease the likelihood of an alcohol withdrawal seizure. Beyond that acute phase, however, these medications should not be used.

Naltrexone was approved by the FDA for the treatment of alcohol dependence. This opioid-antagonist drug was proposed for the treatment of alcoholism after several small studies suggested that it is useful in decreasing alcohol craving, decreasing the probability of relapse, and shortening the time of relapse should it occur; however, experience is very limited with this drug (Schuckit, 2003). Furthermore, a larger study found no significant difference between the naltrexone-treated group and a placebo in the length of time until relapse or the length of the relapse (Krystal, Cramer, Krol, Kirk, & Rosenheck, 2001). Other reviewers of the larger study criticized it for including only patients who were veterans and who had many decades of drinking prior to treatment. The reviewers felt that naltrexone should continue to be recommended to patients who have been alcohol-dependent for less than 20 years and who have good social support and a stable living environment (Engstrom & Hauser, 2003).

The medication acamprosate has been studied in Europe, with similar results to naltrexone, but it is available in the United States only in research studies. The final medication to mention is the oldest one available for the treatment of alcoholism, disulfiram, also known by the brand name of Antabuse. Disulfiram interferes with the metabolism of alcohol, resulting in the accumulation of its first metabolite, acetaldehyde. Acetaldehyde causes very unpleasant symptoms, many of which are potentially life-threatening cardiac and neurologic consequences, including a significant risk of stroke and heart attack. Because the use of disulfiram can be dangerous for patients with heart disease, blood pressure problems, neurological problems, diabetes, and many other medical conditions, and because it has not been shown to be significantly more effective than a placebo, it is rarely used. Most physicians prescribe disulfiram only to patients who have a clear history of successful use of it in the past, and often these patients have used disulfiram successfully to get through holidays or other specific times that are high risk for relapse.

No medication is widely recommended for the treatment of alcoholism per se; each individual patient should be assessed to see if there are other physical and mental conditions that need treatment in order to maximize the probability of sustained recovery from alcoholism. In addition, all patients recovering from alcohol should receive a vitamin supplement that is rich in the B-vitamins, especially thiamine at 50–100 mg/day for the first month of recovery.

ABUSE OF OTHER SUBSTANCES

Selected Features of Other Commonly Abused Substances

Substance abuse should be suspected whenever there are inconsistencies in the person's presentation from time to time. Some of the signs and symptoms that a therapist might observe include the following:

• Patients with *opioid abuse* and dependence may have needle marks ("tracks") at the site of injections (the marks are often hidden in tattoos) and very small pupils. They may complain of chronic constipation. Patients in opiate withdrawal may experience nausea, diarrhea, coughing, teary eyes, runny nose, sweating, muscle twitching, goose bumps, elevated body temperature and blood pressure, diffuse body pain, insomnia, frequent yawning, and craving for the drug of abuse. Opiate withdrawal is very uncomfortable, and the discomfort puts the patients at a high risk of returning to abuse and dependence, but opiate withdrawal does not have the fatal potential that withdrawal from alcohol or benzodiazepines has.

• Patients who abuse *amphetamines* may present with wide mood swings, including euphoria, mood elevation, and a high sense of energy one day; another day they may be exhausted, paranoid, delusional, and psychotic. They may have rapid heart rate, elevated blood pressure, large pupils, weight loss, and complications such as stroke and heart failure or abnormal heart rhythm. Acute amphetamine intoxication can be indistinguishable from schizophrenia at times, and the urine drug screen (UDS) at the time of the psychotic presentation is essential.

• Patients who abuse *cocaine* may appear similar to those using amphetamines. Cocaine is actually an anesthetic that is used on the surface of the membranes inside of the nose, sinuses, and throat so that the surgeon can operate there. Cocaine is considered much too dangerous and toxic to use in the body as a whole, and it is limited to topical application to these small areas. It is considered so dangerous because of its effect on the heart and brain. Cocaine abusers may use it orally, sniffing it into the nose; inhale it into the lungs; and inject it intravenously, sometimes combined with heroin ("speedballing"). Patients may thus have irritation of the inside of the nose, problems with their lungs, or tracks where they injected the drug. Smoking freebase cocaine, which is very potent, leads to the onset of the euphoria in 8 to 10 seconds, but this rapid increase in drug level in the blood also increases the risk of complications, such as irregular heart rhythm, heart failure, and stroke. Often the abuser will try to modulate the effects of cocaine by drinking alcohol at the same time. The use of alcohol and cocaine together results in a compound called ethylcocaine, which has heart and stroke risks similar to cocaine alone, and the toxic consequences to heart and brain can be additive when ethylcocaine and cocaine are present together. Acute cocaine intoxication or overdose is a true medical emergency, and patients should be referred to the emergency department of a hospital. If they have also been drinking alcohol, they will probably be managed in the intensive care unit.

• Patients who use *marijuana* may have red eyes, a rapid heartbeat, and apathy and memory problems. Many daily users of marijuana develop tolerance for the rapid heartbeat, and they may also develop lung disease and chronic bronchial irritation.

• Patients who use *lysergic acid diethylamide (LSD)* will have a rapid heartbeat, large pupils, elevated blood pressure, tremors, and elevated body temperature, along with hallucinations.

• Patients who consume *phencyclidine (PCP)*, a veterinary anesthetic, will appear to be excited and agitated, have difficulty talking, and have poor motor coordination; they may have abnormal eye movements, flushing, sweating, an exaggerated sense of hearing, and changes in mental status; they may proceed to drooling, vomiting, muscle twitching, fever, delirium, and coma. Both LSD and PCP can lead to problems in the circulation of the brain, causing a stroke. Patients who are intoxicated with PCP do not have normal pain sensation, and they may be very seriously injured when they fight those who are trying to bring their dangerous behavior under control. Patients have been known to dig out an eye or scratch out a testicle while under the influence of PCP, and they do not appear to feel the pain involved in these self-inflicted injuries. There are occasional reports of those under the influence of PCP who are threatening police officers with weapons; the officers respond with nonlethal force (bean bag guns, electric shock [Taser], or even a nonlethal bullet wound), but the abusers do not stop their aggression because they do not feel the pain of these interventions. If they continue to attack, they may ultimately be killed. Those under the influence of PCP can be dangerous to manage in the hospital for the same reason; at times they must be placed under general anesthesia for many days in order to keep them and others safe while waiting for the PCP to be cleared from their systems. PCP intoxication can also cause seizures, coma, and respiratory depression, and it often requires management in the intensive care unit of the hospital.

• Patients who are addicted to *nicotine* in the form of cigarette smoking have one of the most common, most expensive, and most deadly addictions. Nicotine addiction is the most common cause of preventable death in the United States. Most smokers started in their teen years, and it is very hard for them to quit—possibly the hardest of all of the addictions. Patients with nicotine addiction are at a much increased risk of a long list of cancers, heart disease, and stroke, but they will definitely develop chronic lung disease if they do not die of one of the other risk factors first.

• Patients with *polydrug* use are so common that even if the therapist or physician is aware of one drug of abuse, there may be others that need attention in the acute management of very ill patients, and the UDS may be essential in establishing that diagnosis.

These signs and symptoms are summarized in Table 7.3.

Intervention and Management of the SUDs

Principles of management of SUDs are very similar to those for the management of alcoholism. The goal is a treatment approach that enhances the probability of abstinence from the substance, assists the patient in rebuilding a life free of substances, and works to prevent relapse. Narcotics Anonymous may be very helpful for some patients.

Detoxification of patients with opioid dependence is usually best done by stopping their drug of abuse and placing them on a long-acting opioid, such as methadone. Once the patient is stable on methadone replacement, the dose is reduced each day by 10–20% of the original day-1 dose until the methadone is stopped. State and federal regulations for the prescription of methadone must be followed. The opioid-antagonist drug, naltrexone, has had varying results in assisting the recovering opiate-dependent person to remain abstinent. When given in

TABLE 7.3. Signs and Symptoms of Substance Abuse

Drug	Signs and symptoms of use
Opioids	Needle marks, small pupils, constipation.
Amphetamines	Wide mood swings: euphoria, mood elevation, and high energy to exhaustion, paranoid, delusional, and psychotic; rapid heart rate, elevated blood pressure, large pupils, weight loss, stroke, heart failure or arrhythmia.
Cocaine	Nose irritation, lung problems, injection marks, heart failure or arrhythmia, stroke.
Marijuana	Red eyes, rapid heartbeat, apathy, memory problems, lung disease, bronchial irritation.
LSD	Rapid heartbeat, large pupils, elevated blood pressure, tremors, elevated body temperature, mental status changes.
PCP	Excited, agitated, difficulty talking, poor motor coordination, abnormal eye movements, flushing, sweating, exaggerated hearing, mental status changes, drooling, vomiting, muscle twitching, fever, delirium, coma, abnormal pain sensation.

sufficient doses and for extended periods, naltrexone blocks the "high" that opiates provide. In the general recovering population, the dropout rate has been high with naltrexone, and the results have been poor. However, it was shown to be helpful in opioid-dependent federal probationers, decreasing the likelihood that they would return to their narcotic of abuse and enhancing the probability that they would stay out of prison (Cornish et al., 1997). One could theorize that the additional motivation of the probation process and the certainty of returning to prison may have enhanced the motivation to use naltrexone and avoid opiate use in that study.

Smoking Cessation

Just as the person with alcoholism needs an intervention to demonstrate the impact of the alcohol use on his or her life, the smoker needs one or more intervention sessions in which education about the impact of smoking on his or her life is presented. Physicians will often use a visit for a sinus complaint, sore throat, or even fatigue as an opportunity to talk about the impact of smoking—for example, "Unless you quit smoking, this is the first of many, many visits you will have for bronchitis; it will become a permanent problem, and we're going to be seeing a lot of you . . . until you need the oxygen tank everyday and then you *have* to quit. . . . "

More than 90% of former smokers quit without formal intervention, and about 80% of those who quit do so cold turkey. For those who utilize the support of others, there are national quit days, 1-800-NO-BUTTS telephone support, and group therapy meetings. Nicotine gum and patches are available without prescription in the drug store; however, the best results will be achieved if the patients use them only in conjunction with a support group. If used alone, the risk is that the patients will use the nicotine replacement patch or gum and will also keep smoking, thus greatly increasing the risk they face from nicotine. For those who are motivated to stop, the nicotine replacement patches and gum can be a very helpful adjunct to their resolve. If in the course of a medical visit, a physician simply says, "You should stop smoking because of your health," that will double the spontaneous stop-smoking rate (Holbrook, 1998). We often utilize a transitional object to reinforce the message to stop smoking by telling the patient that we almost never "guarantee" anything in medicine, but we will give the patient a note written on a prescription, such as the one in Figure 7.1. Patients have taken this home and placed it on the bathroom mirror or the refrigerator as a way to repeatedly deliver the message and the feeling of the inter-

---

Margaret McCahill, MD
123 Any Street
Some Town, CA 90000

Name: Mr. John Q. Patient   **Date:** Today

Rx:
    I guarantee you emphysema and a life of gasping for breath attached to an oxygen tank. You may also get lung cancer, but you will definitely get COPD, emphysema, and heart problems, if the cancer doesn't get you first. This guarantee is only good if you continue to smoke—you could stop smoking NOW and void this guarantee. I hope you will stop smoking.

Signature: M. McCahill, MD   **Refills:**

FIGURE 7.1. Sample "prescription" for smoking cessation.

vention. They have come in weeks to years later to say they have now gotten this message and that they really intend to quit smoking.

PATIENT AND FAMILY EDUCATION

Families are often significantly affected by a family member's SUD. There are few areas in mental health care where patient and family education are as important as they are in the treatment of SUDs. The initial management and intervention described above is focused on educating the patient and family about the nature of SUDs and the need for abstinence. The process of intervention is rarely effective in a single visit, and typically the therapist must conclude the effort with a mutual agreement to keep the door open for future discussion. Referral to AA, Alanon, and Alateen may provide the patient and family with excellent information and educational materials.

As we follow patients who continue to abuse substances, it is important to present the evidence of the illness and need for treatment in a nonjudgmental way with each therapeutic opportunity. We have all heard trainees and colleagues say, and we may have ourselves said, "Why should I waste my time talking to him about alcoholism *again* today? He knows and he continues to drink anyway—why bother?" It would be a sad mistake to give up on a person with an SUD when it may be that for this patient to really hear the problem and enter recovery, he or she needs to hear about it 5,000 times, and today we are on number 2,550. This is not wasted effort; we just need to keep on working with the patient and present our intervention with each opportunity.

PREVENTION OF SUDS

Given the **genetic loading** in the development of SUDs, one might wonder what the mental health professional can do to assist individuals and families in preventing them. We cannot change genetics, but we can educate our patients about genetic influences and encourage them to use the knowledge of these disorders to make healthy choices. We can point out that most of the SUDs begin in childhood, adolescence, or young adulthood and that peer group choice plays an important role for many young people. Parents should be advised to be vigilant about the peer group their children associate with, and youths should be encouraged to "hang out" with academic teams, supervised team sports, scouts, church groups, and family groups, all of which are likely to discourage or clearly forbid substance use. Families should teach their children and adolescents about the norms and appropriateness of alcohol use. Medical personnel usually advise teens and young adults about their family history for diabetes, hypertension, and cancer, and they should also tell them about the possible consequences of any family history of SUDs. Physicians should advise adolescents and young adults that if they have a parent with alcoholism, they have a fourfold increased risk of developing it themselves, and they need to consider that fact in their own decision of whether or not to drink and how to monitor how much they drink. When we see that young man who "holds his liquor well"—that is, he seems to be able to drink more than his friends and not show it or not realize it—we should advise him that research shows that this trait may indicate that he is more vulnerable to developing alcoholism later, and he will need to be extra cautious in his relationship with alcohol. There is no pill to cure alcoholism and other SUDs, but we can help those who are the most vulnerable shape their behavior toward alcohol and other substances in a healthy manner.

CHAPTER 8

Special Populations and Situations

This chapter presents selected background information and clinical pearls that will help therapists collaborate with physicians in caring for patients who suffer from general medical conditions, sleep disorders, obesity, eating disorders, chronic pain, and impulse control disorders. Then we present a brief overview of collaborative issues in the treatment of problems of childhood, problems seen only in women, and special considerations essential to the care of seniors. Finally, we discuss some collaborative considerations about patients with personality disorders. This chapter assumes that the reader has a comprehensive knowledge of all of the clinical syndromes discussed, and it is not a discussion of the disorders themselves. An important caveat: Clinical intervention frequently includes conjoint psychoeducation alongside more traditional therapeutic models. Therapists may be required to solicit additional, external sources of information to supplement their clinical training and support the therapeutic experience of the patient. The overall focus of the chapter is on the specific aspects of the clinical issues and understanding that serve the collaborative work between the therapist and the physician—not a comprehensive treatise of any of the disorders discussed.

PATIENTS TAKING MEDICATIONS
FOR GENERAL MEDICAL CONDITIONS

The focus of our text is the collaboration between therapist and physician and the use of medication to treat psychiatric symptoms. Although we use medications to treat mental illness, it is critical for the therapist to know that the use of certain medications for general medical conditions can cause psychiatric symptoms. The therapist must take a careful history, including knowledge of all of the medications that a person takes for any reason; if it is possible that a medication is causing the mental health problem, the patient must be promptly referred to his or her physician for medication adjustment.

Every time a medication is prescribed, the physician and patient hope that only the desired effect will occur, with no side effects, and certainly not side effects that affect one's mental health. Although side effects are inevitable, they occur inconsistently, and most people get few or none. In particular, most people do not get the type of side effect that affects mental function; if they do, it is mild and transient, and the good of the medication outweighs the temporary inconvenience of the symptom. Detailed knowledge of which medication might cause what kind of psychiatric symptom is the responsibility of the prescribing physician, but we describe here several well-known examples that therapists should know. In addition, therapists may wish to use reference tables, which are published periodically. One table is published as a single issue approximately every 2 years from *The Medical Letter on Drugs and Therapeutics*. It is available online at www.medicalletter.org, where single issues may be purchased. One reference that is usually *not* very helpful for the nonphysician inquiring about side effects is the *Physicians' Desk Reference* (PDR), which is published annually. This widely distributed text contains the pharmaceutical manufacturers' list of everything imaginable that they want to say they have warned against. For example, one can open the PDR to nearly any page or any drug, and it will say that it may cause constipation, diarrhea, headache, dizziness, seizures, coma, death, and so on. The PDR does not help the nonphysician know what is truly a probable side effect for that particular medication.

Antibiotics

One of the early modern medications seen to have psychiatric side effects is the antibiotic isoniazid (also known as INH). Tuberculosis (TB) is usually thought of as a lung infection, but it can spread to any part of the body and, untreated, is often fatal. It has been a scourge on humanity since antiquity, and there were no medications to treat it until streptomycin was developed in the mid-1940s. Although successful at the time, streptomycin came with some toxicity, and because drug resistance developed, new anti-TB drugs were sought. INH was released in 1952, and it is still an important weapon against TB today, used mostly for the prevention of active TB in those who have been exposed to it. In the 1950s, many patients with TB were hospitalized in a sanatorium for many months, where they were isolated from their families and the public, and many of them became depressed. With time, those with strong immune systems contained the tubercular bacillus, became free of symptoms, and were discharged from the sanatorium. In the TB sanatoria, streptomycin, INH, and other early medications were used to speed the recovery from TB, and the staff noted that those patients who were taking INH seemed significantly less depressed than those who were not. This observation gave additional credibility to the suggestion that medications with the tricyclic structure of INH should be further developed as antidepressants. As any medication known for its antidepressant effects, INH can cause mania in those who are vulnerable to it, and it has also been reported to cause psychosis and hallucinations in rare cases. Therapists will treat patients who are taking INH, as this is commonly used today, and they should be aware of its potential to cause psychiatric symptoms.

Many other commonly used antibiotics can cause psychiatric symptoms, for example, clarithromycin (trade name, Biaxin)—which is frequently used to treat respiratory illness, ear infections, and skin infections—has been reported to cause mania in some patients. Metronidazole (trade name Flagyl), which is used to treat many types of infections—from parasites to vaginal infections and abscesses—has been reported to cause depression, agitation, confusion, hallucinations, and mania. Trimethoprim–sulfamethoxazole (trade names Bactrim and Septra)—which is used, for example, for bladder infections and sinus and ear infections—has been reported to cause delirium, psychosis, depression, and hallucinations in rare cases. The fluoroquinolone antibiotics—such as ciprofloxacin (trade name Cipro), levofloxacin (trade name Levaquin), ofloxacin (trade name Floxin), trovafloxacin (trade name Trovan), and others of this class—can cause psychiatric symptoms fairly often, including confusion, agitation, depression, insomnia, mania, paranoia, and psychosis.

Antihypertensives

Many of the medications used to treat high blood pressure can cause psychiatric symptoms, and one of the most common types are the angiotensin-converting enzyme (ACE) inhibitors. ACE inhibitors (ACEIs) are excellent antihypertensives; they are considered first-line therapy for many patients, especially those with diabetes and some with kidney disease. But ACEIs have also been reported to cause depression, anxiety, mania, hallucinations, and psychosis in some patients. Therapists will treat many, many patients who take ACEIs, and in the majority of circumstances, the drug cannot be blamed for their mental health problems. However, the therapist should consider the possibility that the ACEI may be contributing to the problem, especially if it was started about when therapy began. The thiazide diuretics are very commonly prescribed for patients with high blood pressure or heart disease, and patients have developed depression and suicidal ideation after many weeks or months of use. This is an exception to the guideline of considering whether the medication and the psychiatric symptom are linked by the onset of symptoms beginning at or about the time of the start of medication. In the case of the thiazides, the depression and suicidal ideation may come months after the start of the medication.

Benzodiazepines

The benzodiazepines are used to treat anxiety and insomnia, but they can have the unintended effects of disinhibition, rage, hostility, depression, mania, paranoia, hallucinations, nightmares, and amnesia.

Medications to Reduce Stomach Acid

The histamine-2 receptor blockers (H-2 blockers) are used to treat hyperacidity in the stomach, and the most commonly used medications are available over the counter (without prescription). The first one was cimetidine (brand name Tagamet), which is a very common cause of delirium, confusion, psychosis, and aggression in the elderly—especially at night. The other H-2 blockers, such as ranitidine (brand name Zantac) and famotidine (brand name Pepcid), can also cause these symptoms, which are quite rare with these two drugs. Cimetidine should be avoided in the elderly and those with a serious illness. The H-2 blockers can also cause depression, mania, and nightmares. Therapists will see many patients who are taking H-2 blockers, and the patients may not think to mention them because the medications are not "prescribed." Nevertheless, they can be a cause of psychiatric symptoms, and the therapist will need to ask specifically about over-the-counter, nonprescription medication use.

Drugs to Lower Lipids

Modern medical protocols now have millions of patients taking medication to lower their cholesterol and other blood lipids. Although it is not common, there have been several reports that these drugs cause depression, anxiety, delusions, and obsessions.

Anti-Acne Medication

Isotretinoin (brand name Accutane) is used to treat severe acne vulgaris, and it has been reported to cause depression, psychosis, and suicidal ideation. Therapists who treat teens and young adults should ask about medications used for any purpose, and if they take this medication for acne, they need to be referred to their physician for a change.

Miscellaneous Medications

There are many reports of steroids (used in many forms for many conditions) causing depression, mania, psychosis, anxiety, paranoia, and aggressive behavior.

Nonsteroidal anti-inflammatory medications (NSAIDs) are used for many aches and pains and are available over the counter in such forms as ibuprofen (brand names Motrin and Advil, as well as a generic form), naproxen (brand name Aleve and a generic form), and others. There have been reports of depression, anxiety, paranoia, psychosis, and confusion with these medications. Sildenafil (brand name Viagra), used for male sexual dysfunction, has been reported to cause aggression, delusions, hallucinations, mania, paranoia, and confusion in rare cases. Therapists will treat patients who are taking steroids, over-the-counter NSAIDs, and Viagra. When these patients have mental health symptoms, they need to be evaluated by their physician to see if the medication is contributing to the psychiatric symptoms.

The examples above refer to some of the most commonly used medications, and a therapist is certain to encounter many patients every day who are taking at least one of them. Reference charts list many more medications that may cause psychiatric symptoms. Therapists should take a careful history and refer patients to their physician if it seems that a medication might be causing or contributing to the mental illness.

SLEEP DISORDERS

More than one-half of adults in the United States have sleep disturbances, some of them transient and some of them persistent (Czeisler, Winkelman, & Richardson, 2001). If a person consults a physician about insomnia, it will be attributed to a psychiatric disorder approximately 85% of the time (Kroenke & Price, 1993). Although this may be an accurate conclusion for many patients, it is certainly not always correct to presume that insomnia is due to a mental disorder. The therapist can assist the patient in monitoring the degree of sleep disturbance over time, referring the patient back to the physician for additional evaluation and treatment if the insomnia does not improve as expected when mental health improves. For example, some of the more common causes of sleep disturbance that are *not* primarily due to a psychiatric disorder are listed in Table 8.1. It is especially important to obtain the sleep history from the bed partner or other appropriate family member when the patient complains of sleep symptoms because the patient will often be an unintentionally unreliable historian.

Regardless of the cause of insomnia, proper sleep hygiene is always a good initial step in its management. The therapist may often be the first to provide education to the patient and make some recommendations for lifestyle change. For example, patients should be advised to avoid all drugs of abuse, and they should limit, and preferably stop, the use of alcohol, nicotine, and caffeine. As few as three to five cups of coffee early in the day can result in insomnia in some patients, and it may take 1–2 months of abstinence from caffeine to see an improvement (Czeisler et al., 2001). Although most patients realize that coffee is a significant source of caffeine, they often do not realize that caffeine is also found in various forms of cola, chocolate, and tea. Additional sleep hygiene instructions are shown in Table 8.2.

If the therapist has educated the patient about sleep hygiene and has assessed the patient for mental disorders, which are being treated, but the sleep symptoms continue, then medications are often considered. There are over-the-counter sleep aids (including herbals), and although they are often used, many physicians feel that they are less reliable and sometimes present more risk than prescription medications, which have

TABLE 8.1. Common Causes of Sleep Disturbance That Are Not Primarily Due to a Psychiatric Disorder

- Transient situational insomnia—sleep difficulty that is acute in onset and directly related to a stressor.
- Inadequate sleep hygiene (good sleep hygiene is discussed in the text).
- Psychophysiological insomnia—may have started with transient situational insomnia but persisted after the stressor was resolved.
- Sleep apnea syndrome—a serious structural, medical problem.
- Periodic limb movement disorder—previously called nocturnal myoclonus.
- Restless legs syndrome.
- Altitude insomnia.
- Drug- or alcohol-dependent insomnia.
- Sleep disorders associated with neurological disorders.
- Sleep disorders associated with other chronic medical conditions, for example, asthma, chronic lung disease, cystic fibrosis, chronic pain, kidney and liver failure, congestive heart failure, gastroesophageal reflux, thyroid disorders, and menopause.
- Shift work sleep disorder.
- Sleep disturbance due to parasomnias, such as sleepwalking, sleep terrors, bruxism (teeth grinding), and enuresis (bedwetting). Note that family members may need to provide history about these behaviors, which are probably unknown to the patient.

TABLE 8.2. Useful Sleep Hygiene Instructions

- Have a regular schedule for retiring to bed and getting up in the morning.
- Avoid large meals or vigorous exercise for several hours before sleep.
- Do not watch television or read in bed—the bed is used only for sleep and sexual activity.
- Go to bed only when sleepy, and if unable to get to sleep in approximately 20 minutes, get up and do some very routine, boring activity. Do not read or do anything that requires intellectual activity—folding laundry is an example given by many people as a fairly nonstimulating task. Go back to bed when feeling sleepy, and if sleep does not come in another short period, get up again and repeat this sequence.
- Get up at the same time each day, even if not much sleep was obtained during the night—it is important to establish a regular schedule.
- Do not take naps during the day.
- Avoid the use of caffeine in any form (coffee, tea, chocolate, or cola).
- Avoid the use of alcohol, nicotine, and recreational drugs.

Note. Data from Pagel (1994).

been rigorously tested. If any sleep aid is used, whether it is prescription, over the counter, or herbal, it should only be used as needed for 3 or 4 consecutive days, at the most. Use beyond that time increases the probability of dependence, and it also suggests that there may be more to the insomnia than situational stress. If the patient has insomnia that persists beyond treatment of any identified mental disorder, he or she should be referred to a physician (often a primary care physician) for a medical evaluation to look for an underlying medical condition as the cause.

OBESITY

Before we discuss the classically described eating disorders (anorexia nervosa and bulimia), let us begin with a discussion of one of the most common medical conditions in the United States, and it is *not* an eating disorder—obesity. As many as 50% of adults in the United States are overweight, and this has been increasing in the last 50 years (Flier, 2001). Obesity, which is a state of excess fat tissue in the body, is best defined through the body mass index (BMI), which is equal to weight in kilograms divided by height in meters squared. A BMI of 30 or more is generally considered obesity, and a BMI of 25–30 is usually considered medically significant. The consequences of obesity are legion and include high blood pressure, arthritis (especially in weight-bearing joints), diabetes, lung disorders, gallstones, certain cancers, and premature death due to heart attack and stroke. In addition to these well-known physical consequences, obese people face prejudice in the workplace and other areas and challenges to one's self-image, as we all live in a society that generally regards thinness as the only acceptable standard for everyone. Physical consequences, prejudice, and lack of self-esteem work against the obese person, and they are enhanced by a great deal of misinformation about obesity. Therapists can help their patients by providing common-sense, accurate information in a setting of psychological support.

Much research has been done on the causes of obesity—and it is "causes" (plural) because this is a multifactorial problem. We know that if people consume more calories than they utilize in energy, they will gain weight. In fact, if they take in an average of 3,400 kilocalories (which we commonly refer to as, simply, "calories") above the amount they need, they will gain 1 pound of weight. The problem is that how many calories a person needs varies from person to person. Consider this example: two women, each 5 feet, 6 inches tall, both weigh 140 pounds, and they both have similar job activities that they do all day;

they both do only a bit of housework at night before retiring at about the same time, and neither does any other exercise. However, one of them requires many *fewer* calories than the other to do the same activities, so when she eats the same as her peer, she will gain weight. Genetics has allowed one woman to survive with scarce food, whereas the other woman will lose weight quickly when she has less to eat. If the woman who is able to tolerate less food for the same activity level "overeats" by eating the "normal" amount that her peer does, she will gain weight and find it a challenge to shed those pounds. However, her peer may be able to eat a piece of pizza and compensate easily, and she will gain no weight over the week. The genetic factors contributing to obesity are complex and not fully known, but it is believed that there is a subset of obese individuals who are predisposed to obesity and have the capacity to become obese initially without an absolute increase in caloric consumption (Flier, 2001). Obesity is due to *both* genetic and environmental (diet and exercise) factors, and not realizing this fact leads to great discouragement for many obese patients; it also leads to arrogance among the genetically thin, as well as a lack of sustained weight loss among those who have succeeded in a weight loss program (see Table 8.3).

Currently available drugs for weight loss are all aimed at reducing appetite. None of them addresses the issue of the varying utilization of energy from one person to another, and the appetite suppressants all have risks, especially to the cardiovascular system. Sometimes the risk is worthwhile because the obesity itself is causing a more life-threatening risk than the drugs, but for most patients who consult a therapist about their weight, the risk of weight loss drugs is not worth taking. The fundamental issue of how the cells of the body use energy will remain, and the patient would be better off learning how to balance diet and exer-

---

TABLE 8.3. *Just* an Apple a Day . . .

We have all heard the saying "An apple a day keeps the doctor away." However, if you are genetically vulnerable to obesity, and you eat just one apple a day (80–85 calories) more than your (lower than most people's) caloric need, you will be consuming enough extra calories in a year to gain about 9 pounds. It does not take much to gain steadily, and for those with obesity genes, that weight gain over the years stays with them. Their best strategy is to understand what is going on and to work rigorously and continuously to develop a lifestyle of vigorous diet and exercise that is much more intense than their genetically thin peers.

---

cise. In cases of extreme, morbid (life-threatening) obesity, surgical procedures are sometimes considered. Surgery such as gastric stapling and
various other approaches carry very serious risk, and patients who have
had these procedures will have serious side effects for the rest of their
lives. Psychiatric consultation is always indicated prior to any consideration of the surgical management of morbid obesity.

For the typical obese patients, therapists can help tremendously by
revealing the complex nature of obesity—the fact that it *really is true*
that they did not eat more than their peers in a day but still gained
weight, and thus the fact that they are not at fault. By the time the
patients are talking to a therapist about obesity, they have usually lis-
tened to decades of this: "If you would just control yourself and stop
eating so much, you wouldn't be fat!" Obesity is regarded as a character
weakness in our culture, and this does not help the obese patient lose
weight. In many cases, the patients did not create the problem, but they
must take charge of the solution with diet and exercise and a very long-
term view. The therapist can also help their patients understand that
drugs do not work on a long-term basis for most obese people, and the
most effective tools are a diet that leads to gradual weight loss—and sus-
tains that loss for a lifetime—and sensible, aerobic exercise. In addition,
drinking plenty of water while losing weight will help keep the blood
concentration of ketone bodies (a normal byproduct of converting fat
into energy) at a relatively low level. Preventing a high concentration of
ketone bodies in the blood by staying well hydrated may help avoid the
implementation of the fat and weight conservation measures that the
genetically obese are especially gifted with. Thus the therapist can be a
very effective educator and supporter of an obese person who is resolv-
ing to lose weight by teaching the genetic components of obesity, relieving guilt when appropriate, addressing the stigma that obese persons
face, and teaching behavioral strategies for sustained weight loss.

EATING DISORDERS

Anorexia Nervosa

With a typical onset in midadolescence, this predominantly female disorder has a lifetime prevalence of approximately 0.5% (Walsh, 2001).
Patients who suffer with anorexia nervosa fail to maintain at least 85%
of their expected weight; they have great fear of gaining weight, and they
resist any treatment that urges them to return to a goal of approximately
90% of predicted weight. The patient appears unduly thin and may have

soft, longer than normal, downy hair growth, especially on the back and the arms. The patient may have prominent-looking cheeks from enlarged salivary glands and a slow pulse, and she may report that her menstrual periods have stopped. There are many physiological signs and symptoms of anorexia nervosa that the physician will look for in a medical evaluation, but they will not be apparent in the therapist's office. One question that may raise the suspicion of anorexia nervosa is asking the unusually thin patient how she feels about her current weight. The patient who is thin because of some other illness will usually reply that she feels she is too thin; however the patient with anorexia nervosa typically responds that she feels that she is "too fat" or obese, even though she is extraordinarily thin. Patients with anorexia do not think they are too thin, even when they are dying of starvation. When anorexia nervosa is suspected, it is very important that the patient (and her family) be served by a multidisciplinary team. This is a very serious illness with a mortality rate of approximately 5% per decade of the patient's life. Patients often require inpatient treatment in order to stabilize them when they are in a life-threatening phase of the illness. No medication has been proven to be of superior efficacy for anorexia nervosa, and long-term psychotherapy for the individual and the family is indicated. This is a specialty area of both psychiatry and psychotherapy, and the therapist who will be working with anorectic patients and their families is encouraged to obtain specialty training in this area.

CASE: ANOREXIA

Case Description

Laura, a 17-year-old dancer and honors student, makes an appointment to see Dr. P because her dance teacher suggested it. Actually, Laura's mother calls to make the appointment because Laura is so reluctant to come. Laura had been diagnosed with anorexia 4 years earlier and was barely able to maintain her minimal weight. She had never had a menstrual period and currently reports numerous symptoms of starvation.

Laura is being treated for the medical aspects of anorexia by a pediatrician who has expertise in this particular eating disorder. Previously, Laura had seen at least five different therapists of various disciplines and specialties, none of whom had been able to treat her anorexia effectively. Two reasons prompted Laura to contact Dr. P. First, her dance teacher (Eren), whom she idolizes, told her she should (Dr. P had helped Eren when she was clinically depressed). Second, Eren thinks that anorexia is

an illness of the "wealthy and privileged class," and Laura feels ashamed
to have an illness of privilege when there are so many starving people in
the world.

During the initial sessions, Dr. P asks Laura about what Eren said
and suggested. In doing so, she is beginning to assess Laura's motivation
for changing her eating behaviors. Laura is ambivalent. In addition, Dr.
P spends a great deal of time asking about other parts of her life. (Dr. P
feels that she has the luxury to spend time on this inquiry because she
knows Laura's condition is being monitored by her pediatrician.) Dr. P
learns that Laura is an honors student who is applying to Harvard College. She loves modern dance and is concerned about social justice. At
Eren's suggestion, Laura had made a list of reasons of why she might
want to "give up my anorexia," and Laura decides to give this list to Dr.
P. Laura and Dr. P look at a BMI scale together, and Laura chooses a target weight gain that would move her into the (barely) normal range.

Dr. P also meets with Laura's parents, who are very concerned
about her eating disorder. They say that they are also worried about
what Laura might do if she isn't accepted into Harvard. They report
being concerned about her ritualized, private eating; the fact that she has
never menstruated; that she doesn't want to see a nutritionist; and that
she is unwilling to give up her exercise and dance routine, even for a day.

Beginning Collaboration

After several sessions (during which Laura turns 18), Laura and Dr. P
begin to establish strong rapport. At this time, Laura tells Dr. P that she
has been "cheating" when she is weighed, in both unscheduled weigh-ins
by her mother at home and at her regularly scheduled appointments at
her pediatrician's office. She does this by adding weights inside her
clothes. Laura says that she hates deceiving her parents and her physician. She forbids Dr. P from telling anyone.

Dr. P decides to go over several treatment options with Laura: setting weekly eating and weight goals; being hospitalized; seeing a nutritionist; bringing Eren into a few sessions to get her perspective; meeting
with Dr. S, a psychiatrist colleague of Dr. P; and other options. Laura
declines medication but likes the ideas of bringing Eren into therapy, setting weekly goals, and possibly seeing a nutritionist. Over the next
month, many of these treatment options take place, and Dr. P's relationship with Laura continues to grow stronger. Laura dismisses the nutritionist as naive after their first meeting but is very responsive to the therapy session with Eren and agrees on some weight gain goals. After much
prodding from Dr. P, Laura agrees to tell her parents that she has been
cheating on her weigh-ins. This leads to a dramatic family session, but

afterward Laura feels free for the first time from the guilt of deceiving her supportive, loving family.

Laura slowly begins to gain weight. She starts eating in public and even starts eating a little sugar. She tells Dr. P about an important success: She allowed her friends at school to observe her eating some sugar. Laura's family, Eren, Dr. P, and a caring English teacher at school become her cheerleaders as they watch her make tentative, small gains. However, several months into the treatment, Laura's progress stalls and she still has not had a menstrual period—the goal she had set.

Ongoing Collaboration and Outcome

Again, Dr. P brings up the idea of trying a psychotropic medication. Dr. P says, "I'm not asking you to agree to *take* medication. I'm asking you to agree to find out if it might help *us* in achieving our goals. I have a colleague that I respect a great deal. She knows a lot about eating disorders, and I'd like to get her opinion. In fact, I'll go with you to see her in her office." Reluctantly, and perhaps to please Dr. P, Laura agrees.

Dr. P calls her colleague Dr. S to talk about the referral. She chooses Dr. S because she is a woman (Laura seems more comfortable with female physicians); because she knows that Dr. S has a warm, caring style and tends to have strong relationships with her patients; and because she knows Dr. S is knowledgeable about eating disorders and doesn't prescribe medication casually. Dr. P knows that she has one chance at helping Laura connect with a psychiatrist and consider medication, so she chooses the psychiatrist carefully.

Dr. S does an outstanding job during the interview. She obtains all of the medical information she needs while keeping the tone conversational, occasionally asking for Dr. P's thoughts or observations on an issue. She acknowledges the gains Laura has made and validates the fact that she is in charge of her body. Toward the end of the session, she suggests that an antidepressant medication could help Laura achieve her goals. Laura and her parents ask several questions about how the medication works, including details about the neuroscience aspects. At the end of the session, Laura agrees to take a "trial dose" of the medication.

Although the medication effects of the next few months are not dramatic, Laura does start slowly achieving her target goals again. She eventually has a menstrual period. Her body changes color, her skin becomes less wrinkled, and she has to buy new clothes. The following September Laura moves to the northeast to start attending an Ivy League university. Before she starts, she visits the counseling center, finds a new therapist that she likes, and reluctantly agrees to stay on her medication during her first semester.

Questions for Consideration

• *Why did Dr. P wait for over a month before she suggested that Laura see her colleague Dr. S for a medication evaluation? What difference does it make legally that Laura turned 18?* Dr. P knew that Laura had already seen numerous physicians and therapists and had little respect for any of them. Dr. P didn't want to be the next therapist on the long list to not help Laura. She knew that establishing a strong relationship was critical to both therapy and the possibility of using medication. She did not jump into treatment options, including medication, until a strong relationship had been established. When Laura initially turned down the possibility of a medication consultation, Dr. P quickly moved on to the treatment options she preferred. Only when the progress stalled did she revisit medication as an option.

Although Laura was financially dependent on her parents, she had mostly done what she wanted about her treatments for anorexia all along. The fact that she turned 18 gave her more legal rights as an adult, which could have affected confidentiality and patient privilege.

• *Why did Dr. P carefully choose the psychiatrist that she sent Laura to see? How might Laura's insurance options affect the choice of psychiatrist?* Dr. P thought the critical importance of the therapeutic relationship extended to the psychiatrist–patient relationship as well. She chose a psychiatrist who had excellent interpersonal skills, as well as clinical competence. Fortunately, Dr. S could be partially paid by Laura's health insurance. If not, Dr. P would have had a dilemma. Should she ask the parents to pay out of pocket because the therapeutic relationship was so critical? Or should she pick another physician on Laura's list of providers and hope for the best?

• *Why did Dr. P attend the first psychiatry session with Laura? Is it worth it for Dr. P to drive 20 minutes to Dr. S's office just so she could attend the session? How might Dr. P's presence affect Dr. S's interview of Laura, both positively and negatively?* Dr. P knew that if Laura did not like the psychiatrist or if she could find anything wrong with the interview, she would negate the entire experience, including the possibility of taking medication. She knew Laura well enough by this time to believe that she could facilitate the interview, reassure Laura by her presence, and help Dr. S obtain the information she needed. Dr. S welcomed Dr. P's input. However, if Dr. S had seemed at all uncomfortable with Dr. P being present, Dr. P would have had to consider another plan. Again, the strong relationship between Dr. S and Dr. P facilitated the first visit and in essence created an empathic setting for Laura.

• *Laura had anorexia and didn't seem outwardly depressed. So why was an antidepressant medication prescribed?* Eating disorders, especially anorexia nervosa, often have obsessive features. The patients obsess over their weight, over what they have eaten, over exercise, and over many other things. They have an abnormal sense of their body image that is similar in some ways to body dysmorphic disorder, which also frequently responds to antiobsessional medication. The target symptom for Laura's treatment with an SSRI antidepressant, which is also an antiobsessional medication, is her obsessive symptoms within her anorexia. She may need antiobsessional doses of the SSRI, which are higher than typical antidepressant doses, to be effective.

Bulimia Nervosa

Although a minority of patients with anorexia nervosa engages in binge eating, it is universal in bulimia nervosa, and this is one of the diagnostic criteria. Binge eating is often followed by some activity to eliminate (or purge) its consequences, such as induced vomiting and the use of laxatives. Others do not purge but engage in fasting or excessive exercise to compensate for the binge eating. Patients are often ashamed of their behavior; they may not easily volunteer information about it, and they may appear to be of normal or even above normal weight. Very few physical signs suggest bulimia, and they occur only in those who induce vomiting. There may be a reddish roughening of the skin around the knuckles of the hand; there may be large cheeks from enlarged salivary glands, and the front teeth may appear discolored or damaged from the stomach acid injury to the dental enamel. The primary way in which a therapist will learn about the existence of bulimia is the development of enough rapport with a patient so that a very candid history can be obtained.

Bulimic patients have a low mortality rate, but they may suffer the consequences of electrolyte disturbances if they engage in frequent and/ or aggressive purges. The electrolyte disturbances can cause fatigue, seizures, and death in extreme cases. Unlike anorexia nervosa, studies have shown that specific treatments can be effective in bulimia nervosa. Cognitive-behavioral therapy (CBT) is one such intervention, with reported remission rates of 25–50% for bulimic patients (Walsh, 2001). The most effective medications are the SSRIs, which typically require antiobsessional doses to be effective. Often the therapist will want to start with CBT, and if this is not sufficiently effective alone, then consultation can be obtained to add an SSRI to the treatment regimen.

CHRONIC PAIN

"Chronic pain" is defined as a pain state that is persistent and for which the cause cannot be removed or otherwise treated and, in the generally accepted course of medical practice, no relief or cure is possible or none has been found after reasonable efforts. Chronic noncancer pain has been getting more attention in recent years—mandated attention. Examples of chronic pain include pain associated with arthritis, neuropathic pain (due to diabetes or other metabolic causes), pain that persists after an injury, and, the most common, low back pain.

A decade of research on the mechanisms of pain transmission to the brain has led to improved understanding and improved methods of pain control. The Joint Commission on Accreditation of Healthcare Organizations (JCAHO) now requires all accredited health care organizations to fully assess pain in all patients, teach them pain management options, provide appropriate pain management, and record the results of that strategy (JCAHO, 1999). Health care providers are now required to consider pain the "fifth vital sign" (the others are temperature, pulse, blood pressure, and respiratory rate), and they are expected to record it in the patient's medical record just as routinely, often using numerical scales to quantitate the degree of pain from one visit to the next. Some states, including California, have enacted legislation that requires physicians to take courses in pain management before they can renew their medical license beyond 2006. Patients can now file a legal complaint against their physicians for inadequate pain management. The care of the chronic pain patient is now legally more important than it was in the past, and the therapist will be asked to be a part of the treatment team for patients who suffer from chronic pain (see Figure 8.1).

Medical	Physical Therapy	Psychological

Medication trials:
  Lidocaine
  Gabapentin
  Mexilitine
  Opioid
Nerve block
neurostimulation
	Active mobilization
	Desensitization
	Myofascial release
	Aerobic conditioning
	
	_____
	Functional improvement
		Support
		Motivation
		Stress management
		Treatment for depression
		Hypnosis
		Imagery
		Biofeedback

FIGURE 8.1. Multidisciplinary treatment of complex regional pain syndrome.

Biology and Biochemistry of Chronic Pain

The biology of pain perception is among the most complex neurological events, but helping patients understand some of the basic elements will help them develop coping strategies. We can easily imagine a simple situation: a person accidentally touches the flame of a candle with his or her hand. Before that person can think about it, he or she has withdrawn the hand away from the flame and, only a second or so later, may say, "Ouch!" The brain did not dictate that defensive movement—the neurons in the hand relayed the message to the spinal cord, and a reflex action was triggered to remove the hand from danger. The nervous system says: Safety first; tell the brain later. We all have many such reflexes. Pain perception plays a major role in preserving our well-being and safety, and those few individuals born without pain perception die prematurely. But what if the neurons that send the pain message to the spinal cord and then to the brain are injured, or they have become errant in their transfer of information? These are among the ways in which a chronic pain syndrome can be perpetuated.

Pain is generally regarded by the brain as a sign of danger, or at least of serious dysfunction. In what is called the dorsal horn of the spinal cord (the back part), some neurons send pain signals toward the brain and other neurons inhibit the sending of those signals. If the pain signals coming into the dorsal horn are of sufficient magnitude (because of tissue injury, nerve injury, metabolic injury, etc.), the neurons that usually suppress some of the pain impulses to the brain are overwhelmed. The inhibitory neurons stop working, and the pain feels even greater than the tissue injury that started the process. In fact, there can be pain signals for such a long time or of such magnitude that neurons nearby in the spinal cord, which are not even involved in the process, can begin sending pain signals to the brain as well. The additional neurons are "recruited" to help send pain impulses to the brain. Thus, a person may have an injured wrist, and if the nerve was injured, he or she may complain of chronic pain in most of the entire arm. The person is not exaggerating or manipulating; he or she has an injured nervous system, as well as an injured wrist. At a higher level, the brain has the opportunity to suppress some incoming pain signals, and there are some ways in which the therapist can help the patient maximize those opportunities.

Other sensations, in addition to pain, can be a consequence of serious injury to nerve tissue:

- **Allodynia:** pain that is elicited by a non-noxious stimulus—such as the touch of clothing, air movement, or a light touch of the hand—or pain when something mildly cool or warm touches the skin.
- **Hyperalgesia:** exaggerated pain response to a mildly noxious (touch or temperature) stimulus.
- **Hyperpathia:** delayed and explosive pain response to a noxious stimulus; this is indicative of sensitization of pain fibers in the CNS.

It is important to know, and to help patients understand that feeling these very odd sensations does not mean any new danger is occurring. This is part and parcel of the injury they sustained. It may improve and hopefully resolve over time, but it may take a very long time (months to years in some cases). The good news is that there is medication management that can help them in the meantime.

Pain Management

As physicians have increased their understanding of the pathophysiology of chronic pain syndromes, so they have developed new strategies to manage them. Some states have mandated new training in the management of chronic pain because there is so very much new information, of which many physicians are uninformed. Some of those approaches include new medications, but rarely is medication the only modality. The patient who suffers chronic pain will be best served by a multidisciplinary team approach, in which medication is used if appropriate, as well as physical therapy aimed at functional improvement and psychological interventions to provide the cognitive skills to understand and set realistic goals.

The Therapist's Role in the Treatment of Chronic Pain

Chronic pain is often a source of tremendous frustration for patients, family members, and health care professionals. Patients with these problems are often tireless in their pursuit of pain relief. When relief is elusive, patients and their family members can experience severe hopelessness and express rage at the medical profession for failing to locate effective treatments. Health care professionals share this helplessness even as they continue to put forth their best efforts to find pain relief (Turk, 1996).

Mind–body dualism has historically undermined effective treatment for chronic pain patients. In the absence of a purely physiological explanation for symptoms, pain has, at times, been explained as simply psychological distress, which leaves patients and family members with the message that "it's all in your head." This kind of message breeds hopelessness and damages the doctor–patient–family relationship. The biomedical model of pain is slowly giving way to integrative models that examine the dynamic interaction among physical, psychological, and social factors in the development of pain.

The gate control theory (Melzack & Casey, 1968; Melzack & Wall, 1965) was the first model to include psychological factors as an integral aspect of the pain experience. Turk and Flor (1999) describe the significance of the model:

> The gate control model describes the integration of peripheral stimuli with cortical variables, such as mood and anxiety, in the perception of pain. This model contradicts the notion that pain is either somatic or psychogenic and instead postulates that both factors have either potentiating or moderating effects on pain perception. In this model, for example, pain is not understood to be the result of depression or vice versa, but rather the two are seen as evolving simultaneously. Any significant change in mood or pain will necessarily alter the others. (p. 21)

Conditions that may increase the effects of pain include an inappropriate activity level, anxiety, depression, focusing on the pain, and boredom. Conditions that moderate the effects of pain include medications, counterstimulation (e.g., massage), positive emotions, relaxation, distraction, and involvement in life activities.

The therapist will be able to help the patient understand that although the team members all hope that he or she will achieve total relief, the recommended *goal is to achieve maximum life function in spite of whatever degree of continued pain he or she may have.* This goal is a revelation for many patients, and often an unpleasant one. Given that goal for the chronic pain patient, there are several specific things the therapist can do:

- Provide invaluable support.
- Strengthen the patient's support system.
- Help the patient grieve the "old me" and accept the pain as chronic, if appropriate.
- Assist with development of motivation.

- Teach the patient skills in stress management (which will raise the pain threshold and lower pain perception); anxiety accentuates pain perception.
- Treat depression that is present in the majority of patients who have suffered more than 6 months of continuous chronic pain; depression also accentuates pain perception.
- In some instances, teach the patient hypnosis, biofeedback, and the use of positive imagery.
- Suggest bibliotherapy that will teach the patient and family much more about the neurology and management of pain than can be presented here; one such example is a text by Fishman and Berger (2000).
- Address potential negative effects of chronic pain on intimate and sexual relationships.
- Use cognitive therapy, which in most cases can help the patient learn to cognitively reframe the pain impulses—that is, learn to understand that the familiar pain he or she perceives each day is not indicative of injury or danger; it is the same errant set of neurons again, and the pain message in itself does not mean that the patient cannot be active. Addressing the patient's and family's beliefs about the meaning of pain is also helpful.

The therapist can play a vital role in the multidisciplinary team approach. As more such teams are formed (by mandate or by choice), there will be increasing need for therapists who have some understanding of the physiology of pain, its medical management, and the therapist's role in helping the patient develop the cognitive skills needed to contain an errant nervous system and still live a full life.

IMPULSE CONTROL DISORDERS

The treatment of intermittent explosive disorder, kleptomania, pyromania, pathological gambling, trichotillomania, and impulse control disorder not otherwise specified is beyond the scope of this text, and we only briefly discuss some key aspects of impulse control disorders, about which the therapist should seek consultation with the psychiatrist. In particular, one must consider whether the person with intermittent problems of impulse control is manifesting a partial complex seizure (rare), or whether the person who habitually or rhythmically pulls his or her hair has a partial complex seizure instead of trichotillomania (unusual).

A psychiatric examination or, in some cases, consultation with a neurologist is indicated in these situations.

When a therapist is evaluating a patient who demonstrates intermittent loss of impulse control, it is important to look for the sequence of events that kindled the condition. Sometimes, one discovers an obsessional antecedent to the loss of control, and this may respond very well to antiobsessional medication. The woman in the example that follows could have had an intermittent explosive disorder, a personality disorder, or other diagnoses; but given her poverty and lack of health care insurance or access, she would probably have received no treatment. Had she been wealthy, she might have received psychotherapy, which may have helped, given time. However, medication management did result in prompt remission of her symptoms, and it may have saved her life and that of her son. In some cases, medication consultation for a patient with one of the impulse control disorders can be a life-saving collaboration between therapist and physician (see case example below).

Ms. R is a 48-year-old woman and the single parent of a 13-year-old son. They both live in a homeless shelter because Ms. R has been unable to hold a job for more than a couple of weeks at a time. She was referred to the psychiatrist by the shelter staff, who said, "We're ready to ask her to leave now, and we just want to be sure she doesn't have any mental illness reason for her behavior." The story was that Ms. R had accumulated four strikes against her because on four occasions she had "gone off on people," yelling and appearing menacing to those who live and work in the shelter. After the fourth strike, Ms. R had been warned that if there was one more, she would be asked to leave and would again be homeless. Today, number 5 occurred, and she was referred to the psychiatrist on the way out the door. The psychiatrist asked the patient what happened today, and Ms. R reported the events leading up to her outburst as follows: She was walking in an area near the shelter, and she saw a stranger take a candy from a toddler in a stroller, which made the toddler cry. She stopped what she was doing and immediately confronted the stranger, and the event escalated into a shouting and shoving match. Security staff responded, and Ms. R was awarded strike number 5, requiring her (and her son) to leave the shelter. The psychiatrist asked, "But Ms. R, *you knew* that if you lost your temper one more time, you and your son would be on the street . . . what happened, why did you do that? Why didn't you just let it go, and the toddler could be given another piece of candy? You had so much at stake here; why not just let it go?" Ms. R responded, "I *just couldn't* let it go! He was *wrong*! What he did was bad; *it's just not right* to let it go!" When reviewing the history of Ms. R's previous episodes of loss of impulse control, virtually all of them were preceded by her recognition of some event in her world or her workplace that *"was just not right"*; she had an obsessive sense of righteousness and an obsessive need to intervene urgently when things were "not right" in her view. She had lost many jobs, and the reason for the dismissals was a history of "butting into the business of coworkers" when she observed them to be doing something she did not think was "right," causing shouting and intrusive behaviors in the workplace. Thus, what appeared to be an episodic loss of impulse control responded very well to antiobsessional doses of an SSRI. On medication, Ms. R was able to maintain control of her behavior in the face of the wrongs in the world; she was able to gain and hold a job and to provide adequately for herself and her son.

COLLABORATIVE OPPORTUNITIES WITH PATIENTS IN SPECIFIC PHASES OF THE LIFE CYCLE

Children

Mental illness in children is a family matter, and it typically comes with a fair measure of guilt and anguish on the part of the adults involved. A therapist provides invaluable assistance to these adults while striving to provide the best treatment possible for the child. Any child who has a serious mental illness should be evaluated by a child psychiatrist, and the therapist may be treating the child as well or possibly assisting the family. There are many serious disorders of childhood, such as autism, developmental disorders, and PTSD, that will absolutely require a multidisciplinary team approach, and in many (not all) cases, a child psychiatric consultation will also be needed. The decision to use psychotropic medications for a child is very complex, and a child psychiatrist should always be consulted, at least in the early stages of establishing the diagnosis and planning the treatment, if not in the ongoing treatment. A discussion of the management of these conditions is beyond the scope of this book.

One exception to the broad recommendation for a child psychiatry referral is that of attention-deficit/hyperactivity disorder (ADHD). ADHD is relatively common, with prevalence estimated at 3–7% of school-age children (American Psychiatric Association, 2000). The therapist can assist in making an accurate diagnosis when ADHD is considered, and if the diagnosis is confirmed, the therapist can provide essential education to the parents and, in many cases, to the child. ADHD holds an interesting position in psychiatric diagnosis in that it is simultaneously widely overdiagnosed and widely underdiagnosed. It is critical that parents, teachers, therapists, and physicians work together to ensure that the correct diagnosis is established. Conners' Rating Scales are commonly used, and there are questionnaires for parents, teachers, adolescents, and adults who might have ADHD themselves. The Conners' Scales are "B-level products," which require documentation of professional licenses and qualifications before ordering them. Most school counselors' offices have Conners' Scales for screening children for ADHD. Some of the conditions to be considered in the differential diagnosis of ADHD are the following:

- Normal variations of temperament—this is perhaps the most common condition that is misunderstood as ADHD.
- Parent–child or environmental problem.
- Conduct disorder.
- Oppositional defiant disorder.
- Disruptive behavior disorder not otherwise specified.
- Bipolar disorder—this will require a psychiatry evaluation.
- Pervasive developmental disorder.
- Other childhood mental illness or medical illness.

If the diagnosis of ADHD is established, the therapist might consult with the child's family physician or pediatrician for medication management, if indicated; a child psychiatrist might only be needed in unusual situations or if the diagnosis is not clear.

The impact of untreated ADHD on a child can be large and enduring; after all, typically a child has only one chance to be in the second grade. Some of the consequences of untreated ADHD are listed in Table 8.4.

In spite of these factors, parents often worry about giving their child a "mind-altering drug." They understandably look for other explanations and interventions. For example, therapists can help parents understand that, although eating too many sweets is not a healthy diet, there is no objective medical evidence that foods high in sugar or carbohydrates cause hyperactive behavior. On the other hand, there is evidence that fetal exposure to alcohol and exposure to lead (eating lead-containing paint chips, inhaling lead-containing fumes, etc.) can predispose a child to behaviors that can be confused with ADHD. Parents will benefit greatly from information about how they can help their child with

TABLE 8.4. Consequences of Untreated ADHD in Children

- Profound effect on all relationships.
- Child's frustration with self, school, life.
- Lost age-appropriate educational opportunities.
- Possible development of externalizing behavior.
- Adult disapproval and peer rejection, leading to poor self-esteem.
- Depression.
- Frustrated, unhappy, guilt-stricken parents.
- Children at higher risk of abuse than peers.
- Decreased hyperactivity with age, but possible persistence of inattentiveness and impulsivity.
- Approximately one-third of children with ADHD having an Axis I disorder as adults.
- Chronic misunderstanding of medications.

hyperactive behaviors, whether the child takes medication or not. Some good sources to recommend can be found on the website of CHADD (Children and Adults with Attention-Deficit/Hyperactivity Disorder; www.chadd.org). This website has helpful educational materials for parents, with such titles as "50 Tips on the Classroom Management of Attention Deficit Disorder" and "50 Tips on the Management of Adult Attention Deficit Disorder," among many others. An excellent overview of the diagnosis and treatment of ADHD entitled "Attention Deficit Hyperactivity Disorder (ADHD)" is available on the website of the National Institute of Mental Health (www.nimh.nih.gov/healthinformation.adhdmenu.cfm). Understandably, parents will look for information on the Internet, and there is a great deal of sensational misinformation out there. Therapists can do a wonderful service to families by steering them in the direction of high-quality, accurate information.

Medication to treat ADHD should generally be used in concert with behavioral, psychological, and educational interventions and support for the child and family; that is, medication alone is not recommended. Although some new nonstimulant medications are coming on the market for the treatment of ADHD, it will be some time until we know how well they work and with what side effects and risks. Meanwhile, the mainstay of medication treatment continues to be the stimulants, such as methylphenidate (trade name Ritalin), dextroamphetamine (trade name Dexedrine), and amphetamine/dextroamphetamine (trade name Adderall). The stimulant drug pemoline (trade name Cylert) is sometimes used, but it is contraindicated if the child has or develops impaired liver function; liver tests must be monitored regularly. Contrary to popular lore, the stimulants do *not* cause a "paradoxical response" in hyperactive children. The stimulants stimulate the brain, including that part of the brain that allows the person to focus, to attend to detail, and to contain impulsive behavior. The antidepressant bupropion (trade name Wellbutrin) is also sometimes used for children with ADHD, particularly if they also have depression and/or conduct disorder, and bupropion is often the first medication tried in the treatment of ADHD in adolescents and adults.

When the therapist refers a patient to a physician for evaluation, the following should be expected to occur at that visit:

- Complete medical history, as well as developmental, learning, discipline, family, and psychosocial history (the primary care physician may appreciate receiving the history that you have obtained for the latter five items).
- Complete physical examination, with emphasis on neurological, vision, and hearing evaluations.
- Laboratory and other studies, including a complete blood count (CBC), LFTs, thyroid-stimulating hormone (TSH) levels, blood lead screen, and possibly an electroencephalogram (EEG), an electrocardiogram (ECG; depending on the medications used), and brain imaging and/or pediatric neurology consultation.
- Information from school must *never* be omitted from the evaluation and should be sent to the physician for the first visit.

After the child has been started on stimulant medication, there should be regularly scheduled follow-up visits with the physician, during which the child's height, weight, pulse, blood pressure, and growth and development are monitored. Growth suppression or weight loss are side effects to watch for, and some children may experience nervousness, gastrointestinal disturbances, or insomnia. Occasionally, a stimulant is prescribed for a child whom the physician (and perhaps even the parents) did not realize had motor tics, vocal tics, or Tourette's syndrome (the combination of multiple motor tics and one or more vocal tics, occurring many times a day, nearly every day, for more than a year). Stimulants often make tic disorders worse, and they are typically avoided in children with these afflictions. Some stimulants have been associated with sudden death in children and adolescents with heart problems or congenital heart defects, so careful evaluation prior to the start of medication, and close early follow-up after starting medication is prudent.

Parents will talk with their physician about dose amounts and intervals and whether the child should be given a "drug holiday," in which the medication for ADHD is stopped for some period of time, be it a weekend or the summer. There are pros and cons to drug holidays. In favor is that parents can observe how the child does while off the medication, which helps validate the need for it or document that it is no longer needed. Drug holidays also mean that the child will probably suffer from the symptoms of ADHD at a time when he or she should be able to enjoy time with family and friends, and those relationships may become strained because of the child's symptoms. Although the prescribing physician will be monitoring the child for all of these parameters, the therapist's observations of the child's behavior and any side effects that occur will bring a valuable perspective to the decision to continue, stop, or adjust dosages.

CASE: ATTENTION DEFICIT DISORDER

Case Description

Mrs. S makes an appointment with her son Michael's pediatrician, Dr. K. During a parent–teacher meeting, Michael's teacher had suggested that Michael have some type of physical and/or academic evaluation. Michael is in fourth grade and, according to his teacher and previous academic reports, is a bright boy, a good reader, and a good athlete. Whereas his academic testing shows him to have been above average in the first three grades, Michael now seems to be struggling with handwriting and punctuation. His writing is often not legible, and his papers are quite messy. Mrs. S is surprised at the request because the only problems Michael ever had at school were on the playground. He often had trouble with anger and could be impulsive during recess. In contrast, in the classroom, Michael could seem spaced out. Michael's teacher, Ms. E, wonders if Michael has some sort of physical limitation that makes good handwriting difficult.

Beginning Collaboration

Dr. K does a physical examination of Michael but, more important, carefully listens to Mrs. S's concerns. He gives her a form for the teacher to complete. Dr. K asks Mrs. S to talk to the psychologist who works in his office. Although Mrs. S does not believe that Michael has any emotional or learning problems that warrant a meeting with a psychologist, she trusts Dr. K and so she agrees.

During the meeting with the psychologist, Dr. W, Mr. and Mrs. S carefully review Michael's physical, social, and academic history. Dr. W asks Mr. and Mrs. S if they are willing to consider having Michael tested for learning issues and possibly emotional issues. Again, Michael's parents reluctantly agree. Dr. K has been Michael's doctor since he was born, and they trust him. They extend that trust to Dr. W because she works with Dr. K.

Unfortunately, testing is not a covered benefit on Mr. and Mrs. S's insurance, but meetings with Dr. W are. Dr. W informs Mr. and Mrs. S that they can get testing by requesting an individualized education plan (IEP) through the school. Mrs. S investigates this option, but there is a 6-month wait and the school year would be over by the time the testing was completed. Thus, Mr. and Mrs. S decide to pay for the testing themselves.

Dr. W tests for intelligence, visual motor skills, academic achievement, and emotional issues. Based on the test results and Michael's history, Dr. W and Dr. K tell Mr. and Mrs. S that Michael has attention deficit disorder (ADHD)—inattentive type. They are surprised to hear this finding since Michael has never been "hyper." Dr. K and Dr. W schedule a joint appointment with Mr. and Mrs. S to go over their questions and concerns.

During the meeting, Dr. K and Dr. W focus on the many strengths that Michael has displayed during the testing and during the years that Dr. K has been his physician. They recommend several books including *The Myth of Laziness* and *A Mind at a Time* by Mel Levine. Dr. W offers to talk to Michael's teacher and has written a summary of specific recommendations for Michael that can be given to his teacher. Michael participates in part of the meeting, and he is given the chance to ask questions or state his perspective. Dr. K and Dr. W summarize aids that might help Michael with both his emotional regulation on the playground and his learning challenges in the classroom. Dr. K gives Mr. and Mrs. S some information on medications used to treat ADHD-inattentive type and summarizes the existing knowledge about both the benefits and risks of medications. Mr. and Mrs. S decide to go home and talk over their decisions, and they agree to meet with Dr. W the following week to implement a plan.

Ongoing Collaboration

At the meeting the following week, Michael and Mr. and Mrs. S tell Dr. W that they would like to try both medication and a learning coach Dr. S knows who works in the community. They also want Dr. W to talk to Ms. E, Michael's teacher. They have many questions and ask Dr. W if they can return for further follow-up meetings over the coming months. Dr. W agrees and tells them that she and Dr. K will be working together to monitor Michael's response to both the medications and the behavioral treatments.

Questions for Consideration

• *How does Dr. K's long-term relationship with the family influence their responses?* No parent is ever happy to learn that one's child has some learning or physical struggles. Parents can easily respond to this information by becoming defensive or criticizing the source. Grief and worry about one's child is another common response. Making an appointment with a psychologist or other mental health provider can be a painful reminder of the child's weaknesses. Because Mr. and Mrs. S trusted Dr. K, they could more easily accept the appointment and recommendations of Dr. W without becoming defensive. In addition, they felt encouraged when they saw Dr. K and Dr. W working closely together to plan Michael's treatment. They knew that treatment involved both medication and behavioral interventions. They felt that they were getting the best possible care by having two experts coordinating it.

• *How did Dr. K's long-term relationship as Michael's doctor help him when he was considering diagnostic options?* Dr. K had detailed records of Michael's development since he was a newborn. In addition, he had tracked Michael's academic progress since he started school. He was able to quickly rule out other possible medical explanations such as hypoglycemia, thyroid disorders, and anemia. In addition, he could give his findings to Dr. W. Together, Dr. K and Dr. W were able to make a genuine biopsychosocial evaluation of Michael that also relied heavily on Michael's history and development.

As with other patient populations, collaborative practice is essential to the care of children, regardless of the disorder. It is important for the therapist to realize that the scope of the collaborative effort is often expansive, encompassing school staff, pediatricians, and others, and therefore can be more challenging.

Women

Whereas 30–80% of ovulating women may experience premenstrual syndrome (PMS) at some time in their lives, premenstrual dysphoric disorder (PMDD) is seen in only 2–9% of ovulating women and is much more severe. PMDD's core symptoms include anger, irritability, depressed mood, and a variable degree of social and occupational impairment; the symptoms occur in the luteal phase (latter half) of the menstrual cycle, and they resolve by the end of the menstrual period. Women who experience PMDD are at increased risk for major depression and postpartum mood disorders. The therapist can help patients differentiate between PMS and PMDD, as the former is not a disease per se, and the latter often responds very well to treatment with SSRIs.

Although pregnancy and postdelivery may be a time of great joy for many women, it may also be a time of significant risk for those who are biologically vulnerable. Women who are vulnerable to major depression are especially likely to experience it during their pregnancy and/or postpartum period, and the decision to use or not to use antidepressant medication during pregnancy is a hard one for many women. Physicians generally prefer to avoid prescribing medications to pregnant women unless absolutely necessary, and there are three considerations concerning medication during pregnancy:

- The **teratogenic effects**, or potential for the medication to cause physical deformity in the infant—the medication must be taken during organogenesis (first 3 months) for this to occur, and delay until after the first 3 months of pregnancy is preferred.
- The potential toxic effects at the time of birth, including withdrawal syndromes in the infant—the medication must be taken at or near time of delivery for this to occur.
- Potential behavioral teratogenicity—the long-term effect of the medication on the functioning and behavior of the child many years later is an unknown factor for most medications used today, but no harm in this area is known for the antidepressants commonly prescribed.

Studies have found that women who were given SSRIs during their pregnancy had no increase in fetal malformations, no increase in prematurity, no increase in miscarriage or stillbirths, and no difference in birth weight of the infants, compared to control women who were not given antidepressants (Kulin et al., 1998). A case report has been written about newborns showing signs of jitteriness, irritability, and vomiting, which was attributed to withdrawal from paroxetine (Stiskal, Kulin, Kiren, Ho, & Ito, 2001), and indeed adults who stop paroxetine abruptly may have these symptoms as well. Although uncomfortable, the symptoms are not life-threatening. Given some of the potential consequences of untreated major depression in the pregnant woman—such as suicide; poor compliance with prenatal care; poor nutrition; sleep problems; increased risk of drug, alcohol, and tobacco use; and the unknown impact of depression on fetal development—the decision to use medication to treat depression in pregnancy, and if so, with which medication, is a complex decision that should be made by each patient and her physician. In this regard, clinicians will find it useful to consult the joint statement produced by the American Psychiatric Association and the American College of Obstetricians and Gynecologists on the management of depression during pregnancy (Yonkers et al., 2009). Whatever is decided, the patient will almost always be advised to continue with psychotherapy; the therapist can monitor the severity of the woman's symptoms and the risk for suicide or behaviors that put the developing baby at risk, as well as alert the physician to the possible need for hospitalization if the pregnant woman's mental health worsens. If a pregnant woman is critically ill with major depression to the extent that her life and her baby's life are at risk, ECT is sometimes safely used in severely ill patients, especially those who continue to be at imminent risk of suicide even while hospitalized.

A majority of women have "baby blues," or transient periods of sadness in the week or two after delivery, and this requires no treatment; the kind support of those whom she loves and trusts is all that is needed. But approximately 10–20% of women will experience postpartum depression, and 0.2% will develop postpartum psychosis. Of those with depression, approximately two-thirds will recover on their own within a year, but some concerns have emerged about the cognitive development of their infants, and these women have an increased risk of depression after subsequent deliveries (Bright, 1994). Women who develop postpartum psychosis may be at risk of harming their infants and/or themselves, and deaths of infants and mothers have occurred. Because of these serious potential outcomes, treatment of postpartum mood disorders is recommended, and women may wish to utilize multiple modalities of therapy, including psychotherapy and medication. All of the antidepressant medications are secreted in breast milk, so the new mother will need to take this into account. Early studies of SSRI use during breastfeeding discouraged mothers from breastfeeding their infants while taking medication (Baum & Misri, 1996). However, more recent studies on sertraline, for example, showed that very little medication was found in the infant's blood after breastfeeding from a mother taking sertraline, and the tool used to measure the clinical activity of the drug (platelet serotonin levels) showed little to no activity in those infants (Epperson et al., 2001). Nevertheless, the new mother will probably be reluctant to expose her infant to any medication, and she will need support from the therapist for the decision that she and her physician decide upon.

The last women's mental health issue discussed here is menopause. Only a few years ago, women thought that taking hormone replacement therapy (HRT) was necessary to prevent every aspect of aging, and the belief that HRT warded off depression in the fifth decade and beyond was just one more element in its assumed panacea. More recent studies have suggested that HRT does not protect against heart disease and dementia, and it does increase the risk for stroke and for certain cancers (Writing Group for the Women's Health Initiative Investigators, 2002). It is unlikely that HRT will provide protection against mental illness, nor does the onset of menopause cause mental illness. Menopause occurs in most women between the ages of 45 and 55, and that age may also be the beginning of losses in a woman's life: childbearing potential; adult children leaving home; parents aging and dying; and one's own aging, bringing with it an altered self-image and an increased awareness of one's own mortality. All of these adult developmental or life-phase issues are very important, and a woman may benefit from psychotherapy at this time if she has symptoms sufficient to cause distress. However, the menopause itself does not cause mental illness or predispose to it, and it is not an indication, in and of itself, for medication.

The Elderly

Just as midlife brings a new awareness of losses in life, the elderly have many ongoing losses, and they may develop major depression. Elderly patients will develop medical problems, and some of these may mimic symptoms of mental illness. Thyroid disease and vitamin B_{12} deficiency are great mimickers of mental illness, for example, and the only way to discover them is by medical examination and laboratory testing. Patients who develop psychosis for the first time in their senior years should always be presumed to have a general medical condition or a neurological disorder that explains the psychotic symptoms, until proven otherwise. They should be referred to their physician immediately. Patients may develop neurological problems, and they may become aware of the development of cognitive decline. Seniors will also go through the grief of losing parents, spouses, and many others to whom they have been very close, leading to episodes of bereavement that may run together. The challenge for the patient and the therapist is to discern what is normal developmental and life-phase psychotherapeutic work and what represents biological illnesses that will affect longevity if not treated. Therapists should be sure that all elderly patients have had a thorough medical evaluation, *and the physician has been informed about the psychiatric target symptoms*, before embarking on therapy. Major depression is an important cause of morbidity in the elderly, and studies have shown that untreated depression increases the vulnerability to heart attacks and the probability of dying in the first 6 months after the attack (Frasure-Smith et al., 1993). Furthermore, studies have demonstrated the safety of antidepressant medication in the time immediately after a heart attack (Glassman et al., 2002). In addition to the interaction between general medical conditions and depression, seniors are more vulnerable to suicide than many younger depressed patients. Seniors represent about 12% of our population but about 25% of completed suicides. One of the highest risk profiles for successful suicide is the elderly white male, widowed, who lives alone, drinks alcohol, has recently developed a serious medical illness, and has a loaded gun in the house. This profile is not rare, and the therapist should be aware of indications for referral of an elderly depressed patient to a doctor with experience in geriatric psychiatry.

If medications are used to treat any disorder in the elderly, mental illness or otherwise, there are a few general principles to keep in mind. First, as we age, our ability to metabolize drugs and clear them from our body decreases; that is, the liver and kidneys have gradually diminishing capacity to clear the drugs. Doses of medication that are acceptable in a young adult may be too high for an elderly patient, and when a starting dose is adjusted upward, the elderly person will be more sensitive to it and may react to the change more acutely. From this comes the clinical adage: "Start low, go slow." For example, the typical adult dose of the antidepressant paroxetine is 20 mg/day. In an elderly person, the fully effective dose may turn out to be 10 mg/day, and we might initiate therapy by prescribing the 10-mg tablet and advising the patient to take half a tablet (5 mg) a day to start.

Second, it takes longer to see a therapeutic effect in an older person than in a younger one. Typically, we think that it takes 2–4 weeks of antidepressant medication to see initial antidepressant efficacy in an adult with straightforward major depression as the only diagnosis. In seniors, 2–3 months may be required before we think that the treatment is clearly not working. The therapist can help the patient understand that it takes longer to see a response and can provide support for the patient to continue medication long enough.

Third, most seniors are taking medications for various general medical conditions, and all of the psychotropic medications may have multiple drug–drug interaction. Some of those interactions are potentially very serious. The therapist can be helpful in reminding patients to inform their prescribing physicians about *all* of the medications that they take, including over-the-counter (nonprescription) medications and any herbal remedies. Today's hand-held computers readily manage drug information programs that include the ability to check up to 30 simultaneous medications (including herbals) for adverse drug–drug interactions. Most physicians today use these programs, which protect patients from serious consequences *if* they tell their physicians what they take.

Fourth, the side effects of certain psychotropic medications are more worrisome in seniors than in younger patients. For example, the anticholinergic side effects of tricyclic antidepressants can cause cardiac problems, urinary retention, and constipation much more easily in the elderly, and the consequences are much more serious. The widespread (and often inappropriate) use of the tricyclic antidepressant amitriptyline is a prominent cause of anticholinergic delirium in the elderly and a leading cause of drug-related falls and hip fractures. Now that we have excellent alternatives, amitriptyline is generally contraindicated in elderly patients. There are exceptions, of course, such as the patient who is already on amitriptyline, is doing very well, and cannot be tapered off. But we generally do not start elderly patients on amitriptyline. Also, seniors are very sensitive to drugs that lower blood pressure. Amitriptyline has already been mentioned in this regard, but the other tricyclics can also cause **hypotension** (nortriptyline is less likely than other tricyclics to do so). Similarly, the MAOIs and the new generation of antipsychotics (risperdal, olanzapine, etc.) can also cause lower blood pressure to the point of falls and/or loss of consciousness, and these drugs must be started cautiously and monitored carefully.

The benzodiazepines are often used for the treatment of anxiety disorders and for short-term management of insomnia. The choice of benzodiazepine is very important for all patients, especially the elderly. These drugs have very different half-lives, and some of them have active metabolites (the metabolic byproducts of the original drug, which are also clinically active compounds in the blood). The best choice is a medication with a relatively short half-life and no active metabolites, especially if the patient (of any age) has liver disease because the liver metabolizes the benzodiazepines. So, for the patient who has serious liver disease, a good choice of benzodiazepine, if one is needed, is lorazepam (trade name Ativan) or oxazepam (trade name Serax) because they both have no known active metabolites and have comparatively shorter half-lives. If an elderly person is going to be taking a benzodiazepine, generally the starting dose is approximately half of the typical adult starting dose. Several benzodiazepines least preferred for seniors because of their long half-lives and active metabolites are diazepam (trade name Valium), chlordiazepoxide (trade name Librium), and clonazepam (trade name Klonopin). Although they may be prescribed for seniors at times, one must weigh the risk–benefit situation for each individual, and shorter half-life drugs are almost always preferred. Two benzodiazepines that are best avoided altogether for the elderly are, first, flurazepam (trade name Dalmane), a drug developed to treat insomnia. The problem is that the half-life is very long

(24–100 hours); if the patient takes it on a daily basis, the blood level continues to climb progressively because the drug is more than half-present in the blood when the patient takes the next dose. The other benzodiazepine to be avoided is triazolam (Halcion), which was also developed as a sleeping medication. The difficulty with triazolam is that its concentration rises very quickly in the bloodstream and also falls rapidly, with a half-life of only 2.5–3.5 hours. The problem here is that the rapid blood level changes interrupt the storage of memory and the transfer of memory from very short term to long term. Triazolam can eliminate the memory of events from some period of time before the medication was taken until some variable time during the next day, and this is especially troublesome for patients with mild cognitive impairment. Again, both flurazepam and triazolam are best avoided for seniors.

The choice of psychotropic medication is also shaped by one's coincident general medical conditions, and the elderly almost always have at least one additional medical problem. The complexity of selecting medication in this situation is beyond our scope here, but the following briefly illustrates the point. Parkinson's disease is a complex neurologic disorder in which tremor and rigidity are prominent features, and depression is also quite common. The neurotransmitters dopamine, norepinephrine, and serotonin are all decreased, and acetylcholine is increased in the CNS of patients with Parkinson's disease. Although tricyclic antidepressants may appear to improve motor symptoms briefly, they worsen cognition, constipation, somnolence, and urinary retention, and they often cause low blood pressure. Based on the underlying pathophysiology of Parkinson's disease, the preferred antidepressants for these patients include bupropion and venlafaxine, which decrease dopamine uptake (thus possibly improving the symptoms slightly or at least not making them worse), and the SSRIs. However, if selegiline is used to treat the primary symptoms of Parkinson's disease, the SSRIs are contraindicated because of adverse drug interactions.

Another example is the patient who has Alzheimer's-type dementia. The preferred available antidepressant medications for patients who have both Alzheimer's disease and depression include the SSRIs and venlafaxine because they have the lowest probability of adverse cognitive side effects. Patients with Alzheimer's disease should generally avoid TCAs (they are too anticholinergic, and they worsen cognitive function, in addition to all of the other TCA side effects); they should avoid bupropion (increased confusion) and fluoxetine (too agitating for seniors generally, especially those with Alzheimer's disease).

PATIENTS WITH PERSONALITY DISORDERS

Collaboration in mental health care is a *good* thing; in most circumstances, it is a rewarding practice for professionals and a benefit to their patients. When more than one person is involved in the treatment of these patients, very close collaboration is *absolutely essential*. No specific medication is approved for the treatment of personality disorders, although there are times when medication for target symptoms should be considered for a seriously ill patient. In addition, those with personality disorders may also develop other mental illness, and the person with an Axis II disorder will be much healthier and exhibit much less disordered behavior if the Axis I disorder is diagnosed and adequately treated. This is true for all of the personality disorders, regardless of cluster membership. When treating an Axis I disorder in the person who also has a serious personality disorder, close collaboration is a must.

The text revision of the fourth edition of the *Diagnostic and Statistical Manual of Mental Disorders* (DSM-IV-TR; American Psychiatric Association, 2000) categorizes the personality disorders into three clusters.

Cluster A, "odd/eccentric" group, includes:

- Paranoid personality disorder: a pattern of distrust and suspiciousness in which others' motives are generally interpreted as malevolent.
- Schizoid personality disorder: a pattern of detachment from social relationships and a restricted range of emotional expression.
- Schizotypal personality disorder: a pattern of acute discomfort in close relationships, cognitive or perceptual distortions, and eccentricities of behavior.

Cluster A patients rarely call attention to themselves and often suffer in isolation for much of their lives. They may be brought to treatment by a family member, or if they are employed, there may be a problem in the workplace that precipitates referral. By their nature, those with Cluster A personality disorders are difficult to engage in any modality of therapy, including medications. If the person has deteriorated in mental health to the point of developing a psychosis, medication may be considered for the specific target symptoms. Also, therapists should carefully consider the possibility that a general medical condition may explain what appears to be a paranoid personality disorder, especially if the behaviors are not a lifelong trait. Cluster A patients rarely engage in both psychotherapy and medication management, so collaboration is not a common opportunity but may be a goal in some cases.

Cluster B includes those whose style is "dramatic, emotional, erratic":

- Antisocial personality disorder: a pattern of disregard for, and violation of, the rights of others, the criminal.
- Borderline personality disorder: a pattern of instability in interpersonal relationships, self-image, and affects, with marked impulsivity.
- Histrionic personality disorder: a pattern of excessive emotionality and attention seeking.
- Narcissistic personality disorder: a pattern of grandiosity, need for admiration, and a lack of empathy.

The Cluster B patients typically engender the desire for effective medical management of personality disorders; however, there is no medication known to manage, much less cure, these personality disorders. However, the patient with borderline personality disorder in particular may develop specific target symptoms that require medication, sometimes emergently (this is discussed below).

Cluster C includes those with an "anxious/fearful" style:

- Avoidant personality disorder: a pattern of social inhibition, feelings of inadequacy, and hypersensitivity to negative evaluation.
- Dependent personality disorder: a pattern of submissive and clinging behavior related to an excessive need to be taken care of.
- Obsessive–compulsive personality disorder: a pattern of preoccupation with orderliness, perfectionism, and control.

Cluster C patients may indeed present for psychotherapy and may improve with that treatment modality alone. However, the therapist should carefully consider the differential diagnosis between avoidant personality disorder and panic disorder or social anxiety disorder, for example, which responds well to SSRI therapy. And the therapist should particularly evaluate the Cluster C patient for obsessional signs and symptoms that may respond well to antiobsessional medication.

Management of the Patient with Borderline Personality Disorder

Borderline personality disorder is complex, and many texts on this subject have been written for clinicians, including the classic *Severe Personality Disorders: Psychotherapeutic Strategies* (Kernberg, 1984), *Cognitive-Behavioral Treatment of Borderline Personality Disorder* (Linehan, 1993a) and *Skills Training Manual for Treating Borderline Personality Disorder* (Linehan, 1993b). A controlled trial of different modalities of psychotherapeutic treatment of borderline personality disorder can be reviewed in Clarkin, Levy, Lenzenweger, and Kernberg (2004), and an inpatient trial of dialectical behavior therapy for borderline personality disorder can be reviewed in Bohus et al. (2004).

There are also texts available for patients and their families, such as *I Hate You, Don't Leave Me: Understanding the Borderline Personality* (Kreisman & Straus, 1991) and *Stop Walking on Eggshells* (Mason, Kreger, & Siever, 1998). A summary of the approach to the crisis management of the patient with borderline personality disorder—what we call *the four Cs of soft-spoken limit setting* (see Table 8.5)—can be illustrated by the following example.

The medical assistant had blood all over the front of her uniform as she ran from the orthopedic surgeon's office into the medical office next door and yelled to the family physician, "Hurry! Hurry! Doctor wants you to come over right away!" As the family physician followed the medical assistant, she noted that there was blood in the waiting room—unusual indeed. A great deal of screaming and breaking of glass were coming from the hallway, and as the family physician walked toward the commotion, she noted dots of blood on the wallpaper just about at eye level—also a bad sign, as venous blood follows gravity and pools on the floor. Only an arterial bleeder will shoot up in spurts. As she got to the door of the

TABLE 8.5. The Four Cs of Soft-Spoken Limit Setting

• Calm:	Try to remain calm throughout the crisis.
• Connection:	Make an empathic, nonjudgmental connection with the patient.
• Choices:	Present the patient with a few clear, concise choices.
• Control:	Let patients choose in order to give them the responsibility to regain control.

room where the noise was coming from, the family physician saw a struggle going on; the orthopedist had his hands on the shoulders of a very upset young woman, and he was yelling, "Calm down! Calm down! It's going to be all right!" As he did this, the young woman screamed more, struggled with him more, broke more equipment, and threw more furniture in the room. When the orthopedist saw the family physician at the door, he said, "Oh good!" and ran out of the room. This left the family physician standing at the door and the young woman in the midst of the rubble—her arm spurting blood with every beat of her heart. Neither the family physician nor the orthopedist had ever met the woman before. She had taken a bottle out of a trash dumpster behind the medical building, smashed the bottom off it, and jabbed it into her arm and wrist deeply, lacerating the radial artery, which was now bleeding briskly. The family physician stood still at the door—the first C is to remain calm. Then, trying to make an empathic connection with the patient (the second C), the family physician quietly said, "Boy, are you pissed!" And the patient replied, "You're damn right!" The family physician thought, this is great, we've got a dialogue going—much better than how it went for the orthopedist! Then the young woman asked, "And what are *you* going to do about it?" To which the family physician replied, "Nothing." The patient replied in astonishment, "Nothing?" The family physician quietly and calmly said, "Yes. The way I see it, we have two choices here (the third C). Either you can sit down on that chair, put your arm out, and let me put a cotton on that artery until we go to the hospital, or you can keep doing what you're doing, you'll pass out from blood loss in a few minutes, and I'll put a cotton on that artery until we go to the hospital." This puts the responsibility on the patient to restore control to the situation (the fourth C). The young woman sat down on the chair, extended her arm to allow the family physician to apply pressure to the bleeding artery while the ambulance came, and proceeded to complain bitterly about the boyfriend who had left her. Notice that the family physician did not threaten to leave, and when giving choices it is very important that they be few in number, that they be very concisely stated (a person in crisis is not thinking clearly), and that all of them must be something that the therapist can feel comfortable with.

"Crisis meets limit setting *without abandonment*"—this is the treatment sequence for those with borderline personality disorder who are in crisis, and it will be repeated in crises large and small, many hundreds of times, over the years of therapy. When the patient is not in crisis, other psychotherapeutic approaches to borderline personality disorder, notably cognitive-behavioral therapy and dialectical behavior therapy, will be the mainstay of treatment. However, there are times when the patient with borderline personality disorder develops specific sets of target symptoms that may warrant medication. The American Psychiatric Association has published a *Practice Guideline for the Treatment of Patients with Borderline Personality Disorder* with psychopharmacological treatment algorithms (available to members at the American Psychiatric Association website, www.psych.org) for the following clusters of borderline personality disorder symptoms:

- Patient exhibits mood lability, rejection sensitivity, inappropriate intense anger, depressive "mood crashes," or outbursts of temper.
- Patient exhibits impulsive aggression, self-mutilation, or self-damaging binge behavior (e.g., promiscuous sex, substance abuse, or reckless spending).
- Patient exhibits suspiciousness, referential thinking, paranoid ideation, illusions, derealization, depersonalization, or hallucination-like symptoms.

For each of these three symptom clusters, there is a specific algorithm of treatment, sequencing various antidepressants, mood stabilizers, and antipsychotics in varying orders of preference, doses, and combinations of use.

When the therapist and patient agree that a medication management consultation is in order, there are several considerations:

- How the therapist presents the consult option is critical—it must not be perceived as an abandonment or as a panacea.
- The therapist, patient, and physician should hold modest expectations with clear goals for the use of medication, based on target symptoms.
- The therapist should anticipate a high placebo effect, especially initially, possibly followed by demonizing of the medication or physician or idealizing them and demonizing the therapist.
- Both therapist and physician must anticipate a split and must work very closely together to prevent it from damaging the treatment of the patient.
- The therapist should realize that benzodiazepines often make borderline personality disorder worse: They disinhibit someone who has fragile boundaries and poor judgment to begin with, and

in general, they should be avoided or minimized as much as possible.

- The therapist should realize that the patient will often have poor medication compliance, hoarding, and control issues.
- The patient may use drug overdose as an expression of anger or revenge; therapists' vacations are a vulnerable time, along with any other real or perceived abandonment.

The following case illustrates many of the considerations, pharmacological and otherwise, that need to be considered in the treatment of the patient with borderline personality disorder.

CASE: BORDERLINE PERSONALITY DISORDER AND SUBSTANCE ABUSE

Case Description

Mr. B makes an initial appointment with Dr. P because his wife told him that she would leave him if he didn't start therapy. During the initial session, he reported that they had a serious fight that had been upsetting and frightening to both of them. Mr. B had come home one evening after a night of social drinking and started arguing with Mrs. B. He became so enraged during the argument that he "started chasing her around the house." She tried to hide in the shower, and he pulled the shower door off its hinges. Mr. B reports that Mrs. B was terrified and that her look of terror finally made him stop.

Mr. B reports feeling remorse and shame about the incident, revealing that violence had occurred three other times in their 15-year marriage. In each fight, Mr. B had been drinking and had become uninhibited and enraged. Most fights were about Mrs. B's flirtatious personality, which made Mr. B feel threatened and jealous. He says that he suspects that she has had several sexual encounters with other men, including her personal trainer and massage therapist, but he has not wanted to address his fears.

Mr. B reports that Mrs. B is fairly volatile and unstable, but that most of the time her passion and dramatic personality are attractive to him. He states that "the good times are so special they can often compensate for the equally bad times." In general, he says his wife has always been "high maintenance." At times Mr. B has wondered if it was worth it to stay in the marriage, and he knows Mrs. B has asked herself the same question.

Mrs. B had been abused as a child and had a history of stormy, volatile relationships with men and women. She had few lasting friendships and had changed jobs and even careers several times. She had experienced a stormy childhood but as an adult had enjoyed several years of "peace" with her mother until she died 2 years earlier. Since her mother died, Mrs. B had felt adrift, both personally and professionally. She feels ongoing grief and even depression about her mother's death and simultaneously is becoming more distant from her father, whom she considers cruel and exploitive.

Dr. P has Mrs. B join them for the second session of therapy. Mrs. B dominates the session with her vivid stories of abuse as a child, descriptions of the pain she felt as her mother was dying of cancer, and her feelings of emptiness and loneliness since her mother's death. Mrs. B reports that she doesn't know how long she can tolerate the intense pain she's feeling; she says that she's experienced it throughout most of her life and even more so since her mother died.

Beginning Collaboration

Dr. P decides to first address the alcohol abuse of Mr. B by asking him to stop drinking completely, which he agrees to do. But Dr. P is less sure about the dramatic presentation of Mrs. B's life story and the intensity of her affect. Although she says she is not suicidal, she does indicate deep despair. Dr. P internally considers possible diagnoses like depression, borderline personality disorder, or histrionic personality disorder. In addition, Dr. P attempts to clarify the terms for therapy: Are they looking for individual or marital therapy? Dr. P decides to address these questions directly with Mr. and Mrs. B. They both say that they want marital therapy but feel that Mrs. B's pain needs prompt attention also. She's looking for some relief.

Dr. P begins to offer many possible options for each problem they are looking to address and asks them what problems they would like to address first. As part of this discussion, Dr. P mentions the possibility of a referral for a medication evaluation even though she is not convinced medication is essential. In addition to other treatment choices, Mrs. B immediately accepts the medication referral.

After the session, Dr. P calls her colleague, Dr. G, an adult psychiatrist. They talk on the phone about the referral. Dr. G and Dr. P have shared several patients in the past and have come to respect each other's work. Dr. P feels comfortable telling Dr. G that she is a little overwhelmed by the multitude of issues the couple presented and is not quite sure what to make of Mrs. B's dramatic presentation. Dr. G agrees to see Mrs. B.

A week later, Dr. G contacts Dr. P to say that he had also been impressed by Mrs. B's dramatic affect. He reports that he had to keep tight boundaries on the content and even then had run over the allotted time. Dr. G confirms Dr. P's hunch that Mrs. B meets criteria for border-line personality disorder. He expresses some concern that Mrs. B might do something dramatic and asks Dr. P to stay frequently connected with her.

Dr. G is ambivalent about prescribing any psychotropic medication, but Mrs. B implores him to give her something to help "lessen my pain." Dr. G decides to prescribe a very low dose of a new antipsychotic medication, but he tells Dr. P and Mrs. B that he thinks Mrs. B needs psychotherapy more than medication.

Ongoing Collaboration and Outcome

The medication turns out to be more effective than either Dr. G or Dr. P had anticipated. Within a week, Mrs. B reports feeling calmer and happier and has more stability and relief than she'd felt in 2 years. The dramatic outbursts and conflicts between Mr. B and her stop occurring. With the hiatus in Mr. B's alcohol use and Mrs. B's dramatic behaviors, Dr. P and the couple are now able to address numerous marital issues. In addition, Dr. P refers both Mr. and Mrs. B to individual therapists. Six months later, the couple reports that their relationship is more fulfilling and stable than it had been since they met.

Questions for Consideration

• *Why did the therapist refer only Mrs. B for a medication evaluation being that she gave both Mr. and Mrs. B individual diagnoses?* Mr. B wasn't seeking individual therapy. Instead, he was seeking ways to make his marriage work and become more fulfilling. Mrs. B was also seeking ways to improve the marriage, but she was most concerned about her own pain and confusion. Of course, the individual issues influenced the marriage and vice versa, but since a marital separation was not imminent, Dr. P decided to focus on the problem that seemed most acute—Mrs. B's intense affect and pain. There were multitudes of ways to address Mrs. B's pain, but Dr. P knew that the treatment(s) that Mrs. B chose were most likely to work simply because she chose them. Thus Mrs. B was sent for a psychotropic medication evaluation.

• *Why did both the therapist and psychiatrist defer to the patient's wishes to have a medication evaluation and eventually be given a prescription for a psychotropic medication?* Initially, both Dr. P and Dr. G were neutral about whether Mrs. B should take a psychotropic medication. Mrs. B's affect did not present like a typical depression, and there were many underlying psychodynamic and interpersonal issues that influenced her mood. In fact, it was really Mrs. B's desire for medication that propelled them to try it. As stated above, treatment options are most likely to work when chosen by the patient; thus Mrs. B's strong desire to try medication was a good indication that the treatment would be at least somewhat successful.

• *How can a therapist use successful medication treatment to enhance marital therapy?* The medication made a difference in Mrs. B's daily mood, which made a difference in her marriage. Consequently, during marital therapy, Mr. and Mrs. B were able to move beyond dealing with the weekly crisis and begin discussing underlying themes and issues in the marriage. Mr. B reported that the intense interpersonal conflict had stopped. The couple and the therapist had the luxury of addressing long-term issues, such as the impact Mrs. B's childhood had on her life choices and on their marriage.

• *Why did the psychiatrist insist on frequent, ongoing collaboration with the therapist? How had their previous collaborations served as a good foundation for starting joint care of Mrs. B?* Although neither Dr. G nor Dr. P considered Mrs. B to be a suicide risk, they were both concerned that she could make other potentially dangerous or damaging decisions in the heat of a dramatic mood. Dr. G, a conscientious psychiatrist, wanted assurances that his patient would receive the care he thought she needed, even if he wasn't providing that care himself. In essence, there was an unstated pact between Dr. G and Dr. P about the quality and frequency of therapy that both would provide to their shared patients and about the respect they would show each other. This established relationship allowed them to collaborate in caring for a challenging patient and to trust each other to provide the quality of care they each expected.

Psychotherapy is the preferred treatment for patients who have borderline personality disorder, but at times medication for these patients can be lifesaving; then the therapist must work very closely with the prescribing physician to assist the patient. The therapist should also be fully aware of local emergency procedures and state laws for emergency involuntary hospitalization for patients with borderline personality disorder who are seriously ill and in a life-threatening crisis. If the therapist and psychiatrist work together to help the patient, he or she will receive the best care and have the opportunity for safety and recovery at the soonest possible time. Although very ill patients with borderline personality disorder can present a challenge, it is also very rewarding to see them benefit from treatment and grow in health over the years of therapy. These patients provide the strongest evidence for the essential nature of practice in collaboration.

PART III

Creative Collaboration

The previous section provided a solid foundation in the content of psychopharmacology and a basic overview of how medications work to expand our readers' understanding of the range of medication options for a variety of presenting problems and populations.

As most therapists know, a single intervention is only part of the therapeutic process. In the case of starting medication it is equally, if not more, important to understand how to talk with your patients about medication, how to engage and collaborate with the medical professionals who prescribe your patients' medication, and how to support your patients and their family members after your patient has started medication. We review these process issues in the following chapters.

When our patients are taking medication, our mission is to form a multidisciplinary healthcare team that will work collaboratively with each other, the patient, and the patient's family members. Forming this kind of team is easiest when the professionals are working in the same location. However, we recognize that most therapists do not work in settings that include primary care physicians and psychiatrists. When professionals who care for the same patient work in distant locations, it is often incumbent on the therapist to build the professional relationships and communication system to foster collaboration. The time spent trying to communicate with other distant professionals can sometimes feel like an added burden with little payoff. We hope you will persevere through apparent inequities and continue to reach out to the professionals who are working with your patients and the family members who care for them. As time passes, you will develop a list of excellent referral sources and, we hope, establish some meaningful professional relationships simultaneously.

CHAPTER 9

Focusing the Lens

THE REFERRAL PROCESS
AND MEDICATION EVALUATION

Mr. B, age 65, and his wife, age 66, have been seeing Dr. G, a family therapist, for several weeks. Although their marital relationship has been improving, evidenced by better communication and increased intimacy, Mrs. B continues to be worried about Mr. B's depressive symptoms, including hypersomnia, little interest in interacting with friends and family, and "grumpiness." When Dr. G asks Mr. B for his perspective on Mrs. B's concerns, Mr. B echoes her concerns but explains that he is "used to feeling down and tired." He says that the biggest drawback to feeling this way is that he sometimes doesn't feel like spending time with his grandkids. He likes being a grandfather but gets easily irritated when in a bad mood. When Dr. G asks Mr. B if he has ever taken medication for these symptoms, Mr. B says he hasn't given it much thought. Mrs. B interjects and says, "He doesn't think it would be the manly thing to do." Mr. B shrugs his shoulders and says, "My dad went through the same stuff and tried to grin and bear it. He worked hard, put food on the table, and would never consider getting any help. I guess I'm using his approach, except he would roll over in his grave if he knew I was seeing a shrink." Between sessions, Dr. G considers ways to discuss with Mr. and Mrs. B the benefits of a medication evaluation and considers possible referral options.

209

When a therapist concludes that a patient would benefit from a medication evaluation, it is not uncommon for the therapist to worry about how the patient will respond to the suggestion. Common responses or beliefs can include such statements as "Even my therapist thinks I'm crazy," "My therapist is going to abandon me," or, as in Mr. B's case, "My therapist thinks I'm too weak to handle this problem on my own." Other, more positive responses could be a sense of relief (because the therapy alone has not resulted in enough improvement) or an inference of care and concern from the therapist (because he or she is considering every option available). If a family member or friend suggests medication, that suggestion could have many meanings for the patient. It may feel like a form of control or feel demeaning.

Perhaps a physician started a patient on medication and simultaneously sent the patient to a therapist. In these situations, the patient can view therapy as the requirement to receive the psychotropic medication. Regardless of who suggested medication, it is important to understand the meaning the patient attaches to the suggestion. The following questions are helpful when medication is being considered.

At what point in therapy was the idea of medication first discussed? If the patient is already on medication at the first visit, starts medication shortly after the first visit, or starts medication midtherapy, the significance to the patient of the medication may vary. For example, if medication begins midtherapy, the patient may believe that medication is being tried because psychotherapy is not working. If the therapy begins at the same time the medication is started, the patient may credit any positive changes to only the medication or only the therapy.

Has the patient ever been on psychotropic medication before? What are his or her attitudes about those experiences? Have any family members or friends ever been on psychotropic medication? If so, what medications did they take? What are the patient's views about those experiences? How educated is the patient? How much information does the patient want about the effects—good and bad—of psychotropic medications? It is important to inquire about any previous experiences the patient has had with psychotropic medication because these experiences will influence the initial response and attitude about taking medication. Previous experiences may include the patient's own personal treatment, another person's treatment, or something that the patient read or heard about on the Internet.

Does the patient have insurance to pay for a psychiatric evaluation? Patients' financial coverage for medications and therapies vary greatly.

Some policies may cover medications but not therapy, and other policies may do the opposite. In addition, patients may be willing to pay out of pocket for some services but not others. Limits or caps may be placed on medication charges or on the number of psychotherapy sessions allowed. Only certain types of providers may be covered by insurance, that is, only a psychiatrist or only certain types of situations, such as "case management" or "crisis intervention only." Some services might require a primary care physician's referral, even when that physician knows very little about the patient or the problem. Finally, the deductible (the amount the patient must pay initially to obtain the service) can vary, depending on the insurance policy.

Probably the most challenging situation is to provide care for a patient who has no insurance. This often means that the patient is unemployed, between jobs, or has suffered a catastrophic loss. Many ethical issues are embedded in financial decisions about providing care. One way to address these issues is to find out what resources exist in the community for medically indigent patients. If it becomes financially impossible to continue treating a patient, therapists can still remain advocates and consultants in helping the patient find the best possible care he or she can afford—regardless of whether the therapists are compensated for their time. Some examples of this type of financial advocacy include the following:

- Helping an uninsured patient join a clinical trial of a medication so that the care and medication are free (assuming the clinical trial involves medication and/or other treatments that are clinically correct for the patient).
- Keeping a list and business cards of low-fee clinics available in the community.
- Referring a patient to a clinic that provides services for free as long as possible. In the meantime, the therapist educates the patient about obtaining free or low-cost services in the community.

Regardless of the clinic's or practice's financial structure, therapists need to be sensitive to their patients' financial situations. The changing financial landscape of health care and the inequity in reimbursement between physicians and therapists can make this aspect of care challenging. Nevertheless, such care and concern can greatly enhance both the therapeutic relationship and the success of the therapy as a whole.

TOWARD A MEDICATION EVALUATION

There are many reasons that a therapist or patient will consider a medication evaluation (see Table 9.1). Even when one or more indicators are present, therapists at all levels of experience know that getting a patient on the path toward a medication evaluation is not always easy. A patient's decision to follow through with a referral for medication evaluation may be a gradual process rather than a single event.

Some researchers have used the transtheoretical model of behavioral change (TTM; Prochaska, DiClemente, & Norcross, 1995) to look at this decision process (see Table 9.2). The authors of the TTM suggest that change is a process that occurs over time. Instead of viewing patients' reluctance or unwillingness to try something new as "resistance" or "noncompliance," their responses are viewed along a continuum of change. Most people weigh the odds of creating change for some time before they actually begin the behaviors necessary to initiate it. Then, once they make the necessary behavioral changes (e.g., exercise, stop smoking, and eat a healthy diet), they probably won't maintain these changes the first time, or even the first several times, they try.

TABLE 9.1. Indications for Referral for Psychotropic Medication Evaluation

- The patient has a serious illness, such as schizophrenia, bipolar disorder, any psychosis, delusions, hallucinations, or any mental illness with suicidal ideation and/or serious impairment of daily life activities.
- The patient has physical symptoms and behaviors suggestive of medical and psychiatric disorders, such as fatigue, concentration and cognitive difficulties, confusion, memory impairment, sleep and appetite disturbance, panic attacks, and ritualistic behaviors.
- The patient is not getting better or perhaps is getting worse, in spite of therapy.
- There is a marked lability in mood or behavior.
- There is a question about diagnosis.
- There is comorbid substance abuse disorder or other multiple conditions.
- There are prominent physical symptoms.
- There is a family history or previous patient history of serious mental illness.
- The patient or family requests consultation.
- A psychopharmacology question arises.
- A second opinion may help the patient to accept diagnosis and comply with psychotherapy and medication treatment.
- It has been a long time since the person has had a medical examination.

TABLE 9.2. Stages of Change

• Precontemplation:	No intention to take action in the foreseeable future.
• Contemplation:	Intention to change in the next 6 months.
• Preparation:	Intention and plan to change in the next month.
• Action:	Specific, overt modifications made in the last 6 months.
• Maintenance:	Working to prevent relapse.

Note. Data from www.uri.edu/research/cprc/TTM/StagesOfChange

Smokers, for example, usually stop several times (and start smoking again) before they finally stop completely, and over half of the people who start psychotropic medication do not keep using it or do not follow the directions.

Prochaska et al. (1995) define readiness as the patient's willingness to (1) work with the health care provider to decide if medication is a good treatment choice; (2) discuss any concerns he or she has about taking the medication with the physician; and (3) contact the physician if the patient has difficulty in taking the medication. Often, patients are initially only willing to *consider* taking psychotropic medication, not actually to start taking it. A patient's decision to start medication is usually a gradual process. It might begin when the physician mentions the possibility. During the next session, the therapist may offer some reading material or Internet site addresses for the patient to learn more. Finally, several weeks later, the patient may actually decide to start the medication. Again, this ambivalence is not uncommon. In fact, it is a great opportunity for therapists to continue building the therapeutic relationship with patients and family members as they take the time they need to make a decision. It is generally better to wait for patients to think through their options rather than rush to a premature decision. In fact, it is not uncommon to have patients initially refuse medication and later bring up the possibility of a medication trial.

Of course, waiting for patients to make their own decisions does not mean that the therapist or physician cannot voice an opinion. If the therapist knows that evidence-based literature suggests that the patients' problem is best treated with medication (i.e., bipolar disorder or OCD), that information should be given to the patients and their families. The patients should have all the necessary information they need to make an informed decision. Family and friends will also influence a patient's initial decision about trying medication, as well as the willingness to comply with the treatment regimen. Therapists should welcome questions from other people in the patient's life. When a question arises that is not within the therapist's scope of practice or knowledge, he or she should help the patient find a physician who can answer the question. Some patients want to do their own research and should be encouraged to do an Internet search, for example.

ENGAGING PROFESSIONALS IN THE MEDICAL SYSTEM

After the therapist and patient have made the decision to pursue a medication evaluation, it is important to understand the medical culture they are attempting to engage (e.g., psychiatrists vs. family physicians vs. nurse practitioners). They will not just be entering medical culture and departing. They will be inviting other professionals into the treatment system and possibly forming lasting relationships. The following description of medical culture begins with an introduction of the key people and continues in the next chapter with a practical guide for engaging them.

Who Prescribes Medication for Psychiatric Disorders?

In the United States, health care providers are licensed to practice medicine by individual states, and it is physicians who typically prescribe medications. The states of New Mexico and Louisiana have passed legislation granting some psychologists prescriptive authority if they complete certain training, which is currently in development. In many areas, physicians' assistants and nurse practitioners may also prescribe some medications. In the overall category of "physicians" in the United States, there are allopathic physicians (those with a **doctor of medicine**, or MD, degree) and osteopathic physicians (those with a **doctor of osteopathy**, or DO, degree). Although historically they come from different approaches to the practice of medicine, in this era, both MDs and DOs provide excellent general health care for patients; they often train together, and they both take specialty training in psychiatry in the same manner. Both MDs and DOs can prescribe medications for mental health needs. When consulting with any health care provider, it is helpful to understand how he or she relates to others in the larger world of medicine.

Consulting with Physicians in Private Practice

In private practice, a physician may be in solo or group practice or work for a large health care organization, health maintenance organization (HMO), or a government agency such as the health department or a public clinic. Who is consulted will probably depend on what health care insurance (or lack thereof) the patient has. If the patient has HMO coverage, he or she must see the designated physician in that HMO or the cost of care will not be covered. Often, the patient will need to see his or her primary care physician first, and a referral will be given to a psychiatrist only in the case of severe illness. Especially for HMOs and public clinics, cost containment is an ever present factor, and many patients will not receive psychiatry consultation.

Some health care coverage arrangements **carve out** mental health care coverage so that patients cannot receive their mental health care in the same place as their primary medical care. They must go to another group practice, clinic, or agency, and that agency is often given "capitated" funding. This means that they are paid a fixed number of dollars per month for each patient enrolled, regardless of how many patients are seen or how often. To survive, such groups or agencies may be understaffed, and patients may have to wait for an initial appointment, be seen at longer than desirable intervals, and be seen for short visits.

Because, historically, mental health care is not funded on a par with general health care, it is no surprise that approximately 75% of the antidepressants prescribed in the United States are prescribed by nonpsychiatric physicians. Furthermore, as previously mentioned, nonphysicians are being legally granted prescription-writing privileges. So, a therapist may be consulting with a psychiatrist, a primary care physician, and perhaps even a psychologist (depending on the state in which one resides), according to the patient's health care insurance and personal preference. The approach may vary slightly, depending on who is consulted.

Psychiatrists

A psychiatrist has completed 4 years of residency training after medical school (or 5 years for child and adolescent psychiatry or geriatric psychiatry), and the focus of the training is diagnosis and treatment of all mental disorders, including the most complicated, severely ill patients. The psychiatrist should be **board eligible** or **board certified**. Board eligible means that the psychiatrist has completed all training in a satisfactory manner and is in the process of registering, taking, and waiting for the results of the two-tier board certification examination process. The fastest time in which a newly graduated psychiatrist can complete this process is approximately 2 years, so it is not unusual to see younger psychiatrists listed as board eligible. A psychiatrist is board certified after both part I and part II of the specialty examination have been passed, and he or she must recertify (take another examination) every 10 years. Board certification is a quality standard that most psychiatrists, and in fact most physicians of every specialty, aspire to.

Primary Care Physicians:
Three Specialties Make Up the Majority

A pediatrician is a specialist physician who provides health care to children. A pediatric residency training program is 3 years in length, and the pediatrician has had training in childhood development and behavior and in the skills of relating to parents. Most pediatricians are comfortable prescribing medication to children who have ADHD, for example, and some will prescribe antidepressants for children with mild to moderate depression. For more serious illnesses, children and adolescents should be referred to a child and adolescent psychiatrist. It is helpful to start with a referral to the pediatrician or family physician to obtain a general medical evaluation prior to the presumption that the child suffers a mental disorder, as well as to obtain that physician's help in locating a child and adolescent psychiatrist if needed.

An internist is a specialist physician who provides health care to adults. Some internists provide a wide range of primary care, and others limit their practice to metabolic disorders and conditions of organs "between the neck and the navel." The internal medicine residency is 3 years long and does not require training in psychiatry or behavioral health per se; however, many internal medicine residents seek out such training by elective experiences and additional study. Many internists feel comfortable treating their patients who suffer from mild to moderate depression, but most will refer patients with more serious mental health care needs.

Family physicians who are certified by the American Board of Family Medicine and have graduated from a 3-year family medicine residency training program have completed a required curriculum in psychiatry and behavioral health. Most family physicians feel very comfortable prescribing most types of psychotropic medications but will refer patients with severe mental illness to a psychiatrist, at least for initial consultation and management direction.

Other Health Care Professionals Who May Be Part of the Team

The physicians' assistant (PA) has had some graduate school training and has worked in clinical settings under the supervision of a physician. In most states, the PA is licensed as a practice partner with the supervising physician, and whatever the PA does is regarded by the state as an action of the physician, who is fully responsible for the PA's action. A **nurse practitioner (NP)** is an advanced practice nurse who has had graduate school training and supervised practice with either NP faculty or physicians. The states vary concerning the autonomy of the NP's practice, and therapists should be familiar with those regulations if they collaborate with a NP in their practice. The NP and the PA can do an excellent job of primary care and health maintenance for many patients. When there is a question of a general medical condition presenting falsely as a mental illness, either may be able to address this problem; however, it is often preferable to consult a physician, as practitioners vary in their interest and skills in this area.

Registered nurses (RNs) are licensed by the state in which they practice, and they have reached their licensing examination through a 2-year associate degree (community college) program, a diploma nurse (hospital-based, usually 3-year) program, or a college/university-based bachelor of nursing (BSN) degree. After initial licensure as an RN, the nurse may take additional graduate training and specialize in an area, such as certified nurse midwife (CNM), family nurse practitioner (FNP), pediatric nurse practitioner (PNP), or mental health nurse practitioner.

The **licensed vocational nurse (LVN)** or licensed practical nurse (LPN) training varies from state to state, but these nurses have often trained in a community college for less than 2 years or in a professional school for health careers. The **medical assistant (MA)** has typically trained 1 year or less in a community college or private training program. The MA usually works in a private doctor's office or clinic and is considered to be acting as an agent of the physician. The certified nursing assistant (CNA) has often trained for one semester in a community college or private training program and typically works in a hospital or extended care facility under the supervision of licensed nurses.

This rather simplistic overview of the hierarchy of health care practitioners should be helpful to the therapist who calls the private physician's office and hears, "This is Dr. Smith's nurse, may I help you?" That person may be an NP, RN, LVN, or MA. In many offices, the term "nurse" is used broadly. How much you rely on that person's advice may be shaped by your knowledge of his or her training and experience.

Because health care practitioners have varying credentials, experience, and levels of interest in mental health care, it is critical for the therapist to develop a trusting relationship with nearby medical colleagues. This is essential to meet the patient's needs, but it is also essential for the therapist to be taken seriously by the medical professionals. Because in some states, physicians have been held responsible for the therapist's actions when they share patients, some physicians are reluctant to collaborate with therapists of any discipline. Finding a supportive and psychologically minded primary care physician or psychiatrist and developing a relationship of mutual trust and respect are paramount in the care of the therapist's seriously ill patients. Building a relationship with medical colleagues is addressed in more detail in Chapter 10.

Health Care Teams: An Ideal Model

The Institute of Medicine, a prestigious group that influences health policy in the United States, has suggested that primary care teams play a central role in the future of health care. A health care team usually involves a group of health care professionals from different disciplines who are committed to enhanced collaboration, a biopsychosocial model, and continuity of care. They are also committed to sharing care and learning from each other. Usually, the best teams deemphasize the traditional health care hierarchy and stress shared learning and respect for multiple perspectives. We have found that the best treatment teams can be interesting and even inspirational at times.

In a *Journal of the American Medical Association* article, Grumbach and Bodenhemer (2004) suggest that health care teams need to earn "true team status by demonstrating teamwork" (p. 1246). The authors identify five characteristics of strong teams:

1. Clear goals with measurable outcomes.
2. Clinical and administrative systems.
3. Division of labor.
4. Training of all team members.
5. Effective communication.

The authors also point out that health care teams with greater cohesiveness have better clinical outcomes and higher patient satisfaction. On the other hand, if health care teams do not work, it is usually because of problems with relationships and personalities. Thus, it isn't enough to simply find a health care team to join. Therapists have to find a health care team that works, and it helps if they like and respect the team members. Grumbach and Bodenhemer note that teams may include "initiators, clarifiers, or encouragers," as well as "dominators, blockers, evaders, and recognition seekers" (pp. 2–3). When therapists are looking for colleagues with which to build collaborative relationships, they can consider both their credentials and their interpersonal qualities.

Deciding Where to Refer a Patient: Psychiatrist or Primary Care Physician?

Tables 9.3 and 9.4 provide some issues to consider when making a referral. Our general philosophy is that it is important to have contact with the patients' primary care physicians. Should the need arise for a

---

TABLE 9.3. Collaboration with a Primary Care Physician or a Psychiatrist?

Advantages of consulting the primary care physician:
- Can do a more thorough evaluation for general medical conditions and/or drugs that may be causing the psychiatric symptoms.
- Might be more readily available to the patient.
- Might already have a treatment relationship with the patient (trust).
- Might carry less stigma than seeing a psychiatrist, so the patient may actually *go* to the appointment.
- Can manage most of the needs of patients with depression, anxiety disorders, and many other mental illnesses.

Advantages of consulting the psychiatrist:
- Should always be the consult of first choice when the diagnosis is in question.
- Can manage even the most severely ill patient.
- Usually can readily arrange psychiatric hospitalization when needed.
- Usually a better consult choice for the patient with multiple conditions, especially an Axis I disorder, personality disorder, and substance abuse.
- Can help the patient who has forensic mental health care needs or disability evaluation because of mental illness.
- Can clarify diagnosis and care for the most severely ill and/or treatment-resistant patients.
- As a psychotherapist, understands the therapy goals better than a primary care physician.

TABLE 9.4. The Timing of the Referral

Emergent reasons to consult a physician (hospital emergency room, calling 911 for ambulance transport, or calling law enforcement for assistance):
- Patient is suicidal or in danger of harming oneself or others because of mental illness.
- Patient is unable to provide food, clothing, shelter, or safety because of mental illness (in some states, this is called "gravely disabled due to a mental disorder").
- Patient appears very ill and may be medically unstable.

Urgent reasons to consult a physician (same-day or next-day visit):
- Patient's illness is getting significantly worse during therapy.
- Patient has some suicidal thoughts but with no plan or intent.
- Therapist is concerned that a serious metabolic problem is developing (e.g., untreated hypothyroidism, causing depression; untreated diabetes, causing confusion; patient is taking a fluroquinolone antibiotic has developed paranoia and is delusional), and the patient needs urgent medical management of that problem.

Routine reasons to consult a physician (within the next 2 weeks):
- Patient has presented for therapy and has not had a recent physical examination.
- Therapist or patient suspects that medications may be contributing to the mental health problem.
- Therapist or patient suspects that mental symptoms seem to be possibly (or definitely) due to a general medical condition.
- Diagnosis is not clear.
- Patient is improving so slowly with psychotherapy alone that life events are compromised, and medication will probably speed recovery.

psychiatrist, it is ideal to coordinate this referral with the primary care physician, who will have a vested interest in the overall care that is being provided to his or her patients. Whether consulting with a primary care physician or a psychiatrist, it is helpful and sometimes critical for a patient to be examined by the primary care physician first because many general medical conditions can masquerade as mental illness.

If therapists refer a patient to a new primary care physician or a psychiatrist, they should contact the physician's office before giving the patient the referral information to ensure that the physician accepts the patient's insurance plan, is accepting new patients, and has available appointments in the near future. One could take the position that the patient should assume this responsibility. However, anything a therapist can do to minimize barriers to psychiatric care will increase the likelihood that the patient will follow through with a referral and display a positive attitude about its potential. We have seen many patients become exasperated with stalled referral because of provider unavailability and problems with insurance reimbursement.

The patient's insurance plan will often dictate the referral options. Even if the patient pays out of pocket for the therapist's services, he or she is unlikely to pay privately for medication evaluation and management. Physician charges are usually more expensive than psychotherapy charges, and appointments with physicians—regardless of whether they are psychiatrists or primary care doctors—are usually paid for by the patient's insurance. Thus, a therapist can usually start the referral process by asking whether the patient has previously seen a primary care physician or psychiatrist whose fees are paid by the patient's insurance. If the patient is comfortable with Dr. X, and the therapist is comfortable with Dr. X, the initial referral decision is made.

Factors that may confound this decision include (1) the match among the patient's preference, the therapist's preference, and the availability of a psychiatrist versus a primary care doctor; (2) differences in the ease of referral, cost, and waiting time for a first appointment; (3) the degree of flexibility of choice the patient's insurance offers; and (4) the influence of preexisting professional relationships that either the therapist or the patient has with specific physicians.

At times, patients want therapists to choose the physician they will see. If their insurance allows that freedom, we are happy to comply. We maintain relationships with different types of physicians, each with different strengths. At times, two psychiatrists may be equally qualified but have different areas of expertise. We hope that our patients benefit from our detailed knowledge of possible referral sources. We try to match the patient with the physician by thinking about the personality of the patient and the physician's interview style. In addition, we often offer to call our colleague, to say that we are sending a specific patient. We hope that this process communicates to the patients that they can expect the same kind of caring, professional behavior from our respected colleague that they have come to expect from us. We find that these personal relationships provide a safe, calm context in which patients can consider their treatment options.

WRITING THE REFERRAL LETTER:
THREE DIFFERENT APPROACHES

After confirming the physician's availability, the therapist can then begin to prepare a referral letter. The type of letter will depend on the audience: a psychiatrist; a primary care physician; or the emergency screening-unit clinician, who may be an MD, nurse, social worker, or psychologist. Regardless of the audience, it is very important to use a professional tone when writing a psychopharmacology consultation request.

When writing anything about a patient, always assume two things will happen: First, assume the patient—who often has a legal right to do so—will read the letter. The written word should contain the truth but be conveyed in a respectful manner, so that if the patient reads it, he or she will not be embarrassed or offended. Second, assume that a plaintiff's attorney will ask the therapist to read his or her written record aloud in front of a court, so the notes must be comprehensive and respectful of the patient.

As obvious and unnecessary as this advice may sound, it is not rare to see a note that is too informal for the task. Sample letter 1 is such a letter (see Figure 9.1). It is too short, too folksy, and too familiar, with the therapist referring to both the patient and the doctor on a first-name basis. Also, it refers to another patient in the same letter. If the patient reads it, he or she would probably see it as something written by a friend rather than a therapist. If it were ever brought to court for any reason, it would seriously undermine the credibility of the therapist in the eyes of a judge and jury.

Sample letter 2 (see Figure 9.2) is written to a family physician, and a similar tone would be appropriate for other primary care physicians. The first paragraph presents an introduction and explains why the referral is coming to Dr. Smith; that is, it explains the relationships. The second paragraph states the target symptoms in sufficient, but not excessive, detail and covers the question of suicide. The third paragraph asks for the consulting note, states support of medication, and offers collaboration. It does not say that the therapist will continue to see the patient, as the family physician will assume this to be the case, but it would be a good idea to say it anyway.

Sample letter 3 (see Figure 9.3) is written to a psychiatrist. The first paragraph tells how long and for how many sessions the therapist has seen the patient and what psychotherapeutic approach has been used. It also says in the first paragraph that this is a psychopharmacology con-

John Doe, MFT
123 Anywhere Street
Some Town, USA 00000
January 5, 2006

Jane Friend, MD
156 Anywhere Street
Some Town, USA 00000

Dear Jane:

I am sending over Susan Jones for meds. I've seen Suzy a half dozen times or so and I think she's not getting anywhere. I have a release (copy attached). Suzy's depressed and has PTSD, and I'll keep seeing her for therapy. No drugs, no suicidal stuff. She'll probably do well with some Prozac. Let me know if you have any questions.

By the way, I sent Frank to see you last month, and he's doing great!

Thanks.

Johnny

FIGURE 9.1. Sample letter 1: too informal.

sultation, and not a referral for the psychiatrist to assume care entirely. The second paragraph provides details, but more concisely than to the family physician. The psychiatrist will be getting these pieces of history from the patient directly, whereas the family physician may not seek all of them herself. The question of suicidal assessment is covered. The third paragraph requests a copy of the consultation note, expresses support for medication, offers collaboration, and also makes it very clear that the therapist intends to continue to see this patient. This is important to state clearly, lest the psychiatrist assume that the referral is intended to transfer psychotherapeutic care, as well as psychopharmacological care. It would also be appropriate to state the assessment of the patient in DSM Multiaxial Classification System, in the letter to the psychiatrist if desired, but this is not essential in most instances.

Sample letter 4 (see Figure 9.4) is written to a mental health care professional who is acting as the screening clinician in the psychiatric emergency department of the county mental hospital. There is no mention of a release of information or consent from the patient, allowing the therapist and screening clinician to speak to each other. It would be good

John Doe, MFT
123 Anywhere Street
Some Town, USA 00000
January 5, 2006

Mary Smith, MD
Family Medicine Center
344 Anywhere Street
Some Town, USA 00000

Dear Dr. Smith:

I am the therapist for Ms. Susan Jones, a 34-year-old woman who receives her primary medical care in your office. Ms. Jones has signed a consent form to allow us to share information about her care (copy enclosed). I have seen Ms. Jones for five sessions in the last month, and I have asked her to make an appointment to see you as soon as possible because I am concerned about her worsening depression.

Ms. Jones has experienced the following symptoms for the last 3 months: insomnia (she can get to sleep okay but wakes up at 3 A.M. and cannot get back to sleep), poor appetite (10-pound weight loss without trying), feels tired all the time, has difficulty getting work done on time because it's hard to keep focused on her work, and has lost several work days because of fatigue and tearfulness. Ms. Jones has a history of a major depressive episode 10 years ago that was not treated, and she blames it for the loss of her job at the time. She also has a history of sexual abuse as a child; she has nightmares about it, startles easily, and sometimes has dissociative episodes when she feels that someone is getting angry at her. Ms. Jones says that she thinks of suicide occasionally but has no plan to act on that because she is aware of the pain that would bring to her family. She has no history of suicide attempts in the past and no history of substance abuse. My working diagnosis is major depression and PTSD.

I would appreciate receiving a copy of your evaluation note regarding Ms. Jones, and I would like to know about any medications chosen, as well as the doses and your follow-up instructions, so that I can help Ms. Jones to comply with the medication you have prescribed for her. Please feel free to call me if I can provide any further assistance, and I look forward to collaborating with you in the care of our mutual patient, Ms. Susan Jones.

Sincerely,

John Doe, MFT

FIGURE 9.2. Sample letter 2: to a family physician.

John Doe, MFT
123 Anywhere Street
Some Town, USA 00000
January 5, 2006

John Adams, MD
Psychiatric Associates of Some Town
443 Anywhere Street
Some Town, USA 00000

Dear Dr. Adams:

I am referring to you Ms. Susan Jones, whom I have seen for five cognitive-behavioral therapy sessions in the last month. I believe she will benefit from a psychopharmacology consultation at this time because we have noted that her depression has increased in severity, in spite of therapy. Ms. Jones has signed a consent for us to share information about her care (copy enclosed). I hope that you will be able to see her within the next 3 or 4 days.

Ms. Jones is a 34-year-old divorced woman who has experienced the following symptoms for the last 3 months: insomnia with early morning awakening, poor appetite (10-pound weight loss without trying), fatigue, and difficulty in concentrating on her work; she has lost several work days because of fatigue and tearfulness. Ms. Jones has a history of a major depressive episode 10 years ago that was not treated, and she blames it for the loss of her job at the time. She also has a history of sexual abuse as a child; she has nightmares about it, startles easily, and sometimes has dissociative episodes when she feels that someone is getting angry at her. Ms. Jones says that she thinks of suicide occasionally but has no plan to act on that because she is aware of the pain it would bring to her family. She has no history of suicide attempts in the past and no history of substance abuse. My working diagnosis is major depression and PTSD.

I would appreciate receiving a copy of your consultation note regarding Ms. Jones, and I would like to know about any medications chosen, as well as the doses and your follow-up instructions, so that I can help Ms. Jones to comply with the medication you have prescribed for her. I plan to continue to see her weekly for therapy. Please feel free to call me if I can provide any further information, and I look forward to collaborating with you in the care of our mutual patient, Ms. Susan Jones.

Sincerely,

John Doe, MFT

FIGURE 9.3. Sample letter 3: to a psychiatrist.

John Doe, MFT
123 Anywhere Street
Some Town, USA 00000
January 5, 2006

Jane Worker, LCSW
Psychiatric Emergency Department
Some County Psychiatric Hospital
156800 Anywhere Street
Some Town, USA 00000

Dear Ms. Worker:

I am referring to you Ms. Susan Jones, whom I have seen for five therapy sessions in the last month. I believe she is in need of hospitalization today because she has suicidal ideation with a clear plan and intent to carry it out. Ms. Jones is coming to see you voluntarily, but I am so concerned about her risk of suicide that I feel she should be hospitalized on an involuntary basis if she declines care at this time.

Ms. Jones is a 34-year-old married woman who has experienced progressively worsening symptoms for the last 3 months, including insomnia, poor appetite (10-pound weight loss without trying), fatigue, and difficulty in concentrating on her work; she has lost several work days because of fatigue and tearfulness. Ms. Jones has a history of major depression 10 years ago that was not treated; she blames it for the loss of her job at the time, and then she made a serious suicide attempt by drug overdose, resulting in several days in the intensive care unit of the hospital. She also has a history of sexual abuse as a child; she has nightmares about it, startles easily, and sometimes has dissociative episodes when she feels that someone is getting angry at her. Ms. Jones says that she thinks of suicide often and has recently purchased a gun, which she keeps loaded in her bedroom. She states that since the drug overdose did not kill her, she will "be sure to do it right this time." Her husband recently left her, her job is in jeopardy, and she feels that she has nothing to live for. Because of the severity of her symptoms, her recent and pending losses, her prior history of a suicide attempt, and her current clear plans, I feel that Ms. Jones needs emergency psychiatric hospitalization at this time.

I would appreciate receiving a copy of your evaluation note regarding Ms. Jones, and I will resume her care, in collaboration with a psychiatrist, after her hospital discharge. Please feel free to call me if I can provide any further information, and thank you for your urgent attention to the needs of Ms. Susan Jones.

Sincerely,

John Doe, MFT

FIGURE 9.4. Sample letter 4: to a screening professional in psychiatric emergency department.

to have consent, of course, but in most states this is not required in such an emergency. In most locales, public hospitals have only a fraction of the number of beds that the community needs to be allocated to the seriously and acutely mentally ill. The staffs are typically hard working, spread too thin, underpaid, and caring for the community's most ill patients. Therefore, unless the screening clinician is convinced that the patient is an imminent danger to oneself and/or others because of the mental disorder, the patient is not seen by the psychiatrist and is not admitted to the hospital. So, if the therapist has a patient who is severely ill and in dire need of admission to a psychiatric hospital, it is essential to convince the screening clinician of the seriousness of the situation—and in one page. Letter 4 presents compelling details concisely and states the opinion that the patient should be involuntarily admitted if necessary, but it does so in a way that does not insult or undermine the decision making of the screening clinician. Also, the letter states that the therapist will be available for follow-up care after hospital discharge. This is very important, as many hospitals feel that seriously ill patients are "dumped" by therapists when treatment has not gone well.

The detail and style of referral letters should be appropriate to the person to whom they are addressed (e.g., the language for the family physician is a little different from that for the psychiatrist; see Table 9.5). They should be absolutely professional and empathic in tone and, if pos-

TABLE 9.5. The Language of the Referral

After you make a referral, the terminology for the timing of the appointment will vary from one community to another. Some examples follow:

- *Routine*—the patient will be seen at the next routinely available appointment, which may be soon or may not occur for 2 months or more.
- *2-week rule*—if mental health clinic patients have to wait more than 2 weeks for their first visit, the probability that they will show up for the appointment approaches zero.
- *Urgent*—should be seen within approximately 72 hours.
- *Emergency/today*—should be seen today; may be referred to a physician's office.
- *Emergency/hospitalize*—often referred to the psychiatric emergency room or community hospital emergency department.
- *Emergency 911*—the patient is severely ill, threatening harm to him- or herself or others and refuses treatment. In many states, the police are called, and they take the patient to a hospital for emergency evaluation and treatment.

sible, no longer than one page. If the patient is very complex or if there are copious data from psychological testing, for example, then there should be a cover letter of one page and an attached copy of the psychological testing report. A copy of the patient's consent to release information should also be included.

THE MEDICATION EVALUATION

Most physicians today are on a professional treadmill. Their employer requires a certain number of patients to be seen per day, regardless of the nature of the patients' needs. Even if the physician is in private practice, it takes a certain (often large) number of patients per day just to pay the overhead. On average and by specialty, the lowest paid physicians in the United States are pediatricians, psychiatrists, and family physicians, so there is little room to maneuver more time per patient. Because a patient is probably happy with the pace and generous time allotment for therapy sessions, it is important to prepare him or her for the often chaotic pace of medicine.

The psychiatrist may have anywhere from 30–50 minutes for an initial evaluation, whereas the primary care physician will probably have 15–30 minutes for the first visit. Both of them will probably have about 15 minutes for follow-up visits, sometimes less. Visits are often rushed, and any patient can look like *anything* for an hour. Patients can look healthy when they are psychotic, they can look happy when they are depressed and suicidal, they can successfully sublimate personality-disordered behavior, and they can (and usually do) hide substance abuse disorders. Whomever is chosen, it is critical to communicate the reasons for referral; never assume that the presenting problem or diagnosis will be obvious in the visit with the physician.

The physician will take a medical history and perform a physical examination. The details of the mental status examination will be greater from a psychiatrist than a primary care physician, and the primary care physician will probably conduct a more thorough physical examination than most psychiatrists. In common, their consultations will usually include the elements in Table 9.6.

Ideally, the therapist will receive a consultation note from the physician, and, if not, he or she should request one if the patient consents. This note is likely to contain the elements listed in Table 9.6 for the first visit only. Follow-up psychotropic medication visits should usually include the following:

TABLE 9.6. Elements of a Basic Medical Initial Diagnostic Evaluation

- **Chief complaint (CC):** the presenting problem that brings the patient to care.
- **History of present illness (HPI):** "The patient was in his or her usual state of health until . . . "; the rest of this paragraph describes the onset of the presenting problem.
- **Past psychiatric history (PPH):** a listing of prior episodes of mental illness, treatment, hospitalizations.
- **Past medical history (PMH):** a listing of significant medical conditions, treatment, hospitalizations.
- **Current medications (meds):** a listing of names, doses, duration of treatment, reason for their use—for example, "HCTZ 25 mg qd [once a day] × 5 years for HTN [hypertension]."
- **Allergies:** particularly to medications.
- **Substances used:** smoking, alcohol, recreational drugs.
- **Family history:** medical and psychiatric.
- **Social history:** living situation, occupation, education, recreational activities, and so on.
- **Review of systems (ROS):** questions asked about each organ system of the body, head to toe.
- **Mental status exam (MSE):** extent of detail varies from psychiatrist to primary care physician.
- Other medical examinations and report of diagnostic test results, if appropriate.
- Psychiatrists may obtain additional or a more detailed history regarding development, relationships, sexual and legal issues, disruptive behavior, and other psychiatric issues.
- **Assessment or diagnosis:** Psychiatrists will use the *Diagnostic and Statistical Manual of Mental Disorders* (DSM) five-axis format, but primary care physicians will usually just list the diagnoses.
- **Plan:** usually includes diagnostic tests as indicated, medications prescribed, referrals written, and follow-up plans; if medication is prescribed, this section often refers to the informed consent that was obtained.

- Patient education regarding illness.
- Medication benefits and side effects, including informed consent.
- Information regarding therapy options, including no medication.
- Planning, adjustments, encouragement.
- Tracking efficacy/necessity of treatment (target symptoms/behaviors).
- "Support."

During both the initial and follow-up visits, the physician's priorities in the crush of the time allowed for the visit include the following:

- Is this patient going to die before he or she even gets back here?
- What medical conditions does this patient have that, although not fatal before the next visit, are critical to manage now?
- What health maintenance matters need to be taken care of (for the patient's benefit and/or to avoid penalty from the HMO)?
- Does the reason for referral fit into one of the first two categories? If it does not, and if there are pressing needs in those areas, then the reason for referral may be only partly addressed.

How Does the Physician Decide Which Medication to Use within a Class?

Psychiatric diagnosis is occasionally obvious, but it is always a work in progress. Some patients clearly have psychosis, and their behavior may indicate that they are suffering from schizophrenia—until the UDS comes back positive for amphetamines, revealing that the underlying problem is amphetamine-induced psychosis. Some people have such obvious depression that everyone around them knows that the diagnosis is major depression. But then, the major depression is only major depression until the patient's first manic episode, which prompts the therapist or the physician to change the diagnosis to bipolar disorder. We have to make the best diagnoses we can make, given the information we have. However, the diagnosis does not dictate what the treatment will be. Treatment is based on many interwoven factors, some of which are described in Table 9.7.

What Are the Criteria for an Adequate Trial of a Psychotropic Medication?

- Accurate diagnosis and/or tracking of target symptoms.
- Appropriate medication class for the target symptom.
- Adequate dose and duration—with particular attention to the variations in the dose and the longer duration of treatment typically required for seniors.
- Monitoring plasma and blood levels of the drug, if indicated, to ensure therapeutic levels and compliance with medication.
- Supporting the patient's compliance with treatment; anticipat-

TABLE 9.7. Some of the Interwoven Factors That Dictate Which Medication within a Class Will Be Used to Treat a Patient for a Given Illness

• *What are the target symptoms and problems that are interfering with the person's life?* Hallucinations may be a target symptom and also one of the elements of the diagnosis; but even if the diagnosis changes from schizophrenia to drug-induced psychosis or to psychosis due to a general medical condition, the target symptom remains the same—hallucinations. Other examples of target symptoms include crying spells, poor concentration, poor appetite, insomnia, anger outbursts, and threatening behavior. The target symptoms are what we want to treat and follow, regardless of the diagnosis.

• *What other medical conditions does the patient have?* Choosing an antidepressant for a healthy young adult may lead to a different choice than an antidepressant for a man in his 60s with diabetes, hypertension, glaucoma, and prostatism. Some psychotropic medications can make the symptoms of other medical conditions worse.

• *What other illness might the patient have that has not yet been diagnosed and may be causing the target symptoms?* For example, thyroid disease more often presents for the first time in a mental health clinic than in primary care, usually as depression or an anxiety disorder. Severe vitamin B_{12} deficiency can cause serious neurological symptoms, including depression, psychosis, and dementia. (This is not due to a poor diet, and vitamin tablets will not help.) A person who has unknowingly been infected with syphilis for decades can present with mental symptoms, and a significant minority of HIV-infected patients (human immunodeficiency, or AIDS, virus) will present with mental symptoms as the very first manifestation of illness. There are many other medical disorders that can masquerade as a mental illness.

• *What medications must the patient take for other medical conditions?* Psychotropic drugs very often have interactions with other medications. Physicians must check for adverse drug–drug interactions before prescribing. When it looks as if an adverse interaction might occur, the physician must change some medication in order to avoid the problem. Also, the prescribing physician must be ready to manage the consequences of unforeseen adverse interactions, which are not rare.

• *What medications have worked for this patient (or for family members with a similar condition) in the past?*

• *What side-effect profile is most desirable for this patient?* All medications have side effects. If the patient is having trouble sleeping, a medication that causes drowsiness and is taken at bedtime might be preferred.

• *If the first medication did not work or was not tolerated, what were the problems?* Knowing the problems with the first medication will help dictate the next one to be tried.

• *Does the patient have a preference for a particular medication?* Media advertisements for medications may convince the patient that a particular drug is the only one that will work. Although this is rarely if ever the case, going against that conviction may doom the treatment to failure.

(continued)

TABLE 9.7. *(continued)*

• *Is the patient restricted to a particular formulary (list of drugs) by his or her insurance plan or HMO?* Prescribing outside of the formulary can sometimes occur, but it may require the patient to pay full cost for the drug. When many medications cost at least $1.00–$2.00 per pill (and some psychotropic medications cost $8.00 or more per pill), and one might take several pills per day, the cost may be prohibitive; thus staying within the formulary may be the only treatment available.

• *How does the patient respond to the informed consent procedure?* All medications have risks and benefits. The only reason to use them is if the benefits outweigh the risks, and this requires predicting the outcome when the drug is first started. Some patients cannot tolerate the uncertainty; they become too anxious and are not able to proceed with a medication trial.

• *Is the patient taking the medication voluntarily or under the order of a guardian/conservator or court?* States have different laws concerning involuntary treatment of those who have a serious mental illness, often presenting a danger to themselves and others, but refuse treatment. The therapist should become familiar with the laws in his or her state. Often the choice of medication is shaped by the degree of cooperation from the patient. For example, a psychotic patient who is being treated voluntarily may be given risperidone pills or oral solution, a modern antipsychotic with relatively fewer side effects. However, a patient who refuses to take medication orally might be cared for by administering long-acting, intramuscular injections of antipsychotic medication (for example, haldol decanoate, fluphenazine decanoate, Risperdal Consta, or paliperidone (Invega Sustenna), even if these may have more potential adverse effects.

---

ing and asking about side effects since this is a major reason that patients stop medications, often without discussing it with their physician or therapist. Patients rarely volunteer information about sexual side effects, a major reason for stopping medication prematurely.

AFTER THE PATIENT STARTS MEDICATION

The research literature on adherence to treatment suggests that the degree to which a patient agrees with a health care decision strongly influences his or her adherence to the treatment regimen. The patient's agreement is especially important when there are challenges and difficulties along the way. Patients often experience the negative side effects of medications before they experience the symptom relief that the medications offer. In addition, there is a "Black Box Warning" on all antidepressant medications prescribed in the United Sates (as well as on some other psychotropic medications) that warns the patient about the possibility of emerging suicidal ideation, especially during the early days of treatment. Patients should be followed very closely during those early days of treatment, to monitor for this very rare but critically important issue. If a therapist has allowed the patients to make the decision about medication themselves in their own time, they are more likely to persevere during this early period.

If we view the decision to take medications as a process, we will not be surprised if, after having decided to begin medication, the patient or a member of the family complains or questions the value of the medication during the first few weeks of treatment. Because it often takes up to 6 weeks for the positive effects of medications to be felt, this early period is a critical time. The patient is waiting for symptom relief but is experiencing some *negative* effects. Patients may complain of feeling dizzy or "spacey," being tired, having trouble sleeping, and having no appetite.

They may wonder aloud whether it is worth the time and expense to take the medication. They may be fearful about how the medication is affecting their bodies. They also worry that they will have to be on medication their entire lives or that they will be the exceptions for whom the medications won't work. If they have kept their decision to try medication a secret, they may worry that their families and friends may find the medication bottles.

It is common for patients initially to experience a change in self-identity. Our culture values the "rugged individual" who can "pull himself up by his bootstraps." Patients may worry that it is a sign of weakness or disability to try medication for an invisible problem. Other patients may express concerns about the cost of medication and wonder how they can afford to pay for it.

Continuing Medications during Therapy

The decision to start medication is only the first step. Issues and questions about the medications often arise in the course of therapy. The therapist's response to these questions may vary, depending on (1) the therapist's scope of knowledge, (2) the proximity and frequency of interaction that the therapist has with the prescribing physician, (3) the severity of the patient's symptoms or responses to medications, and (4) the patient's wishes and attitudes.

In Chapter 10, we discuss how to collaborate with physicians when they are treating patients who are taking psychotropic medications. Therapists face many of these challenging situations because they often see their shared patients more often than the physician sees them. In addition, it is sometimes easier to get an appointment or have a phone conversation with a therapist than with a physician—simply because the physician often has double or even triple the number of patients that a typical therapist sees in a day. Nevertheless, even when it is difficult for the patient (or the therapist) to reach the physician, the therapist must continue to affirm, both verbally and by his or her behavior, that the physician is in charge of prescribing medications and that the patient must consult the physician about treatment changes, including evaluating side effects, changing doses, or discontinuing medication.

We listen carefully as our patients talk about their medications. They seldom want to spend more than 5 or 10 minutes discussing medication issues. Instead, they want to continue working on their therapeutic issues. However, our support and willingness to answer the appropriate questions, find answers to other questions, and help contact their physician for their biomedical questions can make the difference in whether they maintain their medications during the first few difficult weeks or stop taking them before they have experienced the positive and healing effects.

CHAPTER 10

Sharing Care

BUILDING SUCCESSFUL
COLLABORATIVE RELATIONSHIPS

Dr. R, a family physician, is seeing a patient, Mrs. C, who complains of depressed mood, low energy, and decreased appetite. Dr. R prescribed an SSRI, but Mrs. C stopped it after only 2 weeks because she felt "too jittery." Dr. R decides to refer Mrs. C to Dr. W, a family therapist, for further assessment and treatment. Mrs. C had been diagnosed with bipolar disorder many years ago and had seen a psychiatrist, who prescribed medication for the bipolar disorder. She had stopped taking the medication when her symptoms seemed to improve. Mrs. C has not seen a psychiatrist in 2 years. Dr. W's assessment of Mrs. C's depression uncovers a clear pattern: Her bouts with depression typically occur between December and May, followed by manic-like symptoms between June and November. This initial interview is taking place in April, and Mrs. C predicts that her depression will lift in a few weeks. In the second interview, Mrs. C's husband provides another perspective on this cycle of depression and mania: Although he worries about her during the depression cycle, she is more predictable then than during the manic cycle. As predicted, when Mr. and Mrs. C arrive for their third meeting in May with Dr. R, the depression has lifted. Mrs. C reports feeling energetic and enthusiastic about reconnecting with friends and family she has been distancing herself from during her depression. Although Mrs. C is relieved that the depression has dissipated, both Mr. C and Dr. W are concerned about what appears to be mania, evidenced by little sleep, spending binges at the mall, and a general anxious appearance. Dr. W wants to discuss these concerns with Dr. R and ask if a referral to a psychiatrist is warranted, considering the history of her illness and current disconnection from a psychiatrist. Dr. W, who is afraid that Dr. R might take offense by the inclusion of a specialist, asks the question about a psychiatric evaluation with some trepidation. Will Dr. R think Dr. W is disrespectfully questioning her ability to offer ongoing mental health care to Mrs. C? If Dr. R agrees to a psychiatric evaluation, Dr. W wonders, will the three health care professionals be able to work together in an effective way, or will there be disagreements? How will the professionals communicate, with Drs. W and R in one location and the psychiatrist in another? Will Mr. and Mrs. C be overwhelmed by the addition of another physician?

THE NEW ROLE OF COLLABORATOR: ESSENTIAL SKILLS

In our roles as educators, we have noticed that there is little guidance for therapists interested in answering the questions above. Instead, most students are busy learning the language, skills, and paradigm of their own discipline. To collaborate successfully with physicians, including psychiatric physicians, most therapists will have to relinquish some ideas they learned in training and embrace new ideas and skills. However, many skills that therapists already possess in their work with patients can be transferred to their collaborative work with other professionals. This chapter identifies the essential skills for collaboration (McDaniel, Hepworth, & Doherty, 1992; Seaburn et al., 1996).

Redefine the Role

Successful collaboration often demands a shift in attitude. Patterson, Peek, Heinrich, Bishoff, and Scherger (2002) summarize the differences between viewing oneself as a traditional mental health specialist and as a member of a collaborative team (see Table 10.1). In general, the therapist relinquishes the role of expert on the mental health and emotions of a shared patient and instead embraces a more holistic view of the patient's problems—medical and mental health. In this model, the thera-

TABLE 10.1. Traditional and Integrated Behavioral Health: A Contrast in Focus and Purpose

Behavioral health as a specialty (traditional mental health)	Behavioral health integrated into medical care (integrated mental health)

Professional model

Behavioral health as a specialty service for referral and consultation.	Behavioral health services integrated into medical care (mental health provider as a member of a medical team).

Clinical focus

Mental health care	Medical and all health care

Mental health care	Medical and all health care
• Separate mental health problems. • Considered the mental health care plan. • Care of mental illnesses and conditions such as • Major mental illness and chemical dependency • Diagnosable mental health conditions • Specialty treatment groups and programs • Hospital, day treatment • Psychiatric emergency, triage • Evaluation for any mental health–related complaint • Coordination with medical care, nursing homes, other venues for care	• Intertwined medical and mental health problems. • Considered part of medical care plan. • Psychological aspects of care for any illness or complaint, such as • Common depression and anxiety, comorbidity • Somatic symptoms, psychophysiological symptoms • Rehabilitation, back to work • Complex cases, "thick charts," difficult patients • Family distress that complicates medical care • Chronic illnesses of all kinds • Adjustment to illness, adherence to treatment • Evaluation and referral for any mental health–related complaint, even if not appropriate for follow-up care in medical setting • Coordination with specialty mental health care, hospital, nursing homes, other care venues

Patient view

• Patient sees it as "mental health care." • Patient expects exclusive relationship with little coordination or information sharing. • Patient self-refers for mental health care or comes to treatment via a referral.	• Patient sees it as "health care." • Patient expects team-based medical coordination and information sharing. • Patient can call in for medical and mental health care.

(continued)

TABLE 10.1. *(continued)*

Behavioral health as a specialty (traditional mental health)	Behavioral health integrated into medical care (integrated mental health)
Offices and working culture	
• Mental health clinic space and therapy offices. • Mental health chart. • Mental health clinic systems and support staff. • Culture of traditional mental health clinic and professions.	• Medical clinic space and exam rooms. • Medical chart or quick access to therapist notes. • Medical clinic systems and support staff. • Culture of medical clinic and professions.
Covered benefits and financing	
• Care limited to diagnosable and covered mental health conditions, as per patient's mental health insurance coverage. • Considered part of mental health costs; another referral specialty.	• Care of any covered health care condition, regardless of mental health insurance coverage. • Considered a part of medical costs; a member of the in-house medical team.

Note. Reprinted from Patterson et al. (2002). Copyright 2002 by Norton. Reprinted by permission.

pist acknowledges that all areas related to health are inextricably intertwined. In redefining one's role as a therapist who collaborates with other professionals, a therapist will probably have to make some basic changes in the way he or she works. Some possible changes are listed in Table 10.2.

We realize the process implied in these changes can take more time, thought, and energy than simply telling the patient to "go see your doctor for medication." But we believe this initial extra time can lead to better patient care and more fulfilling clinical work. It also gives the therapist the chance to learn knowledge outside of the usual discipline. To that end, it is important to reiterate that effective collaboration often requires concise, specific, and to-the-point communication with the physician. Furthermore, consultations are often brief (e.g., phone calls and hallway discussions between patients), in keeping with the often fast-paced primary care setting and contrary to the more traditional consultation parameters to which many therapists are accustomed. Ultimately, working collaboratively will save time because of the streamlined process established with the physician.

TABLE 10.2. Tips for Working with Physicians

- Become more succinct, use less theoretical jargon, and talk about your patients' symptoms such as loss of sleep or change in appetite.
- Respond quickly to any initiatives to communicate that the physician makes and initiate the exchange of information with the physician (within the confines of medical confidentiality).
- Accept all "comers." We have noticed that physicians often enthusiastically refer their most difficult, challenging patients to us once they have confidence in our work.
- Accept the patient's and physician's conceptualization of the problem and the referral. Try to use the patient's language when you are describing the problem, not your traditional mental health language.
- Align with the patients' strengths, including their reasons for not needing therapy or medication.
- Help the patient identify social support. Think about the patient's social system, not just the patient. Enlist the family, friends, or medical team in the treatment.
- If you work in an integrated, on-site system, put yourself in the traffic pattern of the clinic, where staff and physicians are constantly running into you.
- Understand and accept the fact that the financial constraints and administrative concerns are as important and influential as the clinical concerns. For example, if the patients' potential medication is not on their formulary they may not be able to obtain it.

Note. Physicians also have to make changes to effectively collaborate. But here our focus is on the changes that therapists must make. Data from Patterson et al. (2002).

Become Culturally Competent

Therapists train and practice in a world that is very different from that of physicians. Because therapists' contact with physicians is often limited, they rarely have opportunities to immerse themselves in the culture of medicine in order to learn about the roles, customs, and beliefs of its members. Just as it is important to be culturally competent with patients from ethnically diverse backgrounds, knowledge of and appreciation for medical culture is also helpful and can strengthen collaborative relationships.

Therapists are sometimes discouraged from pursuing collaboration with primary care physicians who are intimidating or unresponsive (e.g., by failing to return a phone call). Therapists' negative beliefs about physicians and medication can also contribute to a lack of collaboration.

These negative beliefs are formed by stereotypes of physicians, particularly psychiatrists, as "controlling," "egotistical," and "reductionistic." Physicians carry their own stereotypes of therapist, viewing them as too "touchy-feely," "flaky," and "cerebral" (McDaniel, Campbell, & Seaburn, 1995). Although there may be a grain of truth in these stereotypes, believing them will interfere with your ability to form a relationship with other professionals.

The Culture of Primary Care

There are very real differences between the medical cultures of mental health and primary care. As mentioned in the previous chapter, physicians are under severe time constraints, which should be respected. For example, telephone conversations with physicians rarely last longer than 5 minutes without interfering with the physician's responsibilities for patient care. A physician may appreciate a two- or three-sentence note or e-mail, providing a brief update on a patient, rather than having to find time to return a phone call.

Another cultural difference is how therapists and primary physicians view patient responsibility. Because physicians' greatest fear is missing something potentially life threatening, they are loyal to the adage "Don't just stand there, do something" (Bray & Rogers, 1997). Physicians take a tremendous amount of responsibility for their patients' well-being and in facilitating change in their patients' behavior. In contrast, therapists are often trained in the adage "Don't just do something, stand there" (Bray & Rogers, 1997). That is, therapists often place responsibility for change on the shoulders of their patients. This difference can create conflict between therapists and physicians when, for example, physicians expect therapists to intervene more aggressively with patients or when therapists expect physicians to listen to their patients concerns about medication side effects rather than just changing the medication. Recognizing and appreciating the different roles therapists and physicians play can be a helpful step in working collaboratively.

Finally, therapists and primary care physicians have different approaches to confidentiality. Sometimes there are signs in the elevators of hospitals or medical offices reminding physicians to maintain patient confidentiality. Whereas primary care physicians routinely and informally discuss patients with one another, therapists view patient information as sacred. One of the biggest complaints physicians have about therapists is their protectiveness of information, which at times can dramatically impede collaboration.

If a therapist and physician are located in different settings, a signed release of information will allow them to communicate. In addition, a conversation about the boundaries of disclosure with the patient and the family avoids misunderstandings that could later lead to problems. For example, a patient may not want a history of sexual abuse to be discussed with other members of the treatment team.

For professionals who work in the same setting, the rules around confidentiality are less clear, particularly when patient charts contain both medical and mental health notes. Treatment teams in the same setting could assume that a free exchange of information is allowed and necessary. We agree, but we also believe that making this policy explicit to the patient and family is important. Case notes are especially vulnerable to mishandling. For example, there is always a chance that mental health notes that are part of the medical record could be unintentionally released to a third party. If expectations are communicated and understood among the patient, family, therapist, and physicians, confidentiality need not impede collaboration (see Tables 10.3 and 10.4). Furthermore, collaboration need not violate confidentiality.

The Culture of Psychiatry

Many characteristics of primary care are equally true of psychiatry. Primary care doctors and psychiatrists both go to medical school and train in general medicine during their internships. However, after their internships, doctors in different specialties become increasingly focused on their particular area of expertise.

TABLE 10.3. What the Physician Needs from the Therapist

- Obtain proper release of information and consent to share information from patient prior to contact (unless dire emergency).
- Present patient history with appropriate degree of detail . . . and *target symptoms*.
- Present specific questions or problems that prompted the consultation request.
- Leave the practice of medicine to the physician. Most physicians do not appreciate a referral such as "I'm sending you this patient to get him started on Prozac . . . " (or any other named medication). However, some physicians, especially those who have had limited training in mental health care, do appreciate the therapist's suggestion. Learn who does and does not.
- Keep apprised of medication treatment and support it.

TABLE 10.4. What the Therapist Should Receive from the Physician

- Access/availability—especially emergency contact procedure.
- Consultation/collaboration.
- Information about medications used (to support treatment and help the patient understand and cope with side effects).

Since the 1970s, the culture of psychiatry has become increasingly focused on the science of the brain and on psychopharmacology. During the last 50 years, psychiatry has undergone a significant shift. Historically, theory, especially psychoanalytic theory, guided the work of psychiatrists. Compared to other medical colleagues, psychiatrists did few physical exams, little lab work, and few surgical procedures. Instead, they became experts on talking to patients and trying to match signs and symptoms with descriptions of specific syndromes.

Today, psychiatrists are equally interested in signs and symptoms (observable and reported changes in the patient's behavior, thoughts, and feelings) so they can identify a specific diagnosis. But, once they have made the diagnosis, the treatment options have greatly expanded. Today, many psychiatrists focus on using psychotropic medications to treat specific clinical syndromes. They are likely to have a wealth of evidence-based research to guide their treatment decisions, which often involve one or two specific medications to treat specific symptoms.

As a result of these changes, newly trained psychiatrists may have intricate, sophisticated knowledge about psychotropic medications, DSM diagnoses, and drug interactions. But they may have less time to simply listen to the patient's story, or they may feel that they have little to offer a patient who doesn't need psychotropic medications. In addition, they are often employed in systems that reimburse them for medication evaluations and little else. Although many psychiatrists chose their specialty because they enjoyed talking to patients, they may find themselves in professional settings where they are evaluated primarily on their "productivity"—that is, how many patients they can interview, diagnose, and prescribe medication for in a specific amount of time. Therapists can build stronger collaborative relationships with psychiatrists when they understand the unique pressures on them in today's health care environment.

By overcoming cultural differences and successfully managing cross-disciplinary relationships, therapists can help improve a patient's adherence to a treatment regimen that includes medication (Frank, 1997). Patients often appreciate the collaboration of their doctors because it is such a stark contrast to what they are accustomed to in health care.

Build a Relationship

A good relationship with the physician paves the way to effective collaboration (Seaburn et al., 1996). As in work with a new patient, "joining" is the most critical task in building a good relationship. Minuchin and Fishman (1981) define joining as "the glue that holds the therapeutic system together" (p. 32). This is equally true for the professionals in the therapeutic system. Collaboration is much easier if professionals like one another and have confidence in one another's abilities.

It is easy to move too fast through this relationship-building phase or to neglect it because contacts with physicians take place in formats—referral letters, brief telephone conversations, and hallway chats—that therapists may not associate with the process of joining. This is a mistake. Basic joining skills—such as listening; expressing empathy, respect, and concern; and asking questions for better understanding—will make all communications with the physician more effective. Using joining skills allows therapists to understand more fully unique clinical perspectives, as well as the needs and hopes of other professionals.

However, the relationship-building phase often contains two inequalities. The first, described earlier, is a sense that collaboration is more important to the therapist than to the physician, which means that the therapist works harder to make contact with the physician than vice versa. The second inequality is related to decision making about medications because the physician has the final say about treatment. Both of these inequalities are related to hierarchies that exist between different disciplines, which collaboration does not change. These contrasting positions demand that professionals in collaborative relationships become familiar with each other's role in patient care and respect the validity of each other's opinions and ideas. So, although the physician may still have decision-making power, the therapist should offer diagnostic observations and medication inquiries without fear. Respect for the hierarchy and respect for perspective are the key features in building a relationship.

Clarify Frequency and Form of Communication

After release-of-information forms are signed and there is agreement with the patient and family about what can and cannot be told to other professionals, it is important to contact the involved health care providers as soon as possible (Seaburn et al., 1996). During the initial contact, preferably in person or over the phone, the therapist should introduce him- or herself and ask the physician about his or her goals for the shared patient. In addition to the initial impressions and preliminary goals, it is helpful to clarify the frequency and form of future communications.

The frequency of communication often depends on the seriousness of the patient's problem. For example, a patient may be suicidal or have complex medical concerns that require more frequent contact, which will benefit all professionals. At the very least, the therapist should make contact with the physician at the time of referral and the time of termination (Seaburn et al., 1996).

Face-to-face communication is ideal, but such an expectation is unrealistic if professionals work in different locations. Most communication between professionals takes place on the phone. E-mail is another option and is becoming a popular form of communication between physicians and patients and physicians and other professionals. Although e-mail is convenient and provides greater flexibility for responding, it also raises serious questions about confidentiality (Seaburn et al., 1996). If used to provide brief updates, ask questions, or plan a meeting, we endorse the use of e-mail. However, we strongly suggest that any sensitive information be communicated in person or over the phone and that lengthy reports be sent in sealed envelopes through the mail. As electronic medical records become more common and security is improved, e-mail may provide greater options.

Clarify Boundaries

Boundary clarification is a requirement to successful collaboration (McDaniel et al., 1992), particularly when multiple mental health providers participate in one case. Regardless of the degree one has earned, patients and family members may refer to all health care professionals as "doctor" and have skewed expectations about who is responsible for what. For example, patients commonly discuss medication with their nonprescribing therapist and occasionally solicit advice on how much medication to take, when to take it, and whether to discontinue its use. Similarly, patients report the progress of a therapy intervention with their psychiatrist or family physician.

Avoid Triangulation

As with any triad, avoiding triangulation can be a bit like avoiding breathing. A physician, therapist, and patient can form a natural triangle that can be very functional and healthy. We have noticed that our patients are often willing to try medication or at least talk to a physician about medication because they want to help us. They know that we are trying to provide good care. In essence, they are willing to try anything that we think might help because they trust us. The goodwill they feel toward us spills over into their initial visit with the physician. The respect and goodwill that a particular physician and therapist have for each other facilitates the care of a mutual patient. Such a triangle of patient care can be quite effective.

However, this triangle is not without its risks. Because of their trust of one another, a physician and therapist may become more lax about evaluating or continually assessing a shared patient. For example, Dr. Patterson asked a close colleague to provide medication to a patient during the session with the patient. She felt that the patient needed medication immediately and knew there were no openings in the doctor's schedule for several days. Catching the doctor in the hall, she asked him to talk to the patient for a few minutes. In less than 5 minutes, the physician asked a few brief questions and gave the patient some medication samples to start. The physician told the patient to make an appointment for a full evaluation and mentioned that he would start a patient chart later in the day. By providing only medication samples, he felt that he could ensure the patient's quick return for an office visit.

This situation was full of good intentions and full of ethical and legal risks. Dr. Patterson was trying to be an advocate for the patient and obtain access to care as quickly as possible. The physician was trying to please his colleague and respond to her request. The patient was trying to please the therapist by responding to the therapist's suggestions. However, the patient could not get an appointment for several weeks because the physician had no openings. At the end of his overwhelmingly busy day, the physician forgot to start a chart for Dr. Patterson's patient. There was no documentation of the visit or of the physician providing medication samples to the patient. In this situation, the lack of openings in the physician's schedule and his demanding caseload led to compromised patient care.

Sometimes patients and their family members recruit therapists or physicians into an alignment against other professionals. For example, patients may tell the therapist that the psychiatrist does not spend enough time with them and is not as caring as the therapist. Then the patients might ask the therapist for advice on whether to fire the psychiatrist. The therapist could feel flattered by such a comparison and agree with the description of the uncaring psychiatrist. Such a move would damage the collaborative relationship between the therapist and psychiatrist and would be therapeutically counterproductive for many reasons.

Triangulation comes in many different forms. Avoiding this trap is easier with strong, unified, collaborative relationships. With that aim, it may prove beneficial to have an initial joint session with the physician and/or patient to prevent triangulation and cultivate communication. Fostering the collaborative relationship allows a therapist or physician to respond to triangulation attempts with a restatement of the treatment mission, a recommendation to the patient to direct concerns to the appropriate person, or in the above example, education about the differences between psychiatric evaluation and therapy.

COLLABORATION IN ACTION

To illustrate these collaborative skills, we return to the case presented at the beginning of this chapter. Mrs. C's case is a common example of a therapist and physician who are working together in a family medicine setting and seeking consultation from a psychiatrist in a different setting. Although it would be more challenging, a similar process and outcome could be achieved with each professional working in a different setting.

> Dr. F decides to inform Dr. R about the changes in Mrs. C's mood. Although both express relief that the depression has lifted, they also express concern about her current manic symptoms. Since Mrs. C has experienced similar cycles over the years, Dr. F wonders aloud if it might be helpful to get the input of a psychiatrist, who could offer another perspective on Mrs. C and the long-held diagnosis of bipolar disorder. Since she has not been in touch with a psychiatrist in many years, Dr. F suggests it might be time for a checkup to make sure they are on the right track. Dr. R agrees that such an evaluation will be helpful. Dr. F meets Mr. and Mrs. C to discuss a referral to a psychiatrist concerning her current manic symptoms. Mr. C states that this manic cycle is familiar and often worries him more than the depression cycle because of Mrs. C's unpredictability. Mrs. C agrees to the referral and is given the name and number of a reputable psychiatrist. A release-of-information form is signed, giving Drs. F and R permission to speak to the psychiatrist. Drs. F and R write a letter to the psychiatrist, Dr. O, before Mrs. C's appointment to provide a brief history of her illness and their current questions. Following the evaluation, Dr. O sends Dr. R a written summary, which includes his treatment

recommendations. Because of Mrs. C's clear descriptions of her mood cycle and attention to detail in her yearly calendar, it is not a surprise that Dr. O changes her diagnosis from bipolar disorder to seasonal affective disorder. Consistent with this diagnosis, Dr. O stops Mrs. C's medication and recommends light treatment, which serves as a preventive measure in preparation for the shorter days of winter. In a therapy session after the evaluation, Mr. and Mrs. C are cautiously optimistic and ready to begin the light treatment. During a routine medical visit 3 months after the evaluation, Dr. R notices symptoms that appear consistent with mania. Dr. R consults with Dr. F, and both agree that Mrs. C needs to see Dr. O again. Dr. O decides to start her on 600 mg. of Lithium and schedules regular monthly appointments to monitor her progress. The combination of medication, light treatment, and individual and family therapy significantly improve Mrs. C's mood disorder. Although she experiences a reemergence of depression as the winter months approach, the depression arrives late in the year and is much less severe. Mrs. C says, "I feel so blessed to have the three of you working together on my behalf!"

This case is a common scenario for therapists: A patient is referred who is currently on medication or needs medication and multiple professionals become involved, usually a family physician and a psychiatrist. When therapists refer to a physician for assistance with the care of their patients, they are influencing the treatment plan in significant ways. First, and most obvious, is the possible addition of medication. Second, and equally important, is the expansion of the treatment system to include other professionals, who will have some say in the care of a particular patient and family. If the patient was already taking medication when therapy started, the therapist is in the position of a newcomer to the treatment system. It is not uncommon for a patient and physician to have a long-standing relationship, which will continue after the therapist discontinues work with the patient and family. Regardless of the timing of a medical intervention, the patient will benefit from a good collaborative relationship between the therapist and other health care professionals. Medication is a common intervention; good collaborative relationships are rare.

CHAPTER 11

Strengthening Bonds

COLLABORATING
WITH THE FAMILY

Mrs. J has been coming to see Ms. T, a family therapist, for treatment of depression for the last 6 weeks. Ms. T understands the current life stressors that Mrs. J faces. She also knows that Mrs. J has struggled with depression on and off for many years and that Mrs. J's mother also struggled with depression. Ms. T has come to believe that Mrs. J might benefit from medication and wants to send her for a medication consultation.

When Ms. T broaches the subject of medication as a possible treatment, Mrs. J reacts strongly. She explains that she is already concerned about the dissipating intimacy in her marriage and that medication could make it worse. Mrs. J explains that her cousin Sally, who also suffers from depression, had tried medication. Her cousin's husband did not support his wife's decision because he believed she should be emotionally stronger. He did not want her to try medication that might "change her personality and mess with her head." In spite of her husband's objections, Sally tried an antidepressant. About 6 weeks later she felt much better, but she also gained 5 pounds, needed more sleep, and became inorgasmic. Although she was feeling better, her husband was increasingly distant and angry about the changes in their sex life. He was also angry that he had to get up earlier to care for their two small children so Sally could get the extra sleep she now needed. According to Sally's husband, "Sally might be feeling better, but I'm feeling worse every day." Mrs. J told Ms. T that she would rather live with her depression than risk further disrupting her already strained marital relationship. She saw how "medication affected my cousin's marriage and I don't need those problems."

There is very little information to guide Ms. T's next move. She could try to talk Mrs. J into trying the medication, but doing so risks creating another area of conflict for her patient. She could ask Mrs. J to bring in her husband so Ms. T can talk to him about psychotropic medications, but he may be unwilling to come. She could try to find a medication that does not affect sex, sleep, and weight, but she knows that all medications have some side effects. Finally, she could give up on the idea of medication even though she thinks drug therapy will help her patient. Although Mrs. J is the individual patient who takes the pills and experiences the side effects, the implications of the medication extend to her family, which will be affected by the changes, positive or negative, that the medication creates.

Ms. T's next patients are a father and stepmother, Mr. and Mrs. H, of a 9-year-old boy, Tommy. Mr. and Mrs. H have demanding jobs as attorneys and have been married only a year. Tommy lives with them full-time and spends a lot of time alone in his room, playing video games on his computer. He has gotten in trouble at school for aggressive behavior on the playground, leaves his room a mess, easily loses his homework, and fails to do his chores without multiple reminders. Mrs. H is clearly frustrated and angry about Tommy's disruptive behavior, and Mr. H is sympathetic to his wife's frustrations. They bring Ms. T a list of Tommy's infractions during the previous week. After reciting each problem, they conclude by saying that the therapy isn't working and that a friend said that her son with attention deficit disorder got better with Ritalin. Mr. and Mrs. H want to try Ritalin or some other drug that will calm Tommy down and make him behave.

Ms. T is again unsure about what to do next. She has not even considered medication for Tommy and had ruled out the diagnosis of attention deficit disorder several weeks earlier. What Ms. T does know is that Mrs. H is ambivalent about caring for Tommy and would prefer more time alone with her new husband and a more orderly, calm household. In addition, Tommy does not go to bed until almost midnight many nights, and the exhausted parents have been unwilling to enforce Ms. T's recommendation of an earlier bedtime. Tommy is angry with his dad for getting married when he thought their living situation was fine with just the two of them, especially after the painful adjustment to his mother's departure. Tommy is completely uninterested in his schoolwork, and his main source of pleasure is playing his video games, which he does for 3 or 4 hours per day.

Scientific literature about the biochemical impact of medications, their positive and negative effects, and basic neuroscience may be of little value to Ms. T in these situations. It may also be of little use to Tommy because someone else in the family is going to make the decision about medication use. For Mrs. J, her husband's fear of the unknown will ultimately determine her medication question, and for Tommy, Mrs. H's difficulties in adjusting to a new life might lead to his inappropriate use of medication.

We have seen situations like these many times, but there is little discussion in the literature of the family's impact on an individual psychotropic medication decision or the impact of the medication on the family. Perhaps because some mental health professionals have been reluctant to embrace medication's growing influence (Sparks, 2002), they have also not applied their knowledge about families to clinical situations involving medication decisions. In a study on practice patterns of marriage and family therapists, Hernandez and Doherty (2005) report that 24% of cases involving medication include a spouse or partner, and 8.5% include other family members.

In similar manner, physicians prescribe medication for an individual patient and target individual symptoms. It may seem irrelevant to most physicians to consider the impact of the medication on the family and vice versa. But most patients live in families, and they are concerned about their family members' responses to their choices. In addition, decision-making power and influence are not evenly distributed among family members. Often other family members make decisions, including medication decisions, for the very young and the very old as can be seen in the literature concerning the increase of antipsychotic medications for elderly patients with dementia or agitation. At the opposite end of the life cycle, an alarming trend may be occurring: Family members increasingly demanding medications for their young children, especially for children with disruptive behaviors. An editorial in the *Journal of the American Medical Association* (Coyne, 2000) notes the trend of seeking medications as quick fixes to children's problems:

It should be emphasized that most of the drugs prescribed [for young children] involve off-label use because efficacy of psychotropic drugs has not been demonstrated in very young children. . . . Thus, it would seem prudent to carry out much more extensive studies to determine the long-term consequences of the use of psychotropic drugs. (p. 1059)

The editorial laments one cause of this alarming trend, the lack of collaboration between mental health professionals:

Thus, the multidisciplinary clinics of the past that brought together pediatric, psychiatric, behavioral, and family expertise for difficult cases have largely ceased to exist. As a consequence, it appears that behaviorally disturbed children are now increasingly subjected to quick and inexpensive pharmacologic fixes as opposed to informed, multimodal therapy, associated with optimal outcomes. These disturbing prescription practices suggest a growing crisis in mental health services to children. (p. 1060)

Family members are an essential part of any collaborative team (McDaniel et al., 1995). We involve family members early and consult with them often because they have an enormous impact on health and illness and on how the patient relates to the collaborative team (McDaniel et al., 1995). When a patient with depression or anxiety is seen for the first time, the family members have been on the front lines as the de facto health care specialists. They have been witness to the unpredictability and anguish associated with mental illness and have probably adjusted their behaviors in many ways to accommodate and change the course of the illness. They may have been the reason a patient is seeking treatment. Family members are a source of valuable information and play a critical role as partners in treatment.

FAMILIES, MENTAL ILLNESS, AND MEDICATION

The limited literature on families and psychotropic medications comes from families coping with serious mental illness. As early as the 1970s, researchers interested in schizophrenia began looking at the effects of medication not only on the schizophrenic patient but also on the family. In addition, they looked at the impact of family therapy on the patient's medication compliance (McFarlane, Dixon, Lukens, & Lucksted, 2002; Sprenkle, 2003).

In 1981, Michael Goldstein, PhD, and his colleagues at UCLA published a study whose purpose was to "determine whether family therapy increases compliance (compared to individual therapy) and whether this may account for the added effectiveness of the approach" (p. 87). According to Goldstein, "the data are consistent in suggesting that family therapy led to enhanced compliance with pharmacological interventions. The degree to which this improved compliance accounts for better clinical outcome is a difficult issue to unravel" (p. 88). Over 20 years later, a review of the family schizophrenia literature answers Goldstein's question.

> Overall, the relapse rate for schizophrenic patients provided family psychoeducation has hovered around 15% per year, compared to a consistent 30–40% for individual therapy and medication or medication alone. It is important to note that medication is not a variable in these studies: the design of family psychoeducational approaches has medication adherence and its value in promoting recovery as a central element. Therefore, medication is provided in both the experimental and control conditions in every instance. (McFarlane et al., 2002, pp. 229–230)

In another study of schizophrenic patients and their families, the authors conclude that psychoeducational family groups help family members make "significant gains in their knowledge about schizophrenia, particularly about medication. Patients whose relatives attended the group had significantly fewer days in hospital . . . compared to controls . . . but the effect waned" by the second year (Cassidy, Hill, & O'Callaghan, 2001, p. 446). Another study confirms this finding. Family intervention and regular use of medication had independent and additive effects on the outcome. During the 18 months after the index discharge, patients who did not take medication regularly and who did not receive family intervention were 7.9 times as likely to be readmitted to the hospital as patients who took medication regularly and received family intervention (Zhang, Wang, Jianjun, & Phillips, 1994). A more recent study on the impact of family intervention compared the effects of culturally modified family therapy (intervention group) with those of behavioral family therapy (control group) in the management of schizophrenia. After 1 year, the intervention group had significantly less of a family burden, a reduction in the number of exacerbated cases, and improvement in global functioning (Razali, 2000).

Family interventions led to improvements not only in the patients' symptoms but also in the relationships between patients and family members. In a study on the impact of medication on the families of schizophrenic patients, the authors concluded that all family members interviewed felt that their relative had responded positively to the medication (Najarian, 1995). Family members also stated that their relationships improved as a result of the patient's positive response to the medication. The patient could relate better to other family members and had increased interest and ability to participate in social activities.

Another study interviewed families of schizophrenic patients, asking specific questions about the families' responses to the medications and the medication's effects on the families. Families hope that the medications will lessen their relatives' suffering and ease the burden of care (Stebbin, 1995). In a similar study, the researchers concluded that medication had a small but significant effect on the patients' families (Rosenheck et al., 2000). The primary impact was to help reduce negative symptoms in the patient and thus reduce the family's burden. However, the schizophrenic patient who has reduced symptoms may then be released from the hospital and placed in the care of the family, thus transferring the responsibility for the patient from the hospital to the family.

What can we learn from this research? When we expand our target patient to include the family, how do our treatment goals change? Table 11.1 summarizes answers to these questions.

A CLINICAL GUIDE TO COLLABORATING WITH FAMILIES

Although there are few studies of the interaction between families and psychotropic medications, and the few existing studies focus on severe mental illness, we can still glean clinical wisdom from the literature. It makes sense that families would be concerned about their ill family member and that they would be affected by his or her behavior. Although inclusion of the family seems to be a simple guideline, we have been surprised at how seldom families are consulted about treatment decisions or educated about the illness. We have also been surprised by how infrequently therapists and physicians utilize family members as sources of information about the patient's history and progress. Finally, we are often surprised to find that some therapists and physicians are treating seriously ill adult parents, often single parents, and failing to inquire about the welfare of their dependent children.

If we know that a collaborative approach that includes family members works best, why aren't we using it? Our best guess is that family work takes more time, is more complicated, and can provoke more anxiety in therapists and physicians. If we are already feeling pressed for

TABLE 11.1. A Summary of Family Research

- Psychoeducation for family members can increase the patient's compliance with taking the medications.
- Even when the family interventions or therapy are not specifically focused on the medications, one effect of the therapy can be increased adherence to medication regimens.
- Medication adherence decreases as the complexity, cost, and duration of the regimen increases, even with supportive families that encourage compliance.
- Families with members with serious mental illnesses, such as schizophrenia, may be more pleased with the effects of medication because it can lessen the family's burden.
- Families' hidden agendas or expectations about the medications can vary widely. Family members may hope that the medication "cures" the troubled family member and rescues the family from the overwhelming caretaking burden.
- Power struggles and conflicts in the family can erupt over the individual member's decision about taking medication and his or her compliance.
- Both therapy and medication compliance can improve when the family therapist and physician have a collaborative alliance with the family, not simply the patient, and can manage the varying responses of family members over time to the patient, the illness, and the medication.
- Interdisciplinary communication and more consistent patient care, including frequent communication with the family, make the burden of caring for the troubled family member easier. One study concludes by stating, "An alliance between professionals and families holds great potential for maximizing the positive effects of [medication] therapy" (Stebbin, 1995).

Note. Data from Coldham, Addington, and Addington (2002); Dickson, Williams, and Dalby (1995); Haynes, McDonald, and Garg (2002); Kotcher and Smith (1993); McDonald, Garg, and Haynes (2002); Olfson et al. (2000); Ran and Xiang (1995); Smith, Barzam, and Pristach (1997); Stebbin (1995); and Wysocki, Greceo, Harris, Bubb, and White (2001).

time, it is easy to overlook family members' input. Below are suggestions for therapists who want to practice in a collaborative care context and simultaneously expand the scope of care to the patient and family.

Think Systemically

Systems theory provides a lens both to understand the relational context of patients' lives and to predict issues that might arise during the course of treatment. Cole-Kelly and Seaburn (1999) suggest the following family-oriented questions to better understand a patient's illness:

- Has anyone else in the family had this problem?
- What do family members believe caused the problem or could treat the problem?
- Who in the family is most concerned about the problem?
- Along with the illness and symptoms, have there been any other recent changes in the family?
- How can the family be helpful in dealing with this problem?

Additional questions to consider include the following:

- How is decision making balanced in the family? Who will make the decisions for the ill family member if the patient cannot?
- Who in the family wants the patient to try psychotropic medication? Who opposes the medication option? Why? Try to obtain a family history of medication issues.
- What are the effects of the member's illness on the family? The more the family is affected by stressors such as financial costs, time demands, or the patient's inability to contribute to family tasks, the more the family members might want to influence medication decisions.
- Are there influences from outside the family to be considered? The family may experience some pressure to create change in a member's behavior. For example, an employer or school official might notify a family that there are problems with a family member's behavior. The family may be expected to solve these problems. Also, are income, insurance status, or other financial factors likely to influence medication decisions?
- Are any dependent family members strongly influenced by the ill member's functioning, for example, dependent children or dependent elderly adults? Does anything need to be done to ensure their care as well?

These are just a few questions a therapist can consider in understanding the family structure, particularly the interactional patterns that help shape it. For example, an overfunctioning spouse may be attempting to make a treatment decision for an underfunctioning patient. In such a case, a therapist would not want to alienate the spouse or support the patient's sense of powerlessness in the relationship. The therapist would want to acknowledge the spouse's efforts to be helpful and attempt to give the patient a voice in his or her own care.

Include the Family on the Collaborative Care Team

The responsibility of caring for a patient usually falls on members of the family. Thus, they are not simply uninvolved bystanders. For example, it is not unusual for family members to prompt the patient to make the initial appointment with the therapist or physician. Because of the stigma of mental illness and the patient's worries about burdening family members, the family may not be fully informed on the health status of the patient. This lack of knowledge may be related to conflictual relationships in the family and a patient's preference to keep family members uninformed.

Understand the Unique Demands of the Illness

John Rolland (1994), describing a typology of illness to understand the diverse ways in which families cope with a variety of physical illnesses, identified the following variables: onset, course, outcome, and degree of incapacitation. "Onset" of illness refers to whether it is acute, like a stroke, or gradual, like Alzheimer's disease. A family will probably respond to an acute illness differently from a gradual onset illness. For example, an acute illness will quickly mobilize the family and force them to create and implement crisis-management skills. Some families will handle this rapid change better than others. The "course" of an illness can be progressive (type 1 diabetes), constant (spinal cord injury), or relapsing-episodic (asthma). Relapsing illnesses create tremendous unpredictability in families. Furthermore, they demand flexibility in the family structure because of the transitions between crisis and noncrisis periods and the ongoing worry about when the next crisis will occur. The "outcome" refers to a continuum of possibilities—of whether it will shorten the lifespan or quickly cause the patient's death. Of course, some illnesses are nonfatal, such as arthritis, and others are fatal, such as Huntington's disease. "Incapacitation" refers to the degree of a patient's disability—incapacitating (Alzheimer's disease) or nonincapacitating (lung cancer).

Although Rolland's (1994) model is focused on chronic, physical illness, the spirit of his model fits in understanding how families cope with mental illness as well. For example, the demands associated with caring for a family member with a chronic depression are very different from those facing the family of a person who suffers from an acute panic attack, and these are different from the demands created by ADHD.

Similarly, some psychiatric disorders are characterized by more predictability than others. Alcoholism, for example, will probably breed more unpredictability for the family than generalized anxiety disorder.

Another helpful aspect of Rolland's (1994) model is the interaction between the illness and the family's developmental stage. Using Combrinck-Graham's (1985) family life spiral as a backdrop, Rolland states that families naturally oscillate through periods of greater closeness (centripetal periods), as when a baby is born, and periods of greater distance (centrifugal periods), as when a child leaves home after adolescence. Centripetal periods are characterized by greater family cohesion and greater focus on internal family life. Centrifugal periods display a loosening of family boundaries, allowing individual members to pursue goals and interactions with the extrafamilial environment. According to Rolland, the onset of physical illness generally has a centripetal pull on families. An illness that emerges during a centripetal period may prolong the period, or the family may get stuck in this phase. When an illness strikes during a centrifugal period, it can interrupt a family's natural developmental progression and force family members to redirect their attention back to the family. For example, an adolescent may remain at home later than originally expected to help care for an ill parent.

The onset or exacerbation of a mental illness can also have a centripetal pull on families. However, because of its stigma, it can also have a centrifugal effect. For example, many patients attempt to hide their depression or anxiety to avoid burdening their families or to protect a secret, such as an affair, that is associated with the distress. Whereas a physical illness, like cancer, can lead to an outpouring of family support, the shame that accompanies mental illness can often fracture relationships and contribute to significant loneliness. When we encounter these fractured relationships, we attempt to open communication, educate the family, and increase social support.

Address the Family's Belief System

Family members come to treatment with a variety of beliefs about mental illness and medication. These beliefs play a significant role in shaping a family's response to illness and the willingness to support a treatment regiment that has been recommended by a collaborative team of professionals (Rolland, 1995). For example, family members may come to therapy with one of the following beliefs:

- "Mental illness is a character flaw."
- "Everyone gets depressed; why should he receive special attention?"
- "Medication is only for crazy people."
- "Medication doesn't work. My mother took several medications for depression and each medication made it worse."

These beliefs often develop over many years and can be influenced by many ethnic, cultural, and religious traditions. For treatment to move forward successfully, it is important to explore their effects.

Often the family's beliefs about the medication are as important in the treatment as its actual effects. Medicine has long recognized this fact, as seen in the discussions of the "placebo effect." Thus, a therapist is juggling multiple meanings about the *purpose*, *effects*, and *risks* of the medications. At times, the therapist won't recognize family members' beliefs or hidden agendas concerning psychotropic medications. In addition, the therapist needs to be aware of his or her own beliefs about the role of medications. Is medication essential? Optional? Dangerous? Demeaning? Redemptive? There are as many possibilities for the beliefs about psychotropic medications in the family–therapist–doctor–patient system as there are medications. It is hoped that the skilled therapist can make the covert beliefs overt. Peoples' fears and concerns can be addressed. When there is scientific evidence to guide a decision, that evidence can be related and applied to the unique situation. When there is little evidence, the therapist can be frank about the limits of our knowledge and help the family, the patient, and the physician make as informed a decision as possible.

Elicit the Goals of Each Family Member

In clinical practice, one caveat in considering the applicability of the outcome research is the question of whose goals are being measured. Different members of the treatment system may have different goals. The family may want specific symptom amelioration. For example, family members may want the patient to be less agitated or more able to perform the daily tasks of family life. The physician may want better medication compliance or major clinical outcomes such as reductions in psychopathology and increases in functioning. The patient may just want to be left alone.

These numerous and often unspoken agendas about the goals and impact of medications have to be considered; otherwise, disappointment when the expectations are not met could overshadow other positive effects. For example, in one study of the effects of a psychoeducational intervention for married patients with bipolar disorder and their spouses, medication *plus* a marital intervention led to better overall functioning and better medication compliance but not ultimately to better overall symptom reduction (Clarkin, Carpenter, Hull, Wilner, & Glick, 1998). Depending on each participant's goals, the marital intervention may or may not have been viewed as a success.

CONCLUSION

The explosion of knowledge in biology, neuroscience, and technology means that psychotherapists of the future cannot work in the same ways we have worked in the last decade. Our scope of knowledge has to expand, and we have to work more closely with health professionals from other fields who have different expertise.

As we train new therapists, we are aware that many of our students chose the mental health field because they wanted to "help people" and found themselves at home in the social sciences (and, often, did not feel comfortable in their biology, physics, and chemistry classes). They knew that a career in mental health seldom offers fame, glory, and wealth, and they accepted these limitations. What they did expect from their careers was a sense of personal satisfaction and pride in helping people change their lives for the better.

When they began their graduate training programs, they immersed themselves in the knowledge, culture, and clinical work of their specific disciplines. They became experts in cognitive behavioral therapy, family systems work, or developmental psychopathology. For the most part, their training occurred in settings where they would be exposed to other students and faculty who were similar in training and clinical practice. But new forms of practice require that we all begin to learn and communicate across the boundaries of our various disciplines.

We hope this book has filled an important gap by making the scientific information user friendly and by pointing out the strengths and pleasures of working with colleagues from other disciplines. In addition, we hope this book has made you think more about your patients' families and their impact on treatment.

Although this book has focused on imparting to therapists scientific information about psychotropic medications and practical guidelines for collaboration with families and other professionals, we are aware that for a collaborative care model to work, other changes must be made. Ideally, physicians need to know more about psychotherapy so they can have a better appreciation for what a therapist can offer to shared patients—and what the therapist cannot supply.

In this book we have focused treatment discussions on psychotropic medications. But bear in mind that however remarkable the advances in drug therapy may be, the traditional knowledge and skills of psychotherapy practice remain vitally important. In fact, research suggests that an ideal treatment often occurs when both psychotherapy and psychotropic medications are part of the treatment plan. In addition, services and interventions that enhance social support, such as group therapy, family psychoeducation, and Internet chat groups, are often critical to the success of the therapy.

We have suggested that therapists must expand their interests and influence to other factors that have an impact on clinical care: the patient's family, the clinic's organizational structure, the finances of therapy, and the physician–therapist–patient relationships. These factors can influence the outcome of therapy as much as the specific medication or specific psychotherapy techniques used.

Our overall goal in writing this book is to improve the clinical care of patients with mental health problems. We encourage the reader to stay focused on this goal and to measure every new intervention, idea, or technique by asking, "How will this information help me provide better care for my patients?" If better care is our ultimate outcome and measure of success, therapists will continue to learn and to adapt the way they practice as new knowledge is added. We will learn from our colleagues in different disciplines. We will consider the multitude of influences on our patients' care. In the end, not only will patients prosper, but also the therapist's attitude of curiosity and openness will lead to a more rewarding career.

How Drugs Are Developed

On the way home from a doctor's visit, where you just have been diagnosed with an upper respiratory infection that has been making you miserable for the past few days, you stop at your neighborhood supermarket or drugstore to pick up some last-minute groceries. While you shop, the pharmacist is filling some of your prescriptions. You will take those medications, feeling confident that they will safely restore you to health. Though you may not think of it at the time, you are acting on faith—faith in your physician, pharmacist, pharmaceutical company, and the developers, researchers, and regulators of the drug you take—and you are confident that before you put that foreign substance into your body, someone has determined that it is indeed safe (or at least, the result of a favorable risk–benefit analysis) and effective.

The pharmaceutical industry is, arguably, the most regulated industry in the world. Painful lessons of the past have gradually shaped the development of new drugs into a methodical, meticulous, systematic—and still quite imperfect—process that takes many years at a cost of hundreds of millions of dollars. It is estimated that the cost of developing one single drug, from synthesis to market release, exceeds $850 million.

As you read these lines, dozens, perhaps hundreds, of compounds for the treatment of CNS diseases are in different stages of development. Almost every year a new antidepressant, antipsychotic, or anxiolytic drug is released to the market after the U.S. Federal Drug Administration (FDA) has given its stamp of approval. This is the guarantee (of sorts, as we shall see next) to all of us, both prescribers and users, that the medication in question provides reasonable efficacy and safety in treating a certain condition. But in spite of all the safeguards and regulatory controls introduced over the years, the system is far from perfect. Consider, for example, the incidents in 2005, when Vioxx, Bextra, and other nonsteroidal anti-inflammatories were linked to an increased risk of heart attacks, prompting some manufacturers to withdraw their products from the market. There were even charges that some of the drugs were kept in the market for consumption by unsuspecting patients well after the manufacturers became aware of the increased risk. The resolution of this particular affair was still pending in court at press time. Whether due to corporate greed, the limitations of current research technologies, or idiosynratic individual responses, the fact is that there is an element of unknown risk whenever a medication is authorized for marketing. In an attempt to identify potential complications not recognized during the drug development process, postmarketing surveillance studies (see below, phase IV) are being conducted with increased frequency by the manufacturers in response to demands by the FDA.

The laborious process of drug development occurs in two different, successive stages: preclinical and clinical. In the preclinical stage, a potential drug is subjected to a series of standardized tests aimed at elucidating its pharmacological characteristics, its safety, and its therapeutic potential. The process calls for careful and systematic studies in tissues and in laboratory animals. For example, the development of fluoxetine included 4 years of laboratory work, where, among other procedures, its ability to increase levels of serotonin in the synaptic cleft was tested. It was already known by then (1980s) that certain depressed patients, especially those with a significant risk for suicide, had reduced levels of serotonin in some areas of the CNS. It was therefore hypothesized that a "good" antidepressant medication should be capable of increasing serotonin levels. Fluoxetine, by virtue of blocking the transporter that removes serotonin from the synapse, produces a net increase in serotonin in this location. The preclinical stage of drug development has a very low yield because the large majority of possible drugs fails to pass these "screens," and literally thousands are rejected. It is estimated that less than 1% of preclinical drugs actually make it to the clinical stage of testing.

Once a drug has cleared the preclinical stage, it is ready to enter the clinical stage of testing and its highly regulated set of requirements instituted by the FDA. These requirements are intended to subject the drug to very careful testing in human beings. The clinical stage of development, in fact, comprises several substages known as phases. By far, this is the most expensive part of the drug development process, with costs reaching several hundred million dollars. Let's, then, use a fictitious drug, an antidepressant, and follow its journey through the four formal FDA phases of development. Our promising antidepressant, which at this point is usually known only by a number—for example, XYZ-0987654—has already passed the preclinical stage. So we know that its pharmacological characteristics are compatible with mechanisms of action known to be associated with antidepressant effects (e.g., it blocks the reuptake of serotonin at certain neuroreceptors). We also know, through animal testing, that the compound produces desired effects in laboratory animal models of depression (e.g., it has a beneficial effect on learned helplessness). Finally, and most important, it produces no life-threatening or otherwise serious or intolerable side effects in animals. Now our antidepressant is ready for clinical stage testing.

- *Phase I*. During this phase, the drug is tested in a small number of healthy, nondepressed human volunteers (college students are the usual guinea pigs in these cases). Safety and tolerability are the main focus at this stage; the usual testing doses in phase I are a very small fraction of the toxic (i.e., lethal) dose identified during the preclinical stage. During phase I, pharmacological and behavioral data are recorded. For example, how much of the drug is absorbed? How long does it take to reach certain blood concentrations? Does it have any effects on alertness, thinking, or motor behavior? Typically, phase I studies utilize several dozen volunteers and take approximately 1 year to complete. It is estimated that about 70% of the drugs satisfy phase I requirements, thereby becoming candidates for phase II studies.
- *Phase II*. Our drug is now ready for testing in a small number (a few hundred) of depressed subjects. Depending on the design, the study may be conducted in an inpatient or outpatient setting, usually the latter. Subjects are recruited from the clinical practices of the psychiatric investigators and from the community at large, usually by television, radio, and newspaper advertising. After a careful informed-consent process, subjects begin participation in the study proper. Initial studies in this phase are single-blinded: Each subject is randomly assigned to receive the study drug or a placebo, an inert substance devoid of pharmacological activity, without knowing which of the two is being given. Later studies in phase II have a **double-blind** design, in which neither the sub-

jects nor the researchers know whether the study drug or the placebo is being given (of course, measures are in place to immediately "break" the blind should safety considerations so require). The purpose of double-blind studies is to eliminate investigators' bias in the evaluation of clinical results. In this phase, further testing is done on safety and tolerability, but now we also look at efficacy. Does the drug relieve depression in the test subjects? Does it target all or only some symptoms of the depressive syndrome? How long does it take for the antidepressant effect to become apparent? Phase II studies take 1–2 years. About 50% of the candidate drugs fail this stage. But let us assume our new drug proves to be safe and efficacious, and so we now move to the next phase.

• *Phase III.* In this phase, studies are conducted in hundreds to a few thousand subjects. With safety and tolerability presumably established in phase II, attention is now shifted to efficacy evaluation. In addition to placebo-controlled studies, some will include "active comparators," that is, medications already in general use for the indication being studied. In our example, a study would include comparisons of our antidepressant at two or three different doses, a placebo, and another antidepressant currently in use. These studies help to determine the optimal doses of our drug and, in some study designs, whether the new drug represents an improvement over drugs already on the market. Phase III studies last 2–3 years. Since the information on the study drug already amassed by this time is quite voluminous, most drugs, about four out of five, successfully complete this phase and are then submitted to the FDA for approval of general release. Once the FDA approves the drug and the contents of the package insert—that piece of paper, with extensive information in small print, included with the medication samples that sales representatives leave at the doctors' offices—is completed, the drug is now ready for general use.

• *Phase IV.* These studies, also known as postmarketing studies, are typically conducted after the drug has been available for general prescription for a year or more. Since now thousands of patients are or have been on the drug, additional information becomes available. At this stage, the FDA may require the pharmaceutical company to conduct additional studies, for example, to evaluate a worrisome or even potentially fatal but infrequent side effect that may have come to light since release to the market. Although uncommon, there are instances in which drugs have been withdrawn from the market as a result of these studies. For example, several years ago the antidepressant nomifensine was withdrawn because of unexplained occurrences of blood cell abnormalities. Sometimes, reevaluation of available data can also lead to hitherto unrecognized problems. For example, antidepressants now carry a "black-box" warning that they may increase the risk of suicide among children and teenagers.

With so many steps and trials along the way, it is no surprise that the costs of developing new drugs are staggering. Of course, this is not an apology for the controversial practice of drug pricing, a process that goes well beyond actual drug development costs and that is outside the scope of this discussion. In many cases, the development fails because of unexpected safety issues, poor tolerability, insufficient efficacy, or a combination thereof. All this, of course, has a direct impact on the final cost of the drug. Pharmaceutical companies have exclusive rights to manufacture and market their drugs for a certain number of years, the patent life of the drug. During this period, companies aim to recoup their development costs and, of course, to make a profit. Upon completion of this exclusivity period, any company can then produce the drug under its generic name. The original company retains full rights to the brand name in perpetuity. For example, fluoxetine can be, and in fact is, marketed as fluoxetine by several companies worldwide. However, only Eli Lilly and Co. can use the registered name Prozac to label the drug. Because patients may know their drugs by either name, it is useful to be aware of both the brand and generic names of the commonly used psychiatric medications.

Future Trends

NOVEL RESEARCH METHODOLOGY

As we have seen in Appendix A, the development of psychiatric drugs has been very productive and has had a very significant impact on our ability to treat psychiatric illness and substantially decrease patients' disability and suffering. The clinician must be aware of the fact that the drugs currently in the market were developed and studied in a patient population that, because of methodological constraints, does not really reflect the reality of clinical care in the real world. For example, much of the diversity found in the general population is not necessarily represented in the samples of patients who participate in phase II and III of drug research. We do know that there is great variability in the population seen in the course of clinical practice: Genetic traits separate patients from each other, as does the environment in which they were raised, both socioeconomically and culturally, ethnically, and religiously. Different patients become ill at different stages in their life cycles, have a different family history, and have a different array of past and current medical problems. The subject who participates in drug studies is carefully selected according to very strict inclusion and exclusion criteria, which produce a homogeneous set of individuals that is hardly representative of the general population.

This is a serious limitation but one that, for a number of methodological and economic reasons (some required by the FDA), has been unavoidable. To illustrate the problem, imagine that we are planning a study for a new antidepressant drug, and we will screen all depressed patients who are seeking treatment at our clinic. If we gradually apply the criteria usually used for this purpose in drug studies, many of our potential subjects will be "screened-fail." Some will not be entered because they are reluctant to participate in drug studies. Others will be screened out because of age (for adult studies, the limits typically are between 18 and 65 years of age). A number will have either bipolar disorder or other comorbid Axis I diagnoses (e.g., social phobia and panic attacks). Some will meet probable criteria for borderline personality disorder. All these will be eliminated from the pool. Some will be depressed, but not severely so; others will have significant suicidal ideation. Some will have been depressed for too long (e.g., > 2 years), others not long enough (e.g., < 1 month). Some will be rapid cyclers; others will have taken antidepressants recently. Some will be suffering from medical conditions that preclude their participation, perhaps a history of cancer. Others will have laboratory test or electrocardiogram abnormalities. And so on. All these potential patients, very typical in clinical practices, are not offered participation in drug studies. It is estimated that for every 100 patients screened in a typical outpatient clinic, only 5–10 will actually become appropriate candidates for the study. Also, most drug studies are of brief duration (typically, 4–6 weeks) and cross-sectional. In real life, patients often need treatment for extended periods of time and throughout different stages in their lives.

Cultural and ethnic differences are more important than we would initially suspect: Psychiatric syndromes present differently in different cultures—cultural and ethnic pathoplastic effects; different attitudes toward medications; and variations in pharmacokinetics and pharmacodynamics, depending on genetics and ethnic origin. Even when we examine the response to treatment in genders, the results differ. For example, women will do better than men when treated for depression with SSRIs than with TCAs.

Although this approach produces a homogeneous study sample and makes the studies considerably safer (after all, not much is known about how the new drug will affect a number of diverse psychological and medical characteristics), there are clear disadvantages: Results are less generalizable, and the drug will go into general use without really knowing how different patients will be affected by it.

Recently, in recognition of these limitations, several modifications in methodology have been introduced. For example, we now have more studies specifically aimed at the pediatric and geriatric populations, and certain studies require, for validity, the inclusion of minimal percentages of subjects from different ethnic or cultural groups.

Drug studies conducted by pharmaceutical companies are usually designed to compare their drug with a placebo, and only very infrequently are these drugs compared to others used for the same indications. Consider, for example, antidepressant medications. More than 25 such agents are available in the market, yet we know very little of how they compare to each other in effectiveness.

Nowhere are these transitions more apparent than in the design of three important studies sponsored by the National Institute of Mental Health. One—the STAR*D study—is discussed in detail in Chapter 3. The other two, the CATIE study and the STEP-BD study, are reviewed briefly here as an illustration of current trends in psychiatric research. These three studies break new ground in the sense that they go beyond the concept of "efficacy" that is established in the industry-sponsored studies: The drug is shown to be efficacious for a certain disorder, but in the real world, will physicians prescribe it and will patients take it and stay on it? The answer to these questions centers on the concept of "effectiveness." An effective drug is one that not only has efficacy against a certain malady but also is accepted by patients because its safety, tolerability, mode and frequency of administration, price, taste, appearance, and so on. These issues are commonly left unexamined in the classic drug trials.

The CATIE Study

The CATIE project evaluated the clinical effectiveness of atypical antipsychotics in the treatment of schizophrenia and of Alzheimer's disease. Although antipsychotics were first introduced for the treatment of schizophrenia, they are now used for many other disorders. It is unclear how effective they are and, most important, in view of their rather high cost, how favorably they compare to the first generation of antipsychotics, all of which are available in generic (and thus much less expensive) forms. The CATIE (Clinical Antipsychotic Trials in Intervention Effectiveness) study has specific aims, including the determination of long-term effectiveness and tolerability of the atypical antipsychotics, compared to each and to a typical or "classic" antipsychotic. At this stage, the study enrolled a rather large sample of schizophrenic patients (about 1,500 subjects who were followed for 18 months), with exclusion criteria that were much less restrictive than in classical studies (Lieberman et al., 2006). For additional validity, a broad range of treatment settings have been included so that samples will be more representative of the real world. The CATIE study data and results are being analyzed at the time of publication of this text.

The STEP-BD Study

The STEP-BD study (Systematic Treatment Enhancement Program for Bipolar Disorder) planned to enroll 5,000 patients in about 20 centers nationwide (the reader will be reminded that pharmaceutical company studies typically enroll several dozen subjects in phase II studies and several hundreds in phase III studies). It includes all bipolar subtypes, various ethnic groups, and a variety of treatment settings. Several aims are pursued in this study: the implementation of common clinical practice procedures in diverse settings, the determination of effective strategies for bipolar depression, and the determination of the most effective strategies in preventing relapses. A number of publications have started to appear with results of this study. For an updated list, the interested reader is referred to the STEP-BD section in *www.clinicaltrials.gov.*

The breadth, scope, and novel methodology of STAR★D, CATIE, and STEP-BD are expected to have a huge influence on the way medications are used for the treatment of depression, schizophrenia, and bipolar disorder and, by extension, to the overall attitude with which both patients and clinicians approach the treatment of psychiatric disorders.

NEW MEDICATIONS IN DEVELOPMENT

The search for new pharmacological treatments in psychiatry is intense and productive. Several dozen pharmaceutical companies are currently involved in various stages of drug development, and the next few years will see several new medications available for prescription. Altogether, more than 100 medications have completed the preclinical stage and are now in phases I, II, and III of clinical development (see Table B.1).

A few examples will illustrate the current trends: New medications with a novel mechanism of action, unavailable until now, are in the pipe-

TABLE B.1. Medicines in Development for Mental Illness

Indication	Medications in development
• Anxiety disorders	18
• Attention-deficit/hyperactivity disorder	6
• Dementias	25
• Depression	14
• Eating disorders	5
• Premenstrual disorders	4
• Schizophrenia	15
• Sleep disorders	11
• Substance use disorders	24

Note. As of December 2004, some medicines are in development for more than one disorder. Data from Pharmaceutical Research and Manufacturers of America (2004).

line for the treatment of depression. These include medications that antagonize the NK-1 receptor and at least one antidepressant that is given by subcutaneous injection and may have a noticeably strong onset of action in only a few days; a new class of drugs for Alzheimer's disease that modulates **glutamate** levels in the brain, a neurotransmitter that in some conditions may be neurotoxic; a vaccine that promotes the development of anticocaine antibodies; and a cannabinoid receptor antagonist for appetite suppression.

As discussed earlier, some of these medications will never reach the pharmacies, as unexpected findings related to poor efficacy or intolerable and/or dangerous side effects are not infrequently identified during phase II and III trials. However, the sheer volume of potential agents, formulations, and administration routes being investigated bodes well for the near future.

SOME NOVEL NONPHARMACOLOGICAL TREATMENTS FOR DEPRESSION

Repetitive Transcranial Magnetic Stimulation

Repetitive Transcranial Magnetic Stimulation (rTMS) was initially introduced as a neurophysiologic tool in neurology. It became apparent that some patients exposed to it experienced positive mood changes reminiscent of the effects of antidepressants. Further research confirmed that biochemical, endocrine, and sleep physiology changes induced by all effective antidepressants, including antidepressant medications and ECT, were also observed in subjects treated with rTMS. Currently, several research centers in Israel, Spain, and the United States, among other countries, are actively involved in exploring the full potential of this form of treatment. Some have suggested that it may replace ECT, although this prediction is premature at this time.

rTMS is the application of an electromagnetic coil to the scalp to create a strong pulsatile magnetic field, which after entering the brain, can produce neuron activation in localized areas. Repeated applications have had antidepressant effects. The procedure is administered for a few weeks in an outpatient setting, on a fully awake patient, for sessions lasting 15–30 minutes several times a week. The optimal frequency and intensity of the stimulus, frequency of treatments, coil placement, and other technical aspects are still being investigated (see Figure B.1).

rTMS appears to be a well-tolerated and benign form of treatment, at least based on the research to date. The most common side effects are headaches, localized discomfort (e.g., tingling or a buzz feeling), and localized muscle twitching. A few patients have developed seizures. The long-term risks of rTMS, if any, are not known, although data available at this time suggest that they may not be significant. In 2008 the FDA approved the use of a rTMS device for use in patients with major depression who have failed to respond to antidepressant medication treatment.

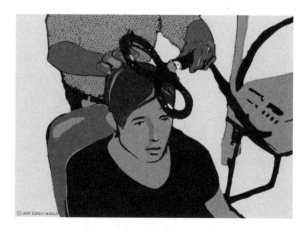

FIGURE B.1. Repetitive transcranial magnetic stimulation (rTMS). Illustration copyright 2005 by Keren Albala. Used with permission.

In addition to depression, rTMS is being investigated for its potential in the treatment of schizophrenia, anxiety disorders, and chronic pain, and even as a potential performance booster.

Vagus Nerve Stimulation

Vagus nerve stimulation (VNS) comes to psychiatry after being used as an effective treatment in certain forms of seizure disorder, and more that 10,000 patients worldwide have received the surgical procedure needed for electrode placement and implantation of the stimulus pacemaker generator. Mood elevations were noticed on some of the epileptic patients being treated with VNS, and its potential as an antidepressant treatment was quickly recognized. There are, in fact, a number of elements that support this contention, including the effects of VNS on the limbic system (the dysfunction of which has been associated with mood disorders), the fact that the vagus nerve projects to brain areas involved in depression, and PET (positron-emission tomography) data showing effects on mood-regulating regions of the brain.

A pacemaker generator is implanted under the skin in the chest wall, and it is connected to an electrode attached to the vagus nerve in the neck area, which has direct extensions into the brain. The pacemaker is receptive to programming and instructions given externally by computer, and thus specific parameters of intensity and frequency, as well as other technical variables, can be controlled and adjusted according to the specific needs of the patient (Figure B.2).

Research on VNS is still in the early stages, but early trials in patients with severely refractory depression have been encouraging, and many patients appear to have benefited from the treatment, some of them experiencing full remission of their symptoms. Some patients continued to improve as months passed, and the beneficial effects lasted through the follow-up period (George et al., 2005; Rush, Marangell, et al., 2005; Rush, Sackheim, et al., 2005). Most of the side effects reported by depressed patients are similar to those reported by patients with epilepsy, and these are related to the actual stimulation periods; they include voice alteration, coughing, difficulty in swallowing, and pain. VNS was approved by the FDA in 2005 "as an adjunctive long-term treatment for chronic or recurrent depression for patients 18 years of age and older who are experiencing a major depressive episode and have not had an adequate response to four or more adequate antidepressant treatments" (U.S. FDA, 2005).

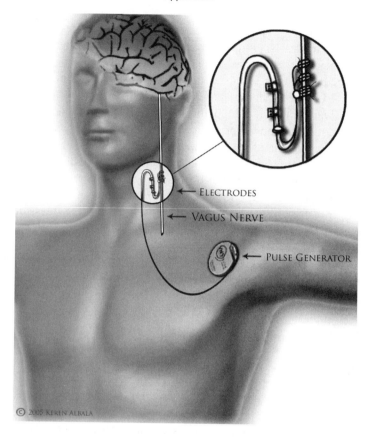

FIGURE B.2. Vagus nerve stimulation (VNS). Illustration copyright 2005 by Keren Albala. Used with permission.

Because of the invasive (surgical) nature of the procedure, it will take some time to discover the actual therapeutic potential and clinical applicability of this technique in the treatment of depression.

Deep Brain Stimulation

The use of deep brain stimulation (DBS) as a therapeutic tool in psychiatry is in the early stages of development. The treatment has been used for several years as a neurosurgical procedure, especially in the treatment of movement disorders (e.g., Parkinson's disease), and it is considered by some to be quite revolutionary (Kopell, Greenberg, & Rezai, 2004). DBS is a neurosurgical technique whereby electrodes are implanted, with great precision, in predetermined areas of the brain thought to be the seat of neurocircuitry involved in the medical condition targeted for treatment. The electrodes are connected to a stimulator about the size of a pocket watch, which is implanted surgically in the chest under the skin. This stimulator is programmable, so the operator can control— among other parameters—the frequency and intensity of the electrical stimulus (including shutting off the stimulation altogether).

The psychiatric application of this technique has its origins in previous neurosurgical experience in the treatment of several nonresponsive psychiatric conditions, especially refractory depression and refractory obsessive–compulsive disorder. The neurosurgical procedures used in these cases (termed "psychosurgery"), which are performed in very few sites in the world—including the United States and parts of Europe—consist of the causation of lesions in specific brain areas thought to be involved in causing the symptoms in question. The reader may have become acquainted with the names of some of these procedures—anterior capsulotomy, subcaudate tractotomy, cingulotomy, and limbic leucotomy—which refer to the site and type of lesion induced. These psychosurgical procedures, much more refined than the crude "lobotomies" practiced in the 1940s and 1950s, provide some severely disabled and suffering patients who are otherwise untreatable with substantial relief and a very low side-effect burden. The main limitation of psychosurgery, of course, is its irreversibility: there is no way to correct the lesion if, for example, a certain side effect was produced or the lesion has caused a worsening rather than an improvement in the symptoms, as occurs sometimes in the imprecise world of medicine. DBS causes—as far as we know at the present time— minimal brain tissue damage during electrode implantation, and the procedure is fully reversible in the sense that the stimulation can be set on or off at will, and if necessary, the electrodes can be removed. DBS's reversibility also offers the opportunity for the introduction of placebo study designs, where in the same patient, in a blind research fashion, the stimulation can be present or absent without the subject's knowledge. Finally, through its ability to stimulate specific brain circuits, DBS may develop into a formidable research tool.

At the present time we are just beginning to learn about the potential that DBS may have in psychiatry. Case reports and a few small patient series have shown encouraging results for the treatment of refractory depression and obsessive–compulsive disorder (Abelson et al., 2005; Aquizerate et al., 2004; Mayberg et al., 2005). However, much more research will be necessary before we learn the true therapeutic value of this technique.

SINGLE-ENANTIOMER MEDICATION COMPOUNDS

Strictly speaking, the availability of single-enantiomer compounds is not a future trend since some of them have already made an entry into clinical medicine. However, this technique's full potential is still unrealized, and it may lead to increased availability of many better and safer medications. The field of stereochemistry, which deals with the three-dimensional structure of molecules, teaches us that chemical compounds, medications included, can occur as a mixture of molecules whose structures are mirror images of each other. This means that two molecules that are otherwise identical may be spatially oriented in opposite directions, say, one to the right, the other to the left. Molecules so characterized are called enantiomers.

The pharmacological significance of enantiomers resides in the fact that many of the receptors, enzymes, and other structures in our bodies are built to react to molecules oriented only in a specific direction (they are said to be chirally sensitive). If a medication has molecules oriented in two directions, only the one oriented in the direction wanted by the targeted receptor will be of value. The receptor will be indifferent to the other molecule, and thus this enantiomer will be therapeutically inactive. Worse yet, in some situations the therapeutically inactive enantiomer may actually interfere with the activity of the therapeutically active enantiomer, essentially reducing the efficacy of the medication. Conversely, an undesired receptor target—for example one that may cause certain side effects—may have spatial affinity for the other enantiomer in the medication, that is, the one devoid of therapeutic benefit. A number of medications contain both the "good" and the "bad" enantiomers in their formulations.

Single-enantiomer technology—which earned its developers the Nobel Prize in Chemistry in 2000—enables the production of commercial quantities of medications that contain only the desired enantiomer, the other having been removed in the production process. Such is the case, for example, in the antidepressant escitalopram (trade name Lexapro) (see Figure B.3). This drug is the successor of citalopram (trade

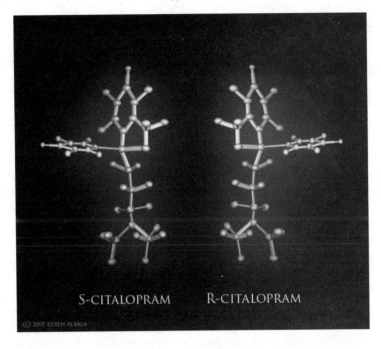

S-CITALOPRAM   R-CITALOPRAM

© 2005 KEREN ALBALA

FIGURE B.3. The chemical structure of citalopram (Celexa), showing its two enantiomers. The S-citalopram enantiomer is escitalopram (Lexapro) (see text). Illustration copyright 2005 by Keren Albala. Used with permission.

name Celexa). Citalopram is a mixture containing identical amounts of two enantiomers: S-citalopram and R-citalopram, the former being the "good" molecule, the latter being responsible, it is thought, for some of citalopram's side effects and, perhaps, interfering with the beneficial effect of its sister enantiomer. Single-enantiomer technology applied to citalopram enabled the development of a "purer" version, containing only the desired enantiomer and eliminating the one thought to be therapeutically inactive and responsible for at least some of the side effects. This purer version is called escitalopram, marketed under the trade name Lexapro and used successfully in the treatment of depressive and anxiety disorders.

Single-enantiomer technology should lead to the development of purer and cleaner medications, which are expected to offer improved efficacy and more benign side effects.

GENETICS, GENOMICS, AND PSYCHIATRY

It has not escaped our notice that the specific pairing we have postulated immediately suggests a possible copying mechanism for the genetic material.

—WATSON AND CRICK (1953)

Prophetic words, indeed. This is the second to last paragraph with which Watson and Crick (1953) closed their brief report, published more than 5 decades ago, in which they described the structure of DNA. Since that time, the growth in the fields of genetics and molecular biology has been nothing short of phenomenal. Its impact in diagnostic and therapeutic medicine is still in its infancy, but now that the human genome has been completed, the potential for very rapid progress is here. The field of genomics—which studies all the genes in the genome and their mode of interaction in the transmission of genetic information—is expected to produce sufficient leads that will enable the development of therapeutic agents for most clinical conditions in which genes play a role. Psychiatry and mental illness are expected to reap extraordinary benefits from this quickened pace of research.

It has been known for quite some time that mental disorders run in families; it has also been suspected that genetic transmission plays an important role in the familial clustering of these disorders. However, higher incidence among family members does not necessarily signify genetic transmission. It is, of course, quite likely that the family environment itself is responsible for the "transmission" of behavioral patterns from one generation to the next. Sophisticated pedigree studies, twin studies, and adoption studies have provided a clearer picture, strongly supporting the contribution of genes to the transmission of mental illnesses. At the present time, certain illnesses, like autism and bipolar disorder, are suspected of having a strong heritability factor, whereas depression has a much smaller one (Table B.2).

Of course, the very existence of a genetic factor that is less than 100% responsible for the generational transmission of disease means that other factors, namely, the environment ("nurture"), must provide the necessary complement for the pathological process to manifest itself. So what in effect is happening is that what is inherited is not really the disease but rather the *vulnerability* to it. An excellent example of this paradigm, of relevance to mental illness, is the report by Caspi et al. (2003), later replicated by Kendler et al. (2005), which examined the moderating effect of genetic polymorphism of the serotonin transporter

TABLE B.2. Relative Risks for Selected Psychiatric Disorders

Disorder	Risk ratio	Heritability estimate
Mood disorders		
Bipolar disorder	7–10	.60–.70
Major depression	2–3	.28–.40
Anxiety disorders		
All	4 6	.30–.40
Panic disorder	3–8	.50–.60
Autism	50–100	.90
Schizophrenia	8–10	.80–.84
Substance dependence	4–8	.30–.50

Note. "Relative risk" = proportion of affected first-degree relatives of affected probands versus the proportion of affected relatives of nonaffected control subjects. Data from Merikangas and Risch (2003).

on the influence that life stress had on the likelihood of developing depression. Individuals who had a certain variation in the genetic structure (one or two short alleles) that governs the function of the serotonin transporter were more likely to develop depression and suicidality in response to stressful life events than individuals equipped with the "normal" genetic structure (two copies of the long allele). This exciting line of research will continue to expand, and studies of the gene–environment interaction in many psychiatric and other medical disorders are being proposed (Moffit, Caspi, & Rutter, 2005).

The therapeutic implications of this finding are important: Genetic manipulation may be capable, at some point in the future, of modifying this genetic vulnerability; conversely, early recognition of individuals made vulnerable by their particular genetic profile can lead to preventive implementation of certain psychosocial interventions (e.g., individual and family therapy), which would be aimed at diminishing the relative impact of stressful events in these genetically susceptible individuals.

Research has produced a group of candidate genes for several mental disorders. For example, for schizophrenia, neuregulin-1, catechol-O-methyltransferase, dysbindin, and G72 are promising leads. The evidence currently available suggests that for most, if not all, psychiatric disorders, not one but many genes will be found to be involved in their heritability risk.

Additional potential benefits of genomics would be the identification of pharmacokinetic and pharmacodynamic patient profiles, which will allow us to tailor medication treatment to a specific patient. No more "average doses" for medications; no more "all antidepressants have equal efficacy." Instead, for example, we might be able to ascertain the patient's likelihood to respond better to a certain antidepressant than to another; or we might be able to predict which patients are more likely to develop certain side effects, like tardive dyskinesia or sexual dysfunction, and thus plan our treatment accordingly. To illustrate the potential of this technology, consider one subset of data from the STAR*D study, which was discussed in detail in Chapter 3, showing that genetic makeup can influence response to antidepressant treatment. Individuals who have two copies of a less common allele of a gene that codes for a serotonin receptor implicated in the regulation of mood increased by 18% the odds of a favorable antidepressant response, compared to having two copies of the more common allele (McMahon et al., 2006). Applied genomics in psychiatry is still many years away.

The areas reviewed in this chapter represent some research trends and directions in psychiatric therapeutics. Some methods, like VNS and a new generation of medications, are just entering clinical practice and only time will tell what their impact will be. Clearly, the bar must be raised so that newer treatments produce stronger beneficial effects, in shorter times, on a wider segment of patients, and with few or no side effects. These challenges, for example, are particularly formidable in disorders like schizophrenia and Alzheimer's disease, which have relatively high prevalence rates, are severely disabling, and current treatments offer only modest results.

In the long run, it would appear that the most potentially fruitful line of research will be in the field of genetics, which is expected to teach us much about the mechanisms of mental illness and, as a result, to steer us in the direction of developing therapeutic tools that will target the specific processes underlying the clinical manifestations of disease.

The psychopharmacology revolution of the 1950s marked a turning point in the treatment of psychiatric disorders, offering hope to patients, families, and clinicians. The genetic revolution in psychiatry currently brewing will have an even more dramatic impact. Indeed, the world of mental illness promises to look quite different in the next decade or two.

Professional Outreach

The following is a list of groups supporting collaborative efforts among health care professionals. We anticipate, with the continued development of the collaborative care movement, that this list will grow over time.

- American Psychological Association Division 38: Health Psychology — www.health-psych.org

- Australian Mental Health Branch of Health Services — www.mentalhealth.gov.au/boimhc/index.htm

- Canadian Collaborative Mental Health Initiative — www.ccmhi.ca

- Collaborative Family Healthcare Association — www.cfha.net

- Counselors and Psychotherapists in Primary Care — www.cpct.co.uk/cpct/

- Cummings Foundation — www.thecummingsfoundation.com

- Integrated Health Care Initiative — www.hogg.utexas.edu/Pages/IHC.html
- Integrated Primary Care — www.integratedprimarycare.com/
- International Society of Behavioral Medicine — www.isbm.info/
- Primary Mental Health Care Australian Resource Centre — www.parc.net.au/
- Society of Behavioral Medicine — www.sbm.org
- Wales Mental Health in Primary Care — www.wales.nhs.uk/sites/home.cfm?orgID=405
- WHO Guide to Mental and Neurological Health in Primary Care — www.mentalneurologicalprmarycare.org

Glossary

absorption: the process of putting drugs into the bloodstream.

acetaldehyde: a metabolite of alcohol.

acetylcholine: a neurotransmitter found diffusely in the nervous system.

agranulocytosis: dangerously low white blood cell count, resulting in compromised ability to fight bacteria.

akathisia: a condition marked by motor restlessness, often with an inability to lie or sit still, which typically prevents rest and sleep.

allodynia: pain elicited by a non-noxious stimulus; for example, the touch of clothing causes pain, or air movement causes a burning sensation on the skin.

antagonist: something that works against something else.

anticholinergic side effects: side effects that occur when a medication is interfering with the normal function of acetylcholine, especially in the brain or parasympathetic nervous system.

anxiolytic: a medication that relieves anxiety.

asymptomatic: lacking symptoms.

augmentation: the process whereby the addition of a second medication enhances the effect of the first.

axon: the part of the neuron that carries the electrical impulse away from the cell body.

barbiturates: a class of anticonvulsants with sedative and anxiolytic properties.

beta-blockers: a class of medications often used to lower blood pressure and heart rate.

board certified: a physician certified as a specialist by the American Board of Medical Specialties.

board eligible: a physician who has completed all postgraduate training in a satisfactory manner and is in the process of registering, taking, and/or waiting for the results of the board certification process.

carve out: an insurance approach to controlling the cost of and access to certain services (mental health care, home care, etc.) by funding only one provider on a capitated basis, and that provider is usually not the primary care provider.

cell: the basic unit of living organisms; the basic building block.

cell membrane: the envelope that contains the contents of a cell and controls what goes into and out of the cell.

cerebral cortex: a higher part of the brain responsible for processes of thought, perception, and memory; it serves as the seat of advanced motor function, social abilities, language, and problem solving.

clearance: elimination of a substance from the bloodstream by breakdown of the substance and/or removal by the liver or kidneys.

collaborative care: health care services that focus on coordinated assessment and treatment by providers from different disciplines so that all aspects of the patient's health—whether biological, psychological, spiritual, or social—can be addressed. Successful collaborative care presumes shared treatment planning and decision making by interdisciplinary teams.

comorbidity: the state of having one or more diagnosable conditions.

concentration: the amount of medication dissolved in the blood.

cytoplasm: the liquid interior of a cell that contains the essential functioning components.

dendrite: the portion of a neuron that carries the electrical impulse toward the cell body.

dependence: any one or a combination of cognitive, behavioral, and physical symptoms indicating that the individual continues to use a substance in spite of significant harm or life problems.

distribution: the process of drugs being transported by the bloodstream to different parts of the body.

dizygotic twins: siblings delivered at the same time, from the same mother, but with their own distinct genetic makeup.

doctor of medicine (MD): a person who graduated from an accredited school of medicine.

doctor of osteopathy (DO): a person who graduated from an accredited school of osteopathic medicine.

dopamine: a neurotransmitter indicated in schizophrenia, other psychoses, and certain neurological disorders.

double blind: a study in which neither the subjects nor the investigators know whether the active drug or the placebo is being given.

drug holiday: deliberate temporary discontinuation of a medication.

DSM: *Diagnostic and Statistical Manual of Mental Disorders*, published by the American Psychiatric Association.

dystonia: muscle tone that is abnormal; a dystonic reaction to psychiatric medications causes involuntary, sudden, and irregular contortions of muscles of the trunk and extremities, which twist the body in various directions, in an often grotesque fashion.

electroconvulsive therapy (ECT): a treatment for depression, mania, and other psychiatric disorders whereby a generalized brain seizure is induced by electrical means in a medically controlled setting.

endocrine system: a system of organs throughout the body that sends chemical messengers (hormones) through the blood to alter the function of various body systems.

enzymes: chemicals that break down proteins and biochemical structures in the body.

epidemiology: the study of the mode of transmission and prevalence of medical disorders in the general population.

ethnopharmacology: the study of drug behavior in different ethnic groups.

etiology: the cause of an occurrence.

extrapyramidal symptoms: side effects of some medications that mimic Parkinson's disease (stiffness, gait disturbance, etc.).

first-pass metabolism: the change that occurs in a substance that was absorbed from the gut into the bloodstream, as that blood passes through the liver *before* it goes to the rest of the body.

GABA (gamma-aminobutyric acid): a neurotransmitter implicated in anxiety modulation.

genetic loading: a term used to describe the risk of developing a disease based only on genetic factors.

gestational period: pregnancy.

glutamate: a neurotransmitter.

habituation: occurs when the effects of a medication decrease as it is taken over time.

half-life: the time required for a medication to decrease its concentration by 50% in relation to its peak level.

hepatocellular injury: damage to liver cells.

HMO: health maintenance organization.

homeostasis: the tendency of a living organism to maintain balanced, constant conditions in its internal environment.

hyperalgesia: a heightened perception of pain.

hyperpathia: a delayed and explosive response to pain.

hypertension: high blood pressure.

hypotension: low blood pressure.

hypothyroidism: low thyroid function.

inhibitory impulses: occur when a receptor activated by a neurotransmitter causes the neuron to not fire off any impulses or to diminish firing.

intramuscular: inside the muscle.

intrauterine: inside the uterus.

licensed vocational nurse (LVN): a person with limited training and licensure to practice certain nursing functions under the supervision of a registered nurse (RN).

MAOIs: monoamine oxidase inhibitors—a class of antidepressants.

medical assistant (MA): a person with minimal training to assist with certain activities in a medical office, such as taking a patient's blood pressure and pulse, under the supervision of the physician and/or nurse.

Medicare: government-funded health care for seniors and disabled persons.

metabolic syndrome: A group of medical conditions (e.g., adult-onset diabetes, obesity, high blood pressure, and cholesterol abnormalities) that increase the risk of developing coronary artery disease.

metabolism: the process of the body's elimination or transformation of a drug.

mitochondria: organelles that provide energy to the cell so that other cell parts can do their work.

monotherapy: therapy with only one drug.

monozygotic twin: twins who are genetically identical.

mortality rates: the likelihood of an illness to cause death.

motor neurons: peripheral nerves that carry orders from the spinal cord and brain, telling a body part to move or to do something else.

neuroleptic: a medication having antipsychotic action, generally the original class of antipsychotics, not the newer "atypical" drugs.

neuroleptic malignant syndrome: a rare complication of treatment with the original antipsychotic medications and an extremely rare complication of treatment with other medications. It includes autonomic instability, rigidity, altered mental status, catatonia, and other symptoms. It is a medical emergency and can be fatal.

neurons: nerve cells.

neuropeptide: a protein with activity in the nervous system.

neurotransmitters: chemicals within a neuron that allow one neuron to transmit an impulse to another.

nonresponse: when a patient does not respond to treatment.

norepinephrine: a neurotransmitter primarily secreted by the sympathetic nervous system.

nucleus: central part of a cell that contains genetic material and controls the function, reproduction, and growth of the cell.

nurse practitioner (NP): a registered nurse with advanced training and licensure; the degree of autonomous practice varies from state to state.

oculogyric crisis: movement of the eyeballs in a sudden, irregular, and involuntary manner, often in a superior and posterior direction with a grotesque appearance; a rare complication of the older generation of antipsychotic medications.

one-way flow: the process, common to most synapses of the central nervous system, of conducting an impulse in one direction only.

organelles: tiny structures in cells responsible for making proteins and other substances that enable the cell to do its job.

organs: collections of tissues, organized into a body part with a unified purpose (e.g., a kidney).

parasympathetic nervous system: the part of the autonomic nervous system that causes a focused response of a particular organ.

parenterally: the administration of a drug by a route other than the digestive system.

parkinsonian symptoms: symptoms similar to Parkinson's disease.

pathophysiology: the physiology that explains the pathology that is observed.

peak concentration: the time required for a drug to go from ingestion to its maximum concentration in the bloodstream.

perinatal: occurring before, during, and soon after the time of birth (literally "surrounding birth").

peripheral nerves: nerves in various regions of the body, such as hands, arms, and legs.

pharmacodynamics: the mechanism of drug action and the relationship between drug concentration and the effects (positive and negative) that it has.

pharmacokinetics: the processes and rates of absorption, metabolism, half-lives, distribution, and elimination of medications in the body.

pharmacopoeia: a book or list of medications, usually with a description of their uses and side effects.

placebo: an inert substance devoid of pharmacological activity.

plasma levels: the concentration of a drug in the plasma.

point of service (POS): the place where a service (care) is provided.

polypharmacy: the use of more than one medication at a time for the same or similar conditions.

postsynaptic neuron: the neuron receiving the impulse from a neurotransmitter in a transmission between neurons.

preferred provider organization (PPO): a health benefit plan between the sponsor and health care providers to treat plan members. A PPO can also be a group of health care providers who contract with an insurer to treat policyholders according to a predetermined fee schedule. PPO contracts typically provide discounts from standard fees, incentives for plan enrollees to use the contracting providers, and other cost-containment methods.

presynaptic neuron: the neuron that makes and releases neurotransmitters in a transmission between neurons.

prognosis: the likely course or outcome of a disease.

prophylactic: preventative.

psychomotor: related to motor (muscle movement) effects of mental activity.

psychotropic medication: medication used for psychiatric conditions.

receptor site: a place on the postsynaptic neuron fit to receive a specific neurotransmitter.

reflex message: a message sent directly from the spinal cord, without consulting the brain, when quick action is needed.

refractory: difficult to control and resistant to treatment.

registered nurse (RN): a nurse who has graduated from an accredited program and has been registered and licensed to practice by a state authority.

relapse: return of illness or symptoms.

remission: complete resolution of illness or symptoms.

reuptake: the process of extra neurotransmitters in the synapse being taken back into the presynaptic neuron.

risk–benefit ratio: the process of selecting a medication that will produce the strongest possible therapeutic effect with the fewest possible side effects.

secrete: to release a neurotransmitter out of a neuron.

sensory gating: the ability of the sensory nervous system to screen incoming sensory information to determine what is significant for higher parts of the brain to focus on.

sensory neurons: peripheral nerves that send information to the spinal cord from various regions of the body.

serotonin: a neurotransmitter.

sign: an observable behavioral or physical change that is characteristic of a particular disorder.

soma: the body; for example, the cell body of a neuron is sometimes called the soma.

split care: patient care provided by two or more providers who have no contact with each other.

spontaneous remissions: the cessation of the symptoms of a disease or disorder without treatment.

SSRIs (selective serotonin reuptake inhibitors): a medication designed to enable more serotonin to remain in the synapse by blocking its reuptake by the presynaptic neuron.

steady state: the amount of time required for a drug to reach a balanced concentration level in the bloodstream.

stimulatory impulses: occur when a terminal activated by a neurotransmitter causes the postsynaptic neuron to fire an impulse to its neighboring neurons.

sympathetic nervous system: the part of the autonomic nervous system that has multiorgan impact, such as the fight-or-flight response.

symptomatology: constellation of symptoms.

symptoms: subjective changes in feeling or behavior reported by a patient that are characteristic of a particular disorder.

synapse: the tiny space between two neurons.

syndromes: a distinctive patterns of symptoms that, taken together, are indicative of a disease or condition.

systems: groups of related things or parts that function together as a whole.

tardive dyskinesia: the abnormal involuntary movements, especially of the tongue, mouth, and face, that can occur after the use of antipsychotic medications. Commonly occurs after years of medication use. ("Tardive" means late; "dyskinesia" means abnormal movements.)

target symptoms: symptoms and problems that are interfering with the patient's life.

TCAs (tricyclic antidepressants): antidepressant medications that have three rings in its chemical structure.

telemedicine: the use of the telephone to practice medicine.

teratogenic effects: causing harm or deformity to a developing fetus.

therapeutic index: the difference in doses of medication between a dose that produces serious side effects and the dose needed for therapeutic effectiveness.

therapeutic window: the blood level below and above which a drug does not work well.

tolerability: capacity for being tolerated or endured.

tolerance: the need to consume progressively larger quantities of a substance to achieve intoxication or the desired effect, or the state of needing a progressively increasing dose to maintain a sense of normality.

torticollis: an involuntary contraction of the muscles of the neck, causing the neck to twist at odd angles. It can occur as a symptom of several illnesses and as a side effect of many medications, not only those used in psychiatry.

toxicity: poisonous, harmful qualities.

treatment adherence: compliance with treatment.

trough levels: the point at which the concentration of a medication in the bloodstream is at its lowest just before the ingestion of the next scheduled dose.

ubiquitous: omnipresent; present in all places; very common.

unipolar depression: depression without mania.

vesicles: sacs in a neuron that are filled with neurotransmitters.

volume of distribution: the volume of blood in which the absorbed and active medication is dissolved.

withdrawal: a syndrome of very unpleasant cognitive, psychological, and physical symptoms that occurs when the amount of a substance declines in the bloodstream.

References

Abelson, J. L., Curtis, G. C., Sagher, O., Albucher, R. C., Harrigan, M., Taylor, S. F., et al. (2005). Deep brain stimulation for refractory obsessive-compulsive disorder. *Biological Psychiatry, 57,* 510–516.

Abramowicz, M. (2000). Rivastigmine (Exelon) for Alzheimer's disease. *Medical Letter on Drugs and Therapeutics, 42,* 93–94.

Abramowicz, M. (2001). Galantamine (Reminyl) for Alzheimer's disease. *Medical Letter on Drugs and Therapeutics, 43,* 53–54.

Abramowicz, M. (2003). Memantine for Alzheimer's disease. *Medical Letter on Drugs and Therapeutics, 45,* 73–74.

American Psychiatric Association. (2000). *Diagnostic and statistical manual of mental disorders* (4th ed., text rev.). Washington, DC: Author.

American Psychiatric Association. (2001). *The practice of electroconvulsive therapy: Recommendations for treatment, training, and privileging* (2nd ed.). Washington, DC: Author.

American Psychological Association. (2002). [Electronic reference on prescription privileges for psychologists.] Retrieved February 14, 2005, from www.apa.org/practice/nm_rxp.html.

Anderson, I. M., & Reid, I. C. (2002). *Fundamentals of clinical pharmacology.* UK: Cromwell Press.

Anderson, R. N., & Smith, B. L. (2003). Deaths: Leading causes for 2001. *National Vital Statistics Report, 52*(9), 1–86.

Aquizerate, B., Cuny, E., Martin-Guehl, C., Guehl, D., Amieva, H., Benazzouz, A., et al. (2004). Deep brain stimulation of the ventral caudate nucleus in the treatment of obsessive–compulsive disorder and major depression. *Journal of Neurosurgery, 101,* 682–686.

Balon, R., & Harvey, K. V. (1995). Clinical implications of antidepressant drug effects on sexual function. *Annals of Clinical Psychiatry, 7*(4), 189–201.

Baucom, D. H., Shoham, V., Mueser, K. T., Daiuto, A. D., & Stickle, T. R. (1998). Empirically supported couple and family interventions for marital distress and adult mental health problems. *Journal of Consulting and Clinical Psychology, 66,* 53–88.

Baum, A. L., & Misri, S. (1996). Selective serotonin-reuptake inhibitors in pregnancy and lactation. *Harvard Review of Psychiatry, 4*(3), 117–125.

Beitman, B. D., Blinder, B. J., Thase, M. E., Riba, M., & Safer, D. L. (2003). *Integrating psychotherapy and pharmacotherapy: Dissolving the mind–brain barrier.* New York: Norton.

Blount, A. (Ed.). (1998). *Integrated primary care: The future of medical and mental health collaboration.* New York: Norton.

Bohus, M., Haff, B., Simms, T., Limberger, M. F., Schamhl, C., Unckel, C., et al. (2004). Effectiveness of impatient dialectical behavioral therapy for borderline personality disorder: A controlled trial. *Behaviour Research and Therapy, 43*(5), 487–499.

Borchert, S. (2004, July 1). Integrated care might fix Medicare. *Family Practice News,* p. 33.

Bray, J. H., & Rogers, J. C. (1997). The linkages project: Training behavioral health professionals for collaborative practice with primary care physicians. *Families, Systems, and Health, 15*(1), 55–63.

Bright, D. A. (1994). Postpartum mental disorders. *American Family Physician, 50*(3), 595–598.

Bruce, M. L., Ten Have, T. R., & Reynolds, C. F. (2004). Reducing suicidal ideation and depressive symptoms in depressed older primary care patients: A reandomized controlled study. *Journal of the American Medical Association, 291,* 1081–1091.

Cade, J. F. J. (1949). Lithium salts in the treatment of psychotic excitement. *Medical Journal of Australia, 36,* 349–352.

Caspi, A., Sugden K., Moffitt, T. E., Taylor, A., Craig, I. W., Harrington, H., et al. (2003). Influence of life stress on depression: Moderation by a polymorphism in the 5-HTT gene. *Science, 301*(5631), 386–389.

Cassidy, E., Hill, S., & O'Callaghan, E. (2001). Efficacy of a psychoeducational intervention in improving relatives' knowledge about schizophrenia and reducing rehospitalisation. *European Psychiatry, 16,* 446–450.

Centers for Disease Control and Prevention, National Center for Health Statistics. (2006). *Self-inflicted injury/suicide.* Retrieved June 6, 2006, from www.cdc.gov/nchs/fastats/suicide.htm

Cipriani, A., Furukawa, T. A., Salanti, G., Geddes, J. R., Higgins, J. P. T., Churchill, R., et al. (2009). Comparative efficacy and acceptability of 12 new-generation antidepressants: A multiple-treatments meta-analysis. *www.thelancet.com.* Published online January 29, 2009. DOI:10.1016/S0140-6736(09)60046-5.

Clark, C. M., Sheppard, L., Fillenbaum, G. G., Galasko, D., Morris, J. C., Koss, E., et al. (1999). Variability in annual Mini-Mental State Examination score in patients with probable Alzheimer's disease: A clinical perspective of data from the Consortium to Establish a Registry for Alzheimer's Disease. *Archives of Neurology, 56*(7), 857–862.

Clarkin, J., Carpenter, D., Hull, J., Wilner, P., & Glick, I. (1998). Effects of psychoeducational intervention for married patients with bipolar disorder and their spouses. *Psychiatric Services, 49*(4), 531–533.

Clarkin, J. F., Levy, K. N., Lezenweger, M. F., & Kernberg, O. F. (2004). The

Personality Disorders Institute/Borderline Personality Disorder Research Foundation randomized control trial for borderline personality disorder: Rationale, methods, and patient characteristics. *Journal of Personality Disorders, 18*(1), 52–72.

Coldham, E., Addington, J., & Addington, D. (2002). Medication adherence of individuals with a first episode of psychosis. *Acta Psychiatrica Scandinavica, 106*(4), 286–290.

Cole-Kelly, K., & Seaburn, D. (1999). Five areas of questioning to promote a family-oriented approach in primary care. *Families, Systems, and Health, 17,* 341–348.

Combrinck-Graham, L. (1985). A developmental model for family systems. *Family Process, 24,* 139–150.

Consensus Development Conference on Antipsychotic Drugs and Obesity and Diabetes. (2004). *Diabetes Care, 27*(2), 596–601.

Cornish, J. W., Metzger, D., Woody, G. E., Wilson, D., McLellan, A. T., Vandergrift, B., et al. (1997). Naltrexone pharmacotherapy for opioid dependent federal probationers. *Journal of Substance Abuse Treatment, 14*(6), 529–534.

Coyne, J. (2000). Psychotropic drug use in very young children. *Journal of the American Medical Association, 283*(8), 1059–1060.

Cukor, J., Spitalnick, J., Difede, J., Rizzo, A., & Rothbaum, B. (2009). Emerging treatments for PTSD. *Clinical Psychology Review.* Available online October 2009. DOI:10.1016/j.cpr.2009.09.001.

Czeisler, C. A., Winkelman, J. W., & Richardson, G. S. (2001). Sleep disorders. In E. Braunwald, A. C. Fauci, D. L. Kasper, S. L. Hauser, & J. L. Jameson (Eds.), *Harrison's principles of internal medicine* (15th ed.). New York: McGraw-Hill.

Davidson, J. R. T. (2003). Pharmacotherapy of social phobia. *Acta Psychiatrica Scandanavica, 108*(417), 65–71.

Depression Guideline Panel. (1993a). *Depression in primary care: Vol. 1. Detection and diagnosis* (Clinical Practice Guideline No. 5; AHCPR Publication No. 93-0550). Rockville, MD: U. S. Department of Health and Human Services, Public Health Service, Agency for Health Care Policy and Research.

Depression Guideline Panel. (1993b). *Depression in primary care: Vol. 2. Treatment of major depression* (Clinical Practice Guideline No. 5; AHCPR Publication No. 93-0551). Rockville, MD: U.S. Department of Health and Human Services, Public Health Service, Agency for Health Care Policy and Research.

DeRubeis, R. J., Hollon, S. D., Amsterdam, J. D., Shelton, R. C., Young, P. R., Salomon, R. M., et al. (2005). Cognitive therapy vs. medications in the treatment of moderate to severe depression. *Archives of General Psychiatry, 62*(4), 409–416.

Dickson, R., Williams, R., & Dalby, J. (1995). The clozapine experience from a family perspective. *Canadian Journal of Psychiatry, 40,* 627–629.

Doherty, W. J. (1995). The why's and levels of collaborative family health care. *Family Systems Medicine, 13*(3–4), 275–281.

Doherty, W. J., & Baird, M. A. (1983). *Family therapy and family medicine: Toward the primary care of families.* New York: Guilford Press.

Engel, G. L. (1980). The clinical application of the biopsychosocial model. *American Journal of Psychiatry, 137*(5), 535–544.

Engstrom, J. W., & Hauser S. L. (2003). Alcohol and alcoholism. In E.

Braunwald, A. S. Fauci, K. J. Isselbacher, et al. (Eds.), *Harrison's online.* New York: McGraw-Hill.

Epperson, N., Czarkowski, K. A., Ward-O'Brien, D., Weiss, E., Gueorguieva, R., Jatlow, P., et al. (2001). Maternal setraline treatment and serotonin transport in breast-feeding mother–infant pairs. *American Journal of Psychiatry,* *158*(10), 1631–1637.

Ezzell, C. (2003). New research addresses the wrenching question when someone ends his or her own life. Why?: The neuroscience of suicide. *Scientific American, 288*(2), 44–51.

Feighner, J. P., Robins, E., Guze, S. B., Woodruff, R. A., Jr., Winokur, G., & Munoz, R. (1972). Diagnostic criteria for use in psychiatric research. *Archives of General Psychiatry, 26*(1), 57–63.

Fishman, S., & Berger, L. (2000). *The war on pain.* New York: HarperCollins.

Flier, J. S. (2001). Obesity. In E. Braunwald, A. C. Fauci, D. L. Kasper, S. L. Hauser, D. L. Longo, & J. L. Jameson (Eds.), *Harrison's principles of internal medicine* (15th ed.). New York: McGraw-Hill.

Folstein, M. F., Folstein, S. E., & McHugh, P. R. (1975). "Mini-mental state": A practical method for grading the cognitive state of patients for the clinician. *Journal of Psychiatry Research, 12*(3), 189–198.

Frank, E. (1997). Enhancing patient outcomes: Treatment adherence. *Journal of Clinical Psychiatry, 58*(Suppl. 1), 11–14.

Frasure-Smith, N., Lesperance, F., & Talajic, M. (1993). Depression following myocardial infarction: Impact on 6-month survival. *Journal of the American Medical Association, 270,* 1819–1825.

Freemantle, N., Anderson, I. M., & Young, P. (2000). Predictive value of pharmacological activity for the relative efficacy of antidepressant drugs. *British Journal of Psychiatry, 177,* 292–302.

Fried, B. J., Rundal, T. G., & Topping, S. (2000). Groups and teams in health services organizations. In S. M. Shortell & A. D. Kaluzny (Eds.), *Health care management.* Albany, NY: Delmar Thomson Learning.

Geddes, J. R., Carney, S. M., Davies, C., Furukawa, T. A., Kupfer, D. J., Frank, E., et al. (2003). Relapse prevention with antidepressant drug treatment in depressive disorders: A systematic review. *Lancet, 361,* 653–661.

George, M. S., Rush, A. J., Marangell, L. B., Sackheim, H. A., Brannan, S. K., Davis, S. M., et al. (2005). A one-year comparison of vagus nerve stimulation with treatment as usual for treatment-resistant depression. *Biological Psychiatry, 58,* 364–373.

Gitlin, M. J. (1996). *The psychotherapist's guide to psychopharmacology* (2nd ed.). New York: Free Press.

Glassman, A. H., O'Connor, C. M., Califf, R., Swedberg, K., Schwartz, P., Bigger, J. T., Jr., et al., for the Sertraline Antidepressant Heart Attack Randomized Trial Group. (2002). Setraline treatment of major depression in patients with acute MI or unstable angina. *Journal of the American Medical Association, 288,* 701–709.

Goldstein, M. (1981). Drug treatment and family intervention during the aftercare treatment of schizophrenics. *Psychopharmacology Bulletin, 17*(3), 87–88.

Goodwin, F. K., & Jamison, K. R. (1990). *Manic–depressive illness.* New York: Oxford University Press.

Gottesman, I. I. (1991). *Schizophrenia genesis: The origins of madness.* New York: Holt.

Green, S. A., & Bloch, S. (2001). Working in a flawed mental health care system: An ethical challenge. *American Journal of Psychiatry, 158*(9), 1378–1383.

Grumbach, K., & Bodenheimer, T. (2004). Can health care teams improve primary care practice? *Journal of the American Medical Association, 291*(10), 1246–1251.

Hamilton, M. (1960). A rating scale for depression. *Journal of Neurology, Neurosurgery, and Psychiatry, 23,* 56–61.

Harvey, K. V., & Balon, R. (1995). Clinical implications of antidepressant drug effects on sexual function. *Annals of Clinical Psychiatry, 7*(4), 189–201.

Haynes, R. B., McDonald, H. P., & Garg, A. X. (2002). Helping patients follow prescribed treatment: Clinical applications. *Journal of the American Medical Association, 288,* 2880–2883.

Henry, C., & Demotes-Mainard, J. (2003). Avoiding drug-induced switching in patients with bipolar depression. *Drug Safety, 26*(5), 337–351.

Hernandez, B. C., & Doherty, W. J. (2005). Marriage and family therapists and psychotropic medications: Practice patterns from a national study. *Journal of Marital and Family Therapy, 31*(3), 177–189.

Holbrook, J. H. (2001). Nicotine addiction. In E. Braunwald, A. C. Fauci, D. L. Kasper, S. L. Hauser, D. L. Longo, & J. L. Jameson (Eds.), *Harrison's priniciples of internal medicine* (14th ed.). New York: McGraw-Hill.

Hollon, S. D., DeRubeis, R. J., Shelton, R. C., Amsterdam, J. D., Salomon, R. M., et al. (2005). Prevention of relapse following cognitive therapy vs. medications in moderate to severe depression. *Archives of General Psychiatry, 62*(4), 417–422.

Institute of Medicine. (2001). *Crossing the quality chasm: A new health system for the 21st century.* Washington, DC: National Academies Press.

Jensen, G. B., & Pakkenberg, B. (1993). Do alcoholics drink their neurons away? *Lancet, 342,* 1201–1204.

Joint Commission on Accreditation of Healthcare Organizations. (1999). [Electronic reference on pain management.] Retrieved September 21, 2004, from www.jcaho.org/news+room/health+care+issues/jcaho+focuses+on+pain+management.htm.

Kahn, D., Gwyther, L. P., Frances, A., Silver, J. M., Alexopoulos, G., & Ross, R. (1998). Treatment of agitation in older persons with dementia. The Expert Consensus Panel for agitation in dementia. *Postgraduate Medicine, Special Report #1,* 81–88.

Kandel, E. R. (1995). Neuropeptides, adenylyl cyclase, and memory storage. *Science, 268,* 825–826.

Kandel, E. R. (1998). A new intellectual framework for psychiatry. *American Journal of Psychiatry, 155,* 457–469.

Kandel, E. R. (2006). *In search of memory.* New York: Norton.

Kane, J. M., Marder, S. R., Schooler, N. R., Wirshing, W. C., Umbricht, D., Baker, R. W., et al. (2001). Clozapine and haloperidol in moderately refractory schizophrenia: A 6-month randomized and double-blind comparison. *Archives of General Psychiatry, 58*(10), 965–972.

Karege, F., Perret, G., Bondolfi, G., Schwald, M., Bertschy, G., & Aubry, J. (2001). Decreased serum brain-derived neurotrophic factor levels in major depressed patients. *Psychiatry Research, 109*(2002), 143–148.

Katon, W., Schoenbaum, M., Fan, M.-Y., Callahan, C. M., Williams, J., Jr., Hunkeler, E., et al. (2005). Cost-effectiveness of improving primary care treatment of late-life depression. *Archives of General Psychiatry, 62,* 1313–1320.

Kendler, K. S., Kuhn, J. W., Vittum, J., Prescott, C. A., & Riley, B. (2005). The interaction of stressful life events and a serotonin transporter polymorphism in the prediction of episodes of major depression. *Archives of General Psychiatry, 62,* 529–535.

Kernberg, O. F. (1984). *Severe personality disorders: Psychotherapeutic strategies.* New Haven, CT: Yale University Press.

Kessler, R. C., Berglund, P., Demler, O., Jin, R., Koretz, D., Merikangas, K. R., et al. (2003). The epidemiology of major depressive disorder: Results from the National Comorbidity Survey Replication (NCS-R). *Journal of the American Medical Association, 289*(23), 3095–3105.

Kessler, R. C., McGonagle, K. A., Zhao, S., Nelson, C. B., Hughes, M., Eshleman, S., et al. (1994). Lifetime and 12-month prevalence of DSM-III-R psychiatric disorders in the United States: Results from the National Comorbidity Survey. *Archives of General Psychiatry, 51*(1), 8–19.

Kessler, R. C., Sonnega, A., Bromet, E., Hughes, M., & Nelson, C. B. (1995). Posttraumatic stress disorder in the National Comorbidity Survey. *Archives of General Psychiatry, 52*(12), 1048–1060.

Kessler, R. C., Stein, M. B., & Berglund, P. (1998). Social phobia subtypes in the National Comorbidity Survey. *American Journal of Psychiatry, 155,* 613–619.

Kessler, R. C., Zhao, S., & Katz, S. J. (1999). Past-year use of outpatient services for psychiatric problems in the National Comorbidity Survey. *American Journal of Psychiatry, 156*(1), 115–123.

Kinney, J. (Ed.). (1989). *The busy physician's five-minute guide to the management of alcohol problems.* Chicago: American Medical Association.

Kissling, W. (1991). The current unsatisfactory state of relapse prevention in schizophrenic psychoses—Suggestions for improvement. *Clinical Neuropharmacology, 14*(Suppl. 2), 33–44.

Koppell, B. H., Greenberg, B., & Rezai, A. R. (2004). Deep brain stimulation for psychiatric disorders. *Journal of Clinical Neurophysiology 21*(1), 5–67.

Kotcher, M., & Smith, T. (1993). Three phases of clozapine treatment and phase-specific issues for patients and families. *Hospital and Community Psychiatry, 44*(8), 744–747.

Kraepelin, E. (1971). *Dementia praecox and paraphenia.* Huntington, NY: Krieger. (Original work published 1919)

Kraepelin, E. (1976). *Manic–depressive insanity and paranoia* (reprint ed.). New York: Arno Press.

Kramer, P. D. (1993). *Listening to Prozac.* New York: Viking.

Kreisman, J. J., & Straus, H. (1991). *I hate you, don't leave me: Understanding the borderline personality.* New York: Morrow/Avon Press.

Kroenke, K., & Price, R. K. (1993). Symptoms in the community: Prevalence, classification, and psychiatric comorbidity. *Archives of Internal Medicine, 153*(21), 2474–2480.

Krystal, J. H., Cramer, J. A., Krol, W. F., Kirk, G. F., & Rosenheck, R. A., Veterans Affairs Naltrexone Cooperative Study 425 Group. (2001). Naltrexone in the treatment of alcohol dependence. *New England Journal of Medicine, 345*(24), 1734–1739.

Kuhn, T. S. (1957). *The structure of scientific revolutions.* Chicago: University of Chicago Press.

Kulin, N. A., Pastuszak, A., Sage, S. R., Schick-Boschetto, B., Spivey, G., Feld-kamp, M., et al. (1998). Pregnancy outcome following maternal use of the new selective serotonin reuptake inhibitors: A prospective controlled multicenter study. *Journal of the American Medical Association, 279*(8), 609–610.

Kupfer, D. J. (1991). Long-term treatment of depression. *Journal of Clinical Psychiatry, 52*(Suppl. 5), 28–34.

Kupfer, D. J. (2005). The increasing medical burden in bipolar disorder. *Journal of the American Medical Association, 293*(20), 2528–2530.

Lieberman, J. A., Stroup, T. S., McEvoy, J. P., Swartz, M. S., Rosenheck, R. A., Perkins, D. O., et al. (2005). Effectiveness of antipsychotic drugs in patients with chronic schizophrenia. *New England Journal of Medicine, 353*(12), 1209–1223.

Lin, E. H. B., Von Korff, M., Katon, W., Bush, T., Simon, G. E., Walker, E., & Robinson, P. (1995). The role of the primary care physician in patients' adherence to antidepressant therapy. *Medical Care, 33*(1), 67–74.

Linehan, M. M. (1993a). *Cognitive-behavioral treatment of borderline personality disorder*. New York: Guilford Press.

Linehan, M. M. (1993b). *Skills training manual for treating borderline personality disorder*. New York: Guilford Press.

Luukinen, H., Viramo, P., Koski, K., Laippala, P., & Kivela, S. L. (1999). Head injuries and cognitive decline among older adults: A population-based study. *Neurology, 52*(3), 557–562.

Marder, S. R., Essock, S. M., Miller, A. L., Buchanan, R. W., Casey, D. E., Davis, J. M., et al. (2004). Physical health monitoring of patients with schizophrenia. *American Journal of Psychiatry, 161*(8), 1334–1349.

Mason, P. T., Kreger, R., & Siever, L. J. (1998). *Stop walking on eggshells: Coping when someone you care about has borderline personality disorder*. Oakland, CA: New Harbinger.

Mayberg, H. S., Lozano, A. M., Voon, V., McNeely, H. E., Seminowicz, D., Hamani, C., et al. (2005). Deep brain stimulation for treatment-resistant depression. *Neuron, 45*, 651– 660.

McDaniel, S. H., Campbell, T. L., & Seaburn, D. B. (1995). Principles for collaboration between health and mental health providers in primary care. *Family Systems Medicine, 13*(3–4), 283–298.

McDaniel, S. H., Hepworth, J., & Doherty, W. J. (1992). *Medical family therapy: A biopsychosocial approach to families with health problems*. New York: Basic Books.

McDonald, H., Garg, A., & Haynes, R. (2002). Interventions to enhance patient adherence to medication prescriptions: Scientific review. *Journal of the American Medical Association, 288*(22), 2868–2879.

McFarlane, W., Dixon, L., Lukens, E., & Luckstead, A. (2002a). *Family psychoeducation and schizophrenia: A review of the literature*. Paper presented at the American Association for Marriage and Family Therapy Research Conference, Reno, NV.

McFarlane, W., Dixon, L., Lukens, E., & Luckstead, A. (2002b). Severe mental illness. In D. H. Sprenkle (Ed.), *Effectiveness in research in marriage and family therapy* (pp. 255–288). Alexandria, VA: American Association for Marriage and Family Therapy.

McGrath, P. J., Stewart, J. W., Fava, M., Trivedi, M. H., Wisniewski, S. R., Nierenberg, A. A., et al. (2006). Tranylcypromine versus venlafaxine plus mirtazapine following three failed antidepressant medication trials for depression: A STAR*D report. *American Journal of Psychiatry, 163*(9), 1531–1541.

McMahon, F. J., Buervenich, S., Manji, H., et al. (2006). *American Journal of Human Genetics.*

Melzack, R., & Casey, K. L. (1968). Sensory, motivational and central control determinants of pain: A new conceptual model. In D. Kenshalo (Ed.), *The skin senses* (pp. 423–443). Springfield, IL: Thomas.

Melzack, R., & Wall, P. D. (1965). Pain mechanisms: A new theory. *Science, 50,* 971–979.

Merikangas, K. R., & Risch, N. (2003). Will the genomics revolution revolutionize psychiatry? *American Journal of Psychiatry, 160,* 625–635.

Messing, R. O. (2001). Biology of addiction. In E. Braunwald, A. C. Fauci, D. L. Kasper, S. L. Hauser, D. L. Longo, & J. L. Jameson (Eds.), *Harrison's principles of internal medicine* (15th ed.). New York: McGraw-Hill.

Minuchin, S., & Fishman, H. C. (1981). *Family therapy techniques.* Boston: Harvard University Press.

Moffitt, T. E., Caspi, A., & Rutter, M. (2005) Strategy for investigating interactions between measured genes and measured environments. *Archives of General Psychiatry 62,* 473–481.

Montgomery, S. A., & Asberg, M. (1979). A new depression scale designed to be sensitive to change. *British Journal of Psychiatry, 134,* 382–389.

Najarian, S. (1995). Family experience with positive patient response to clozapine. *Archives of Psychiatric Nursing, 9*(1), 11–21.

National Coalition for Health Professional Education in Genetics. (2004). [Electronic reference on genetics and psychiatric disorders.] Retrieved September 21, 2004, from www.nchpeg.org/cdrom/empiric.html

Nierenberg, A. A., Fava, M., Trivedi, M. H., Wisniewski, S. T., Thase, M. E., McGrath, P. J., et al. (2006). A comparison of lithium and T3 augmentation following two failed medication treatments for depression: A STAR*D report. *American Journal of Psychiatry, 163*(9), 1519–1530.

Olfson, M., Marcus, S. C., Druss, B., Elinson, L., Tanielian, T., & Pincus, H. A. (2002). National trends in the outpatient treatment of depression. *Journal of the American Medical Association, 287*(2), 203–209.

Olfson, M., Mechanic, D., Hansell, S., Boyer, C., Walkup, J., & Weiden, P. (2000). Predicting medication noncompliance after hospital discharge among patients with schizophrenia. *Psychiatric Services, 52*(2), 216–222.

Osler, W. (1898). *The principles and practice of medicine.* New York: Appleton.

Pagel, J. F. (1994). Treatment of insomnia. *American Family Physician, 49,* 1417–1421.

Pampallona, S., Bollini, P., Tibaldi, G., Kupelnik, B., & Munizza, C. (2004). Combined pharmacology and psychological treatmentfor depression: A systematic review. *Archives of General Psychiatry, 61,* 714–719.

Patterson, J. E., & Magulac, M. (1994). The family therapist's guide to psychopharmacology: A graduate level course. *Journal of Marital and Family Therapy, 20*(2), 151–173.

Patterson, J. E., Peek, C. J., Heinrich, R. L., Bischoff, R. J., & Scherger, J. (2002). *Mental health professionals in medical settings: A primer.* New York: Norton.

Peterson, R. C., Doody, R., Kurz, A., Mohs, R. C., Morris, J. C., & Rabins, P. V. (2001). Current concepts in mild cognitive impairment. *Archives of Neurology, 58,* 1985–1992.

Pharmaceutical Research and Manufacturers of America. (2004). [Electronic reference on new medicines in development for mental illness.] Retrieved on August 30, 2005, from www.phrma.org/newmedicines/surveys.cfm?newmedsrindex=78.

Post, R. M., Roy-Byrne, P. P., & Uhde, T. W. (1988). Graphic representation of the life course of illness in patients with an affective disorder. *American Journal of Psychiatry, 145,* 844–848.

Preskorn, S. H., Feignhner, J. P., Stanga, C. Y., & Ross, R. (Eds.). (2004). *Antidepressants: Past, present, and future.* New York: Springer.

Prochaska, J. O., DiClemente, C. C., & Norcross, J. C. (1995). *Changing for good.* New York: Morrow.

Ran, M., & Xiang, M. (1995). A study of schizophrenic patients' treatment compliance in a rural community. *Journal of Mental Health, 4*(1), 85–89.

Razali, S. M., Hasanah, C. I., Khan, U. A., & Subramaniam, M. (2000). Psychosocial interventions for schizophrenia. *Journal of Mental Health, 9*(3), 283–289.

Riba, M. B., & Balon, R. (1999). *Psychopharmacology and psychotherapy: A collaborative approach.* Washington, DC: American Psychiatric Association.

Richelson, E. (1994). The pharmacology of antidepressants at the synapse: Focus on newer compounds. *Journal of Clinical Psychiatry, 55*(Suppl.), 34–39.

Risch, N., Herrell, R., Lehner, T., Liang, K-Y., Eaves, L., Hoh, J., et al. (2009). Interaction between the serotonin transporter gene (5-HTTLPR), stressful life events, and risk of depression: A meta-analysis. *Journal of the American Medical Association, 301*(23), 2462–2471.

Robinson, D. G., Woerner, M. G., Alvir, J. M., Geisler, S., Koreen, A., Sheitman, B., et al. (1999). Predictors of treatment response from a first episode of schizophrenia or schizoaffective disorder. *American Journal of Psychiatry, 156*(4), 544–549.

Roesler, T. A., Gavin, L. A., & Brenner, A. M. (1995). *Family Systems Medicine, 13*(3–4), 313–318.

Rolland, J. S. (1994). *Families, illness, and disability: An integrative treatment model.* New York: Basic Books.

Rosenheck, R., Cramer, J., Jurgis, G., Perlick, D., Xu, W., Thomas, J., et al. (2000). Clinical and psychopharmocologic factors influencing family burden in refractory schizophrenia. The Department of Veterans Affairs Cooperative Study Group on Clozapine in Refractory Schizophrenia. *Journal of Clinical Psychiatry, 61*(9), 671–676.

Rush, A. J., Marangell, L. B., Sackeim, H. A., George, M. S., Brannan, S. M., Stephen, K., et al. (2005). Vagus nerve stimulation for treatment-resistant depression: A randomized, controlled acute phase trial. *Biological Psychiatry, 58,* 347–354.

Rush, A. J., Sackeim, H. A., Marangell, L. B., George, M. S., Brannan, S., Stephen, K., et al. (2005). Effects of 12 months of vagus nerve stimulation in treatment-resistant depression: A naturalistic study. *Biological Psychiatry, 58,* 355–363.

Rush, A. J., Trivedi, M. H., Wisniewski, S. R., Stewart, J. W., Nierenberg, A. A., Thase, M. F., et al. (2006). Bupropion-SR, sertraline, or venlafaxine-XR after failure of SSRIs for depression. *New England Journal of Medicine, 354,* 1231–1242.

Sammons, M. T., & Schmidt, N. B. (2001). *Combined treatment for mental disorders: A guide to psychological and pharmacological interventions.* Washington, DC: American Psychological Association.

Sapolsky, R. M. (2001). Depression, antidepressants, and the shrinking hippocampus. *Proceedings of the National Academy of Sciences, USA, 98*(22), 12320–12322.

Schuckit, M. A. (1994). Low level of response to alcohol as a predictor of future alcoholism. *American Journal of Psychiatry, 151,* 184–189.

Schuckit, M. A. (1995). Alcohol-related disorders. In H. I. Kaplan & B. J. Sadock (Eds.), *Comprehensive textbook of psychiatry/VI* (6th ed.). Baltimore: Williams & Wilkins.

Schuckit, M. A. (2001). Alcohol and alcoholism. In E. Braunwald, A. C. Fauci, D. L. Kasper, S. L. Hauser, D. L. Longo, & J. L. Jameson (Eds.), *Harrison's principles of internal medicine* (15th ed.). New York: McGraw-Hill.

Schuckit, M. A. (2003). Alcohol and alcoholism. In E. Braunwald, A. S. Fauci, K. J. Isselbacher, D. L. Kasper, S. L. Hauser, D. L. Longo, et al. (Eds.), *Harrison's online.* New York: McGraw-Hill.

Schuckit, M. A., & Segal, D. S. (2001). Opioid drug abuse and dependence. In E. Braunwald, A. C. Fauci, D. L. Kasper, S. L. Hauser, D. L. Longo, & J. L. Jameson (Eds.), *Harrison's principles of internal medicine* (15th ed.). New York: McGraw-Hill.

Schuckit, M. A., & Smith, T. L. (1996). An 8-year follow-up of 450 sons of alcoholic and control subjects. *Archives of General Psychiatry, 53*(3), 202–210.

Seaburn, D. B., Lorenz, A. D., Gunn, W. B., Jr., Gawinski, B. A., & Mauksch, L. B. (1996). *Models of collaboration: A guide for mental health professionals working with health care practitioners.* New York: Basic Books.

Smith, C., Barzam, D., & Pristach, C. (1997). Effect of patient and family insight on compliance of schizophrenic patients. *Journal of Clinical Pharmacology, 37,* 147–154.

Smith, G. R., Monson, R. A., & Ray, D. C. (1986). Psychiatric consultation in somatization disorder: A randomized controlled study. *New England Journal of Medicine, 314*(22), 1407–1413.

Sparks, J. A. (2002). Taking a stand: Challenging medical discourse. *Journal of Marital and Family Therapy, 28*(1), 51–59.

Spitzer, R. L., Endicott, J., & Robins, E. (1975a). Research diagnostic criteria. *Psychopharmacology Bulletin, 11*(3), 22–25.

Spitzer, R. L., Endicott, J., & Robins, E. (1975b). Clinical criteria for psychiatric diagnosis and DSM-III. *American Journal of Psychiatry, 132*(11), 1187–1192.

Sprenkle, D. (2003). Effectiveness research in marriage and family therapy: Introduction. *Journal of Marital and Family Therapy, 29*(1), 85–96.

Stebbin, H. (1995). Families' perspective of clozapine treatment. *Perspectives in Psychiatric Care, 31*(4), 14–18.

Stein, M. B., Torgrud, L. J., & Walker, J. R. (2000). Social phobia symptoms, subtypes, and severity: Findings from a community survey. *Archives of General Psychiatry, 57,* 1047–1052.

Stein, M. B., Walker, J. R., & Forde, D. R. (1996). Public-speaking fears in a community sample: Prevalence, impact on functioning, and diagnostic classification. *Archives of General Psychiatry, 53,* 169–174.

Stiskal, J. A., Kulin, N., Koren, G., Ho, T., & Ito, S. (2001). Neonatal paroxetine withdrawal syndrome. *Archives of Disease in Childhood, Fetal Neonatal Edition, 84*(2), F134–F135.

Trivedi, M. H., Fava, M., Wisniewski, S. R., Thase, M. E., Quitkin, F., Warden,

D., et al. (2006). Medication augmentation after the failure of SSRIs for depression. *New England Journal of Medicine, 354*, 1243–1252.

Trivedi, M. H., Rush, A. J., Wisniewski, S. R., Nierenberg, A. A., Warden, D., Ritz, L., et al. (2006). Evaluation of outcomes with citalopram for depression using measurement-based care in STAR*D: Implications for clinical practice. *American Journal of Psychiatry, 163*, 28–40.

Turk, D. C. (1996). Biopsychosocial perspective on chronic pain. In R. J. Gatchel & D. C. Turk (Eds.), *Psychological approaches to pain management: A practitioner's handbook* (pp. 3–32). New York: Guilford Press.

Turk, D. C., & Flor, H. (1999). Chronic pain: A biobehavioral perspective. In R. J. Gatchel & D. C. Turk (Eds.), *Psychosocial factors in pain: Critical perspectives* (pp. 18–34). New York: Guilford Press.

Unützer, J., Katon, W., & Callahan, C. M. (2002). Collaborative care management of late-life depression in the primary care setting: A randomized controlled trial. *Journal of the American Medical Association, 288*, 2836–2845.

U.S. Food and Drug Administration. (2005). [Electronic reference on VNS Therapy System.] Retrieved on September 8, 2005, from www.fda.gov/cdrh/PDF/p970003s050a.pdf.

Walsh, B. T. (2001). Eating disorders. In E. Braunwald, A. C. Fauci, D. L. Kasper, S. L. Hauser, D. L. Longo, & J. L. Jameson (Eds.), *Harrison's principles of internal medicine* (15th ed., pp. 486–490). New York: McGraw-Hill.

Watson, J. D., & Crick, F. H. C. (1953). Molecular structure of nucleic acids—A structure for deoxyribose nucleic acid. *Nature, 171*, 737–738.

Writing Group for the Women's Health Initiative Investigators. (2002). Risks and benefits of estrogen plus progestin in healthy postmenopausal women: Principal results from the Women's Health Initiative Randomized Controlled Trial. *Journal of the American Medical Association, 288*, 321–333.

Wysocki, T., Greceo, P., Harris, M. A., Bubb, J., & White, N. H. (2001). Behavior therapy for families of adolescents with diabetes: Maintenance of treatment effects. *Diabetes Care, 24*(3), 441–446.

Yonkers, K. A., Wisner, K. L., Stewart, D. E., Oberlander, T. F., Dell, D. L., Stotland, N., et al. (2009). The management of depression during pregnancy: A report from the American Psychiatric Association and the American College of Obstetricians and Gynecologists. *Obstetrics & Gynecology, 114*(3), 703–714.

Yood, M. U., DeLorenze, G., Quesenberry, C. P., Jr., Oliveria, S. A., Tsai, A. L., Willey, V. J., et al. (2009). The incidence of diabetes in atypical antipsychotic users differs according to agents: Results from a multisite epidemiologic study. *Pharmacoepidemiology and Drug Safety, 18*(9), 791–799.

Zhang, M., Wang, M., Jianjun, L., & Phillips, M. (1994). Randomised control trial of family intervention for 78 first episode male schizophrenic patients. *British Journal of Psychiatry, 165*, 96–102.

Index

Page references in **bold** indicate glossary entries; *t* indicates table; *f* indicates figure.